"This guide to our complicated, confusing and often frustrating heource for the general public as well as healthcare providers who may struggle complex system. It covers changes in insurance, hospital and outpatient payment and technology. My long career in clinical and academic social v oritative, well-written and user-friendly book. The clinical examples, Key F and reviews and Appendices will be useful for those seeking greater details. I particularly like the descriptions of the different providers in terms of their training and clinical abilities to help patients know who might be providing care and what to expect from them."

—**Judith Lemberger**, Ph.D., MSW, Clinical Professor (retired), Silver School of Social Work (New York University)

"This book by two experienced and savvy doctors gives wise, practical advice on how to understand and navigate a complicated medical system. The authors offer practical strategies on being a patient in this system that have applicability for citizens in countries throughout the world. With clarity and heart, the authors guide you on how to advocate effectively for the highest quality medical care for yourself and your family, ensure you are seeing the 'right' kind of medical professional, get a second medical opinion that can save your life, reduce your out-of-pocket expenses, and help elderly family members cope successfully with end of life issues. Read it. You will be glad you did!"

— **Joel Sadavoy** MD, FRCP, Founder, Geriatric Psychiatry, FCPA (Distinguished) and Professor of Psychiatry, University of Toronto

"Finally, a user-friendly guide written by two seasoned doctors to help all Americans choose the highest quality health care while containing out-of-pocket costs. Medical and mental health professionals can better understand how the healthcare system really works to help their patients advocate for and participate in their own and their family's health care more effectively."

— **A. John Rush**, MD, Professor Emeritus, Duke-National University of Singapore, Adjunct Professor, Duke and Texas Tech Medical Schools

"The sound recommendations offered by the INSIDER'S GUIDE have the potential of saving money for the individual patient, as well as reducing costs for the healthcare system. Following the authors' sage suggestions is likely to improve outcomes from outpatient and hospital procedures and to enhance satisfaction with the many healthcare provider interactions. This book is as valuable as that GPS system on your cell phone."

— **Constance Holden**, RN, MSN, Co-founder of The Conversation Project and Co-chair of the Clinical Ethics Committee, Boulder Community Health

INSIDER'S GUIDE TO QUALITY, AFFORDABLE HEALTHCARE

Practical Strategies to Navigate our Complex System and Save Money

LAWRENCE LAZARUS, MD

JEFFREY FOSTER, MD

Published by: To Life and Health Publishing

Publisher's Cataloging-in-Publication Data

Names: Lazarus, Lawrence W., 1941-, author. | Foster, Jeffrey R., author.
Title: Insider's guide to quality, affordable healthcare: practical strategies to navigate our complex system and save money / Lawrence Lazarus, MD; Jeffrey Foster, MD.
Description: Includes bibliographical references and index. | Longmont, CO: For Health and Life Publishing LLC, 2019.
Identifiers: LCCN 2019900463 | ISBN 978-1-7335192-0-5 | 978-1-7335192-1-2 (eBook)
Subjects: LCSH Medical care--United States. | Medical care, Cost of--United States. | Delivery of health care--United States--Popular works. | Patients--Legal status, laws, etc. | Medical care--Handbooks, manuals, etc. | Consumer education--Handbooks, manuals, etc. | Medical care, Cost of--Handbooks, manuals, etc. | Health insurance--Handbooks, manuals, etc. | BISAC REFERENCE / Consumer Guides | REFERENCE / Personal & Practical Guides | MEDICAL / Health Care Delivery
Classification: LCC RA776.5 .L36 2019 | DDC 362.1--dc23

ISBN (print): 978-1-7335192-0-5
ISBN (e-book): 978-1-7335192-1-2

Printed in the United States of America

Acknowledgements

First and foremost, we would like to thank our patients and their families who have taught us the challenges they have faced to obtain quality and affordable healthcare from our complex and often times adversarial healthcare system. Together, we have had to figure out innovative strategies to convince insurance companies to pay for important coverage such as for expensive brand name medications and consultations with "out-of-network" specialists. We have had to guide patients in their selection of quality insurance, hospitals and specialists—knowledge we didn't acquire during our medical school and graduate training.

We want to thank our mentors who served as excellent role models during our formative training. They include Drs. Ferdinand Bonan and Jay Fink in Philadelphia; Drs. Roy Grinker, Jack Weinberg, and Jan Fawcett in Chicago; and Dr Alvin Goldfarb in New York City.

Special thanks and appreciation go to Dr. RoseMarie Foster for her encouragement and assistance in completing this project. Special thanks and appreciations also to Dr. Nicole H. Lazarus (researcher in immunology at Stanford University in Palo Alto) and Dr. Mark A. Lazarus (Board certified in internal medicine and hospitalist, Scripps Health in San Diego). He broadened our knowledge about how to benefit from and avoid dangerous errors during periods of transition in the hospital.

We wish to thank our assistants Mary Ellis and Charlotte Schaaf who prepared numerous drafts of our manuscript; Barbara Roth for her editing wizardry; and Cliff Pelloni and Martha Bullen for their publishing and marketing guidance.

We hope you, our readers, will be more empowered to obtain the quality healthcare you deserve from America's complicated and changing healthcare system.

INSIDER'S GUIDE TO

QUALITY, AFFORDABLE HEALTHCARE

Practical Strategies to Navigate our Complex System and Save Money

Contents

Introduction

Take Control and Responsibility to Get the Quality Healthcare You Deserve

We have all been in a quandary trying to obtain quality, reliable, affordable healthcare for ourselves and our families in America's rapidly changing, often dysfunctional healthcare system. Like most Americans, you are probably struggling with increasing healthcare costs (higher premiums and deductibles) and even "surprise" bills that you expected your insurance to pay. And if you or your employer has recently changed to a different health insurance company that your current doctor is not contracted with, you've had to begin the arduous search for a new physician who accepts your new insurance. If you're self-employed or between 50-64 years old (not yet eligible for Medicare), you may be worried that your cost for health insurance will escalate when the tax penalty for going without insurance ends in 2019. Millions of Americans, especially the young and healthy, will decide to go without insurance, raising health insurance premiums for everyone else!

Do you find your doctor spending less time talking and interacting with you and more time glued to a computer screen pounding a keyboard? During your first visit to a new doctor, have you been uncertain whether you're seeing a real physician with the initials M.D. or D.O. after his/her name or a nurse practitioner (NP), clinical nurse specialist (CNS), physician's assistant (PA), or medical assistant (MA) whose role with you is not clear? We explain the differences in their level of training.

It has become more difficult to find a physician or other primary care practitioner (PCP) because of the worsening doctor shortage and because the Affordable Care Act (ACA) has increased the percentage of Americans with insurance to 88 percent, as of 2017. Also, fewer doctors are accepting patients with Medicare and Medicaid and other government insurance. Some no longer accept any insurance, preferring to have a "boutique practice" where patients make full payment directly to the doctor. To make matters worse, doctors are stressed by pressure to see more patients for shorter periods of time, by increased administrative tasks (e.g. paperwork), concern about malpractice suits, and payments from insurers that do not keep up with their increased overhead expenses. We show you how to make use of your doctor's limited time by being thoroughly prepared for each office visit.

If your health problems require seeing several doctors and other health professionals for treatment, is it unclear to you who is the "captain" (coordinator) of your healthcare team? Does this critically important role fall on you or a busy family member? Patients, as well as doctors, often feel that trying to obtain and provide consistent quality healthcare is like landing in the middle of a jungle without an experienced guide or even a map to lead them to safety.

Despite these obstacles, there are many strategies and practical solutions to ensure that you and your family receive the best affordable healthcare possible – the main purpose of our book! We would like to serve as your guides to navigate through the oftentimes dangerous, confusing, rapidly changing landscape of America's healthcare system.

As we begin our journey together, we explain the necessity for you to take a more active role and assume more control and responsibility for your and your family's healthcare. You will see the importance of having a personal patient advocate, we like to call a "guardian angel," to serve as your second set of eyes and ears when you encounter potential landmines in the healthcare terrain (such as doctor, hospital, and medication errors, and billing mistakes). We help you understand why advanced planning is so important should you or a loved one have a medical emergency, why and how to obtain a second medical opinion from a specialist and, should you require hospitalization, what you and your family can do to promote a safe, successful hospital stay and smooth transition home.

Our goal is to increase your knowledge about the real "inside" story of how our healthcare system works, how best to learn about an illness and its treatment and to find the best doctors so you are empowered to make the best healthcare decisions. There are actions you can take to enable your doctors to practice to the best of their abilities. We help you take full advantage of the Affordable Care Act (ACA) and other insurance choices (rather than insurers taking advantage of you). We provide many practical strategies to reduce your healthcare costs. How to benefit from alternative (eastern) healthcare approaches and integrate them with traditional (western) medicine is discussed. We explain ways of adopting a healthier lifestyle in order to stay well and live longer. Your children and grandchildren can emulate your healthy lifestyle so they too can live longer, healthier lives. And they can learn from you ways of avoiding illnesses that "run in the family" (e.g. diabetes). Lastly, we discuss ways of taking full advantage of innovative diagnostic and treatment approaches and future constructive changes in our healthcare system.

We have written this book for all adult Americans: the young, the middle aged, and those in the later phase of life. For example, if you have elderly family members dealing with the challenges and losses associated with aging, you'll become more knowledgeable and effective care providers by better understanding the ins and outs of Medicare, innovative healthcare services available in the community that support independent living at home, and the necessity for them to complete special legal forms like the HIPAA, POLST, living will, healthcare and financial proxy, and a patient advocate form.

Others benefitting from our book are healthcare professionals who work directly with patients: doctors, nurses, social workers, mental health professionals, physical therapists, and others. By teaching their patients and their patients' families to become more assertive and more effective advocates for themselves, and more engaged and cooperative in their treatment, patients and their healthcare professionals can work more effectively together to assure the best possible healthcare results.

We believe that you can benefit most from our book by focusing your attention particularly on chapters most relevant to your current life situation. For example, if you are employed by a large company or self-employed and it's the yearly open enrollment period, we suggest reading *Chapter 3, Taking Advantage of the Affordable Care Act (ACA) and Other Insurance Options* and *Chapter 11, Choosing the Best Insurance and Assuring End of Life Wishes*. If your medical and medication costs have gotten out of hand, read *Chapter 2, Strategies for Keeping Costs Down*.

The book is organized into four main parts, each containing three to four chapters. Most chapters begin with a real-life medical story that you, a family member or friend may be grappling with. Strategies for solving the medical problem are revealed as the chapter unfolds.

- **Part 1** shows you how to develop a personal healthcare record (PHR) for yourself and family members to make coordination and transfer of your medical information to a new physician, a specialist, or a hospital as rapid and seamless as one mouse click on a computer key. The many benefits of having a personal patient advocate are explained. Simple strategies for reducing your healthcare costs before and even after incurring debt and preventing and dealing with "surprise" bills are explained. We guide you to take full advantage of the Affordable Care Act and to reduce your health insurance premiums. If you have insurance with a high deductible, you may be eligible for a Health Savings Account (HSA) where you can invest tax deductible money. The money can be used if necessary to pay out-of-pocket medical costs and also be used as an investment vehicle for an early retirement. We explain traditional and new, innovative ways of getting out-patient medical care (for example, from urgent care centers) in an emergency or when your primary care provider is unavailable.

- **Part 2** guides you to find the best primary care physician (PCPhys.), primary care provider (PCP), medical specialist, hospital, and emergency department. We explain the important role of your PCP as the "captain" (coordinator) of your healthcare team, and ways to encourage and facilitate that role to enable him/her to practice at the highest level. We provide practical ways to obtain a second medical opinion about your diagnosis and treatment, which can save you money and your life, from an excellent board-certified medical specialist so you are assured you're getting the best healthcare possible.

- **Part 3** explains practical ways to prepare for, and promote a safe hospital stay, including what you, your family, and your patient advocate can do to avoid a hospital-acquired infection, medication and other preventable errors, and how best to prepare for a smooth, safe transition home. Should you need surgery, we show you steps you can take before and after surgery to facilitate a successful recovery and outcome. We also discuss the careful, conservative use of prescription medications, effective treatments for those afflicted with opioid dependency, and how to protect against "super-bug" infections.

- **Part 4** discusses the pros and cons of adding a supplemental health insurance policy to protect you from unexpected expenses. We explain strategies for helping older family members to live safely in the natural setting of their home even if they are suffering from chronic medical and emotional problems. We explain why it is so important for most Americans (from teenager to senior citizen) to complete most of the following legal forms – a HIPAA, POLST, living will, healthcare and financial proxy and to enlist the help, if needed, of a patient advocate. We discuss the judicious use of alternative (complementary or eastern) treatment, such as acupuncture, herbal or vitamin remedies and how they can be successfully integrated with traditional (western-style) medicine so you have the advantages of both. Finally, we explain how you and your family can take full advantage of future medical discoveries and changes in how our complicated healthcare system works.

A Note About Chapter Format

At the end of each chapter are four to six informative "key points" that summarize the main topics. It is helpful to review the key points before and after reading the chapter. Appendices at the end of some chapters contain more detail about topics covered in the chapter. The bottom of most pages contains footnotes to provide easy access to additional information and reliable websites. There is a reference list at the end of each chapter should you want to explore a topic in greater depth.

The following is an explanation about our use of the terms primary care provider (PCP) and physicians (PCPhys.). PCP is an all-inclusive term, referring to all health professionals you visit within medical facilities, offices and clinics; they may be physicians, nurses, specialized nurses, or physician assistants. Some of these PCPs function in some ways like your primary care physician (PCPhys.). When we refer specifically to physicians (M.D.s or D.O.s) we'll use the initials PCPhys.

Go to Our Website www.qualityaffordablehealthcare.net

We have also integrated our book with additional information on our website. A special section of our website **www.qualityaffordablehealthcare.net/book** contains a more extensive list of Key Points for each chapter in our book and additional important Appendices, such as health-related legal forms, which were not included in the book. We hope you will take advantage of our website, and use it also to ask us questions about problems you are encountering accessing high quality medical care.

We have established a "healthcare medical forum" on our website for you, our reader, which will keep you up to date every month about important changes to our healthcare system that directly affect you and your family. This is also found on our website. After reading the medical forum, we encourage you to email us with your questions. Answers to your questions may help others. While we cannot answer questions about your medical problems or give medical advice, which is best provided by your doctor, we can provide knowledge and strategies to get the best medical care for you and your loved ones.

About the Authors

The authors are physicians with long careers as teachers, researchers, and clinicians. We have provided medical care to people of all ages, from adolescents to the elderly and their families for many years. We know how important it is to be assertive advocates for our patients. We've argued on behalf of our patients with their insurance companies to pay for needed, expensive, brand name medications, special tests, and to obtain a second medical opinion from even "out-of-network" medical specialists. We've guided patients to understand and successfully challenge "surprise bills". We have integrated our clinical skills with those of other specialists and primary care professionals. We have provided our services in the settings of outpatient offices, acute hospitals, long-term care facilities, and skilled nursing facilities. We have dealt with both patients and their families within the required respect for patient privacy. These professional experiences allow us to share our "insider" knowledge with you about how our healthcare system really works as it continues to change.

Part 1

Dealing with Major Changes in Healthcare

CHAPTER 1

Taking Control of Your Healthcare

Stephen is a successful estate attorney who retired from his law firm in Southern California at age sixty and moved with his young wife to Taos, New Mexico, to live his lifelong dream of becoming a ski instructor and small-town attorney. He always prided himself on his fitness, excellent health, and meticulous planning for his and his wife's future.

Before moving to Taos, Stephen gathered their medical records, personal health records (PHR) – conveniently stored on his smartphone – and copies of their living will, their patient advocate agreement, and their healthcare and financial proxy. He also made an appointment with a Taos internist, Dr. Jonas, who had a reputation for being an excellent coordinator of his patients' healthcare.

During Stephen's initial medical assessment with Dr. Jonas, he was assured that if Dr. Jonas were unavailable, his two partners would take over and have immediate access to his PHR. Dr. Jonas also highly recommended a nearby urgent care center and the best hospital within seventy miles, should that ever become necessary.

Weeks later, Stephen visited the urgent care center and the hospital, and provided both with copies of all of his and his wife's PHRs and legal documents. Stephen also sent this updated information to his two adult children.

Unfortunately, a few years later he developed excruciating pain down his left leg that was unresponsive to multiple conservative treatments and even to back surgery. Stephen became increasingly discouraged. When mild pain medication was ineffective, he was put on hydrocodone, which caused constipation and possibly contributed to a bowel obstruction, which required emergency surgery.

His wife remained with him in the hospital 24/7, protected him from some medication errors and helped him avoid the risk of a hospital-acquired infection by making certain that family and friends with head colds refrained from visiting and reminded all visitors to wash their hands. Stephen's wife won the admiration of the nurses, who referred to her as "Mrs. Nightingale." Stephen recovered, partly due to his wife's vigilance and diligent role as his advocate. The social worker coordinated a smooth transition home. Stephen was skiing again a month later.

This true story demonstrates the necessity of taking a proactive approach to your and your family's health. In this and subsequent chapters, we explain the inside story about how America's complex and often dysfunctional healthcare system really works and the reasons for becoming more knowledgeable and assuming more responsibility for your healthcare. We provide step-by-step strategies for assuming more control so you are empowered to obtain the best healthcare possible.

Four hundred thousand Americans die each year from doctor and hospital preventable errors, making these errors the third most frequent cause of death [1][3]. Every year, medication errors made by doctors, hospitals, pharmacies, and patients cause 1.3 million injuries to Americans [2]. By assuming more responsibility for your healthcare, you can help protect yourself and your family from being a casualty of these errors.

When you have an office visit with a new doctor, do you always know whether you are actually seeing a doctor rather than a clinical nurse specialist, nurse practitioner, or physician's assistant, whose training and experience are vastly different? If you're seeing more than one doctor as well as other health professionals, do you wonder whether they communicate with one another so your care is coordinated? In this chapter we explain many ways to ensure that your care is coordinated, including the benefits of developing your own personal health record (PHR). All your health records and legal documents can easily be stored on your smartphone or other electronic device so they are immediately available should you change to a new physician, move to another city, become ill while traveling, or end up in an emergency department where no one knows you. We also explain ways of improving and strengthening your relationship with your primary care provider (PCP) to enable him/her to practice to the very best of his/her abilities and to be the active captain (coordinator) of your healthcare team.

Let's begin our healthcare journey together by reviewing some of the deficiencies of our current healthcare system and ways for you to take more control and to assume more responsibility so you can obtain the best healthcare possible.

Reasons for Being More Knowledgeable and Assuming More Responsibility

- Doctors spend less time with you in today's healthcare system, which leads to impersonal care.

- There is a shortage of doctors, especially in rural communities.

- Your vigilance and assistance from your family members and patient advocate can lessen the risk of you becoming a victim of medical errors.

- Actively clarify who is the "captain" (coordinator) of your healthcare team and encourage him/her to fulfill the leadership role.

- One way of assuming more responsibility is to ask questions until you truly understand the risks and rewards of medications, tests, and surgery. When necessary, have your advocate assist.

- Active inquiry gives you a clearer understanding of the training, experience, and role of the health professionals taking care of you.

- Your introspection and self-awareness can help you overcome emotional barriers to recognizing and attending to early signs of an illness.

- Adopting a healthier lifestyle will enable you to be healthier and live longer.

- Serving as a good role model will help your children and grandchildren to live healthier and longer lives.

Consequences of Briefer Doctor Office Visits – How You Can Compensate

PCPs today typically spend only ten to fifteen minutes with each patient. During that time, they are often typing medical information about you into their laptop computer and spending less time listening to your concerns and examining you.

Do you remember when your doctor could spend as much time with you as necessary? Your physician felt pride and a sense of responsibility and autonomy in caring for you and your family members. When one of the authors was a youngster, the family physician came to his house (the now almost obsolete "house call") when a family member was too sick to go to the office. Later in life, while practicing medicine for twenty-three years in Chicago, the author had an excellent old-fashioned physician who spent an hour carrying out a yearly medical checkup, including a half-hour physical examination. A follow-up appointment was scheduled and the physician personally called with the results of all tests.

What happened to change the bedside manner of the family physician? Big business happened. It became the intermediary between you – the patient – and your doctor. Insurance companies, the mergers of big medical centers and practices and increasing medical costs are three major reasons why medical care has become more impersonal. Today, doctors who are employees of hospitals and big medical centers are pressured – because of financial and other reasons – by their employers to see more patients for shorter periods of time. Doctors in small private practices, which are quickly disappearing, have increasing overhead expenses (for example, malpractice insurance, staff salaries, electronic health records, and patient portals), but payments from insurers have not kept pace with these expenses. Physicians spend 20 percent or more of their valuable time doing administrative work: telephoning for authorizations, filling out endless paperwork, and practicing defensive medicine to avoid malpractice suits. These pressures account for some of the dissatisfaction and demoralization of physicians and their staff – tension that you sometimes experience as their staff's impatience and harried behavior.

Busy, pressured physicians don't find the time to communicate with your other physicians and health professionals – crucial tasks to ensure coordination of your healthcare. One way for you to compensate for this lack of coordination is to always remind your doctor(s) to send copies of your records to all your other health professionals. Also, keep your own copy of every medical report and all test results to include in your personal health record [5]. If you are under the care of other health professionals, you can ask your PCP or PCPhys., "Since you are my primary care provider (or doctor), can I count on you to discuss with, and send a report of your findings to, my specialists and other providers?"

Doctors' frustration with the rapidly changing healthcare system and demands on their time have led many physicians to retire earlier than planned. Many have reduced the number of patients who have insurance that pays less (for example, Medicare, Medicaid, and managed-care companies). In fact, many physicians have ceased having contracts with any insurance companies, preferring to have what is called a "concierge" or "boutique" practice where patients pay directly to their doctor (see *Chapter 4*). These and other factors have resulted in a shortage of PCPhys.

In the following sections, we explain ways to (1) reduce your risk of medical errors, (2) better understand the risks and rewards of tests and treatments recommended by your doctor, (3) understand the benefits of developing your own personal healthcare record, (4) select a patient advocate, (5) overcome normal psychological barriers to recognizing early signs of a medical illness, (6) adopt a healthier lifestyle, and (7) help your children and grandchildren live healthier and longer lives. We understand that time limitations may allow you to implement only some of our suggestions, but we strongly believe it will be time well spent.

Reducing Your Risk of Medical Errors (Especially During Periods of Transition)

Do you remember when you were a kid and played the game of passing a seven-word message from a friend who then passed it on to six others? You were all probably surprised when the message at the end was so very different from the original. Communication problems during periods of transition contribute to frequent medical errors in our healthcare system. Being aware of this possibility can help you protect yourself and your family from being harmed.

Medical errors occur most frequently when information about you is passed from one health professional to another, such as when your pharmacist tries to understand the scribbled handwriting of your doctor and you return home from the pharmacy to find that you were given the wrong medication or the wrong number of pills. Medical errors also occur frequently when your doctor explains your medical condition and treatment in technical medical terms while you are distracted and unable to listen carefully. Errors can also occur in the hospital when your hospitalist (who is not your PCP but rather a specially trained "hospital" doctor who is assigned to you) passes information about you to another hospitalist coming on duty. Many errors can also occur during your transition from the hospital back to home. For example, patients may not know if they should continue to take the medications taken while in the hospital or resume the medications they were taking at home prior to hospitalization.

In these and many other periods of transition, you and, if necessary, a family member or your patient advocate need to be especially attentive and ask questions until you fully understand the answers. For example, before leaving the pharmacy with your new pills, check and count them carefully to make certain you have the correct kind and number.

If you are feeling ill and not at your best before heading to a doctor's appointment, take a relative or your patient advocate with you. The person accompanying you can even take notes or tape-record the doctor's instructions to make certain that you both understand and follow them correctly. If a harried doctor is talking too fast and using medical terms you don't understand, ask him/her to slow down and use words you can understand.

If hospitalized, have a relative and/or your patient advocate spend as much time with you as possible, just as Stephen's wife, Mrs. Nightingale did, to provide emotional support and help protect you from medication, a hospital-acquired infection, and other errors especially during the first days of your hospitalization. Ask your nurse for a copy of your daily medications, dosage, and time each medication is given so you and/or your advocate can check for accuracy.

Understanding the Risks and Rewards of Suggested Tests and Treatments

We assess the risks and rewards when making decisions in our everyday lives. For example, if you're trying to decide whether to stay later at a Saturday night party, you know that the reward is some additional enjoyment with friends, but the risk is feeling tired the next morning when you've promised your teenage sons to attend their Sunday morning football game.

It's important to fully understand what the risks and rewards (benefits) are when your PCPhys. or PCP recommends a treatment or test so you can make the best decision. For example, if he/she recommends a new medication, the following are some questions worth asking. Your PCPhys. wants you to be fully informed and may ask you to sign a consent form indicating that you understand the risks and rewards and that you agree to take the medication.

Time limitations may not permit you to ask all these questions, so begin with those most important to you.

- What are the benefits and risks (side effects) of this new medication?

- Does this new medication pose a risk of interacting badly with ones I'm currently taking?

- Is there a medication equally effective but less expensive, such as a generic?

- What do I do if a side effect occurs?

The following is an example of a more complicated situation. You may have been taking heart medication for a long time, and then heart surgery is proposed. Your doctor wants you to be fully informed about the risks and rewards and the choices you have, which may include adjusting your current medications, considering the proposed surgery, and perhaps even a third choice so you can carefully weigh the risks and rewards of each option before making your decision. Having a trusted family member or your patient advocate with you to hear and understand the options can help you decide and also provide you with emotional support.

The following is a question the authors like to ask their personal physicians: "If you were my age with the same overall health status and similar insurance and financial limitations, which option would you choose and why?"

The Importance of Having Your Personal Health Record (PHR)

Another important way to assume more responsibility for your and your family's healthcare is by gathering and organizing all your current and past medical records into a personal health record (PHR). Your PHR is a comprehensive health history that you organize, maintain, and keep updated; it is meant to be shared in a team-like fashion with your doctors, other health professionals, and the staff should you be admitted to a healthcare facility [4].

Having your own PHR and one for each family member is especially valuable to ensure continuity and coordination of your healthcare in the following situations:

- Your first visit to a new PCPhys., PCP or a medical specialist.
- If you or a family member becomes ill while traveling.
- If you need to go to an emergency department where no one knows you.
- If you are admitted to a hospital where your medical care is taken over by a hospitalist who doesn't know you.
- Your previous records are not available because your doctor has retired, moved, or died.
- You want more time for discussion during brief visits with your new PCPhys. or PCP.
- You've lived in different parts of the country where your records still reside.
- Your medical records can't be sent electronically from your previous doctor to your new doctor because their computer software is not compatible.

You may be asking yourself, "Why bother doing this if I'm young, healthy, and haven't had any serious medical problems? Should I need to see a doctor, I'm capable of conveying the information needed." You probably don't need a PHR now, but a PHR may be helpful for someone in your family, such as an aging parent, grandparent, or a child with medical problems. You can help them develop their PHR.

How to Construct Your PHR

One basic way to construct your PHR is to begin putting together a file with copies of medical records you currently have and adding all future records chronologically. You may need to request a copy of your past records – including all test results – from your current and previous PCPs and other healthcare professionals. You are legally entitled, under HIPAA (Health Insurance Portability and Accountability Act of 1996) to these records. If you discover diagnostic or other errors while reviewing your records, you are entitled to request that your physician consider making corrections.

If you have had previous hospitalizations, you can write letters requesting a copy of your records. Ask for a written confirmation that your request has been received and keep a list of who you've contacted. Don't be surprised if you need to make follow-up calls after several weeks. And be aware that keeping a paper file of your or a family member's medical records has limitations: Records can be bulky, difficult to carry, misplaced, and not readily available in emergency situations.

A much simpler way of organizing all your medical information is by using any number of Internet sites, such as www.webmd.com/phr, or www.healthvault.com, and just provide the information requested. Some sites charge a nominal fee. Be sure to include in your PHR the names and contact information of those you want called in case of an emergency, for example, family and friends, and include all your legal documents (such as your HIPAA, patient advocate, living will, healthcare and financial proxy.). Also, include contact information about your PCP, specialists, attorney, and (if pertinent) the leader of your place of worship. You can then transfer all the information to your smartphone, laptop, or tablet by emailing the PHR to yourself, locating it on your smartphone (or other electronic device), and then copying and pasting the copy into whatever file system app you use on your phone. In the interest of everyone's time and given problems different software systems have communicating with one another, your doctor and other health professionals may prefer that you print out your PHR to bring to each office visit.

If you carry your phone with you at all times, all your medical and legal records will be readily available when you're traveling or in emergency situations. Keep a note written in large type in your wallet or purse explaining how, in case you are incapacitated, a healthcare professional in an ED can easily access your PHR from your smartphone. And give a copy of your PHR to a nearby reliable family member, your patient advocate, and your healthcare proxy in case of an emergency when your copy is unavailable. Also, periodically update your PHR, including changes of medication and updated contact information about family members and your advocate and healthcare and financial proxy. Once your medical information is assembled, your new PCPhys., a specialist, the hospital team, and anyone you've given permission to can immediately access it.

The following are examples of how having your PHR can be lifesaving, and not having it can be regrettable.

- A sixty-six-year-old woman had severe osteoarthritis and needed a right hip replacement, which she had previously done on her left hip. During the first surgery, she had an allergic reaction to some metal components of the hip prosthesis. Because she kept good records, she printed out from her computer the hospital report from her first operation, which included the allergy doctor's findings concerning which implants were safe to use, along with other parts of her PHR. Her new orthopedist was appreciative because the information expedited her surgery, which was successful.

- John, a sixty-eight-year-old man with multiple medical problems, including debilitating chronic lung disease, moved to another city and consulted a new PCP, who requested that he obtain the medical records of his previous PCP. John never kept copies for himself. Despite several requests to his former doctor, the records were never sent. The new PCP recommended a medication that the patient dimly recalled might have been used before and caused bad side effects. Because his previous records were not available, the same medication was used again. John developed serious side effects that required hospitalization. This could have been avoided if John had had a PHR.

The Importance of Having (and/or Being) a Patient Advocate

A Patient Advocate is a person you choose to serve as a kind of assistant or overseer of your healthcare in specified ways and under specific health-related situations. You and your prospective advocate need to have a lengthy discussion so you both agree what specific responsibilities you want him/her to assume. It's helpful to have an alternate in case your primary advocate is unavailable.

A **patient advocate** is different from your **healthcare power of attorney (proxy)**. Your healthcare proxy is responsible for making healthcare decisions on your behalf only if you become incapacitated and lack the ability to make medical decisions for yourself *[see Chapter 12: Healthcare Power of Attorney (or Proxy)]*. Your Advocate assists you in navigating our complex health system and in you making decisions about your care for which you are quite competent.

If you are young and healthy, you're probably thinking that you don't need an advocate. But one of your family members, perhaps an elderly parent or grandparent with chronic medical problems, could benefit greatly by having you or some other reliable person serve as their advocate. Patient Advocates comprise a diverse group with differing skill sets and sometimes differing responsibilities. There are two large groups of potential Patient advocates: Family and Friends; and professional—even certified—Patient Advocates. Their roles, responsibilities and limitations are discussed in detail in *Chapter 12 Benefits of Having a Patient Advocate.*

As far as we know, there is no standard or universal advocate agreement form, so you can simply write down the specific responsibilities that you and your advocate (and alternate) agree upon. We have developed a simple advocate agreement (see our *website Chapter 1, Appendix: Designation of My Patient Advocate and Alternate).* On that form you will find the usual duties that a Patient Advocate may be asked to perform. We suggest that you have your attorney or estate planner review the draft of your agreement to make certain it will be honored in the state where you live.

If you hire an advocate from a neighborhood agency, they most likely have a standard agreement that can be modified. Make sure the agreement includes everyone's contact information. You, your advocate, and an alternate need to sign the agreement and have your signatures witnessed. According to what's required in your state, you may consider having the document notarized. Make certain you distribute a copy to your advocate, alternate, doctors, hospital administration, selected family members, your lawyer, and others so everyone knows who your advocate and alternate are, their responsibilities and contact information.

Recognizing and Overcoming Emotional Barriers to Early Signs of an Illness

---

"Not me" refers to the deceptive belief that getting sick may happen to others but "not to me" – a notion especially prevalent among the "young and healthy" who understandably may believe they are not mortal and vulnerable like everyone else. Unless you are challenged by personal or family illness or other serious life events earlier in life, this "not-me" belief may quietly extend into mid and later life and prevent you from accepting your vulnerability to illness. You may ignore early signs of a problem, passing it off to "getting older" and delay seeking appropriate medical care. One of the biggest factors in not addressing health problems early on involves the normal psychological and emotional barriers most of us share.

What are some of these emotional barriers? First, it is common and normal to experience anxiety if we suspect we are ill. Fear and anxiety can make us put off getting medical care at the very time it's most needed and the problem is most likely to be remedied.

Second, we all share, in varying degrees, psychological defenses such as denial, suppression, and/or rationalization. All these reinforce the belief that we are not vulnerable to the slings and arrows of misfortune, such as an illness. Denial helps you avoid the awareness of some painful aspect of reality – such as symptoms of a medical illness – by negating sensory data (for example, ignoring discomfort from a persistent cough). Using suppression, we consciously or semiconsciously postpone attention to a conscious concern (for example, the persistent cough). We may acknowledge the discomfort, but we minimize it. Using rationalization, we offer explanations to justify our belief or behavior (for example, "My cough will go away; it's only a cold.") We may procrastinate while using these normal (and – if used excessively – potentially detrimental) defenses to reinforce the "not me" phenomenon. And they can get in the way of a proactive approach to your healthcare.

Third, we all prefer, to varying degrees, to avoid unpleasant situations. It is more fun to plan our vacation, retirement, or our child's upcoming graduation than to address the possibility of a medical illness. However, confidently preparing to deal with adverse situations, such as a medical problem, is constructive and potentially lifesaving. You recall our story at the beginning of this chapter about how Stephen and his wife, Mrs. Nightingale, had carefully planned the transfer of his medical care to a new doctor well in advance of their move from California to New Mexico.

Here's another example of these defenses. A forty-four-year-old woman notices a swelling in her breast but tells herself it's nothing and doesn't give it a second thought (denial). Months later the swelling has increased, but she consciously decides not to give it much thought (suppression). The swelling increases further, but she ascribes it to having bumped into something, which explains the initial swelling (rationalization), so she puts off seeing her doctor (procrastination), much to her detriment.

How can you overcome these emotional barriers that may interfere with getting prompt medical care? First, be more introspective and do an active self-appraisal. Seriously think about your personal, emotional makeup and coping style. Recognize you're like most of us who have a tendency to use these normal emotional mechanisms to avoid recognizing early signs of a health problem. Listen to what your body is telling you. One of the authors had a recurring toothache for two weeks. After reading this part of the chapter several times, he finally overcame his belief that the pain would go away and made an appointment with his dentist who discovered a cavity.

Second, just take care of it! If you notice early signs of an illness, make an appointment with your PC-Phys., PCP, or a nearby outpatient facility (*see Chapter 4*).

Taking a long-term perspective, strive to be as healthy as possible, which also serves as a good model for your family members to follow. This includes finding good healthcare providers who are reliable and invested in your health over the long haul, choosing the best affordable insurance, and following a healthy lifestyle.

Third, complete your and your family members' PHR and carry it with you on your smartphone so it's readily available when you visit your physician or should you have a medical emergency.

Fourth, consider consulting with a health coach or trainer who can help you develop a personalized exercise program, diet, and other ways of adopting a healthier lifestyle. Trainers are available at your neighborhood gym, recommendations from friends, ads in your local newspaper, or via the Internet. When you do your part toward staying healthy, you give the healthcare system, imperfect as it is, the best chance to work for you and your family. You can be the example for those close to you.

Getting and Staying Healthy Throughout All Stages of Life

Perhaps the surest way of not having to deal with an imperfect healthcare system is to stay healthy. We all know that following a healthy lifestyle will reduce your risk for acute and chronic illnesses, help you be more resilient should you become ill, and increase your longevity.

Yet Americans have one of the highest rates of obesity in the world. Many of us do not eat nutritional foods, exercise regularly, sleep seven to eight hours a night, take a multivitamin, or have sufficient meaning and purpose in life. We all have our individual ways of dealing on a daily basis, with significant stresses that are so prevalent in 21st century America.

Adopting a healthy lifestyle can result in less need for doctor visits, medications, and the hospital. So, why don't more of us follow a healthy lifestyle?

The following are some reasons why we don't practice scientifically proven ways for adopting a healthier way of life and living longer. Think seriously about which obstacles stand in your way. It is never too late to change.

1. **Lack of role models**

   If you grew up in a family who didn't practice a healthy lifestyle, you probably didn't eat healthy food, exercise regularly, or get enough sleep, simply because we tend to emulate those closest to us. During adolescence, peer pressure can make you conform to your group's sometimes less than healthy behavior, such as eating fast foods and excessive risk-taking. If these role models exclude principles of healthy living, where will we learn them?

2. **Fast-paced American lifestyle and stressful economic times**

   The pressure on middle-class families to make a living during difficult economic times can lead to shortened mealtimes and choosing inexpensive, non-nutritional fast food high in calories, salt, fat, and sugar – a recipe that can lead to obesity and all its complications.

3. **The desire for instant gratification**

   We all tend to want instant gratification, including denial of the long-term health consequences of an unhealthy lifestyle. We are more apt to order a gooey rich dessert rather than fresh fruit from a restaurant's dessert menu because of wanting some reward after a strenuous week at work. We find ways of rationalizing our less than healthy choices.

4. **Medical and mental health problems**

   Obesity and depression are two of many problems that can deter you from beginning an exercise program at a gym because of self-consciousness and/or apathy. Exercise is known to combat depression by stimulating the brain's production of endorphins and mood-enhancing neurotransmitters. Depression can interfere with medical treatment, such as following your doctor's treatment plan and keeping follow-up appointments. Untreated, depression and obesity can significantly impair quality of life and shorten life expectancy.

The Greatest Gifts You Can Bestow on Your Children and Grandchildren

———————————

As a parent and/or grandparent, you can set a good example for your family by carrying out suggestions offered in this and subsequent chapters. Your children will want to emulate your healthy lifestyle and your strategies for securing good healthcare from our complicated healthcare system.

Another important gift to your children is helping them feel empowered to avoid illnesses that they may be genetically predisposed to (illnesses that "run in the family"). If diabetes is prevalent in older family members, encouraging one's children to adopt a nutritious diet low in sugar and fat, and an exercise program, may lower their risk.

One of the authors developed tinnitus ("ringing in the ears") when he turned sixty-five, about the same age that his father and older sister developed the same problem. Consulting several ear specialists, he learned that there was no effective treatment. But by doing some investigation, he learned about preventative measures that may help his children avoid "inheriting" tinnitus, such as avoiding exposure to loud sounds (such as rock concerts) and avoiding teeth grinding. These preventive measures were shared with his adult children, who were appreciative and agreed to share the information with their children.

Chapter 1 Key Points

Key Points: Reasons for Assuming More Responsibility for Your Healthcare

- America's healthcare system is rapidly changing, dysfunctional, fragmented, and impersonal.
- Healthcare providers spend less time with you and are in short supply.
- Reduce the risk of being a victim of medical, hospital, and medication errors.
- Clarify who's "the captain" (coordinator) of your healthcare team.
- Adopting a healthy lifestyle can serve as a model so you and your children can live healthier, longer lives.

Key Points: Reducing Your Risk of Medical Errors

- Medical errors are a major cause of preventable death and injury.
- Medical errors occur especially during periods of transition (e.g. in hospital settings: shift changes, changes in medication, transition home).
- Fully understanding the risks/rewards of proposed tests/treatments helps your decision making and reduces the risk of errors.
- If hospitalized, have your trusted relative or patient advocate spend time overseeing your care.

Key Points: Personal Health Record (PHR)

- Collect and organize your past and current health data.
- Include contact information about all your doctors, your patient advocate, healthcare and financial proxy, and close relatives.
- Include allergies and blood type.
- To construct your PHR, simply use one of the Internet sites (e.g., www.myPHR.com)
- Maintain and update your records routinely on your computer, tablet, or smartphone.
- Carry it with you on your electronic device. A nearby relative or friend should have a copy.

Key Points: Patient Advocate

- To oversee your healthcare in ways you designate and both agree.
- Is different from a healthcare proxy; the latter assumes responsibility for making decisions on your behalf if you become incapacitated.
- Especially valuable during the first days of hospitalization and during the transition home.
- Can accompany you to tests and treatments and help you follow through with treatment.

Key Points: Recognizing and Overcoming Emotional Barriers to Early Signs of an Illness

- Recognize these normal, emotional barriers – denial, suppression, rationalization – so they don't interfere with obtaining medical assistance at early signs of an illness.

- Adopt a healthier lifestyle. Obtain assistance from your doctor and a trainer (coach).

- One of the greatest gifts you can bestow on your children is adopting a healthy lifestyle for them to emulate.

References

1. Allen, M., *How many die from medical mistakes in U.S. hospitals?* 2013 (accessed 2018 October 10); Available from: http://www.npr.org/sections/health-shots/2013/09/20/224507654/how-many-die-from-medical-mistakes-in-u-s-hospitals.

2. Gwande, A. Being Mortal. New York: Metropolitan Books, 2015-p.79-111.

3. James, J.T., *A new, evidence-based estimate of patient harms associated with hospital care.* Journal of Patient Safety, 2013. 9(3): p. 122-8.

4. Michelson, L.D. Three things you can do right now to be better prepared. in Michelson, L.D. The Patient's Playbook. Alfred A. Knopf. New York 2015-p.62-75.

5. Press, M.F. Instant replay: A quarterback's view of care coordination. New England Journal of Medicine, 371-489-497, 2014.

CHAPTER 2

Strategies for Keeping Costs Down

Introduction

Carol is a forty-year-old married woman who works at a small company. Her husband is self-employed, and the family's health coverage comes from Carol's employer. The economy is weak, and her company is looking to decrease employee costs and overhead. Her boss recently asked if she would be receptive to a decrease in her work hours. That was out of the question since family finances were already spread thin. She feared losing her health insurance if she worked part-time. Her company had just switched to an ACA-compliant insurance policy with a very high deductible but the same premiums. Carol's husband had just left the hospital after a skiing accident that left them with a flood of bills from the ambulance company, hospital, several doctors, and the laboratory. Because he was hospitalized emergently, neither he nor Carol knew that two of his physician specialists were out-of-network. She felt overwhelmed at handling the bills. She was reluctant to ask her boss for help since he was preoccupied with business survival. We'll learn later in this chapter how Carol's resourcefulness helped solve their financial problems.

Americans are burdened with escalating healthcare costs. Medical debt continues as the number one cause of personal bankruptcy in America. Health insurance premiums, especially for those with individual (as compared to group) policies, increased by double digit percentages in 2018, with further increases expected in future years. Employers have shifted more healthcare costs onto employees in the form of higher yearly deductibles, co-pays, and other out-of-pocket costs. What can we Americans do to protect ourselves and actually reduce medical costs?

This chapter offers practical, effective strategies to reduce your medical expenses before and even after you incur them. We explain the inside story about how doctor and hospital billing really work, how to reduce your medical bills, innovative uses of health and flexible savings accounts, and how to avoid expensive, often unnecessary, tests and procedures. We also discuss how you can protect yourself and your family from a healthcare system where doctors and hospitals and even patients unknowingly over-test and over-treat, even in situations when palliative or hospice care may be the more humane approach.

Why Americans Are Burdened by Medical Debt

Chances are that medical debt problems affect you, a family member, or a friend. In 2016, one in five Americans was contacted by bill collectors about their medical debt. We don't want you to be that person. Medical debt accounts for more than one in every three dollars owed in collection accounts, far more than any other type of debt in collections. Once your bill – medical or otherwise – goes to collections, your credit rating can suffer.

There are several reasons why you and many other Americans are saddled with medical debt. Every year, healthcare expenses rise several times greater than the rate of inflation while wages remain stagnant.[1] In the past decade, especially during the economic recession of 2008 to 2011, employers turned to less expensive insurance policies for their employees because of escalating healthcare costs. Employers also shifted more of the burden of healthcare onto employees in the form of higher out-of-pocket expenses.

In 2006, the annual deductible that employees of a large company had to pay out-of-pocket before their health insurance kicked in was $303. In 2015, it more than tripled to $1300, That is seven times higher than wages rose in the same ten-year period. Employees of small businesses in 2015 had an even higher deductible — $1,800. The average employee in 2014 paid $5,000 out-of-pocket for healthcare, which included his/her share of premiums, the deductible, co-pays, and other out-of-pocket medical expenses.[2] But thanks partly to the ACA, even large businesses in the fast-food industry had to provide insurance for their employees. In 2015, 98 percent of firms with two hundred or more employees offered their workers at least one health plan; those companies that didn't had to pay a penalty.

If you are in your fifties to early sixties, you are part of a group that is most vulnerable to unexpected, unplanned medical debt. Check to see if your company's post-retirement insurance benefits can be relied upon to provide coverage for you and your family and whether you can expect Medicare alone, after you reach age 65, to be your healthcare safety net. If not, you may be very disappointed at a time when you most need coverage.

Healthcare needs typically increase as one gets older. Retirees who rely on Medicare alone without a supplemental plan to pay their healthcare expenses should expect that Medicare will cover only about half their medical expenses. The amount of out-of-pocket money that retirees who have only Parts A and B Medicare without a supplemental plan will need to pay for the additional 30 to 50 percent of medical, medication, and other health-related expenses, will continue to rise. For example, the savings that a couple with only Medicare insurance (without a supplement) will need for their healthcare expenses during the twenty-plus post-retirement years was estimated to be $160,000, per a 2002 study. That figure rose to $240,000 in 2009.[3] Extrapolate those figures for another eight years to 2017 and you can estimate, or maybe you prefer

---

1   The Associated Press. "Health care costs projected to grow faster than economy. Obamacare, aging population responsible". *Albuquerque Journal* (July 29, 2015).

2   http://www.forbes.com/sites/brucejapsen/2013/10/17/in2014-workers-share-of-health-co.

3   http://www.cnbc.com/2013/11/04/health-care-costs-can-destroy-all-that-retirement-planning.html.

not to, what amount of money might be needed. So, you can see why it is very important to have a good supplemental insurance plan in addition to Medicare Parts A, B, and D.

A colleague of one of the authors learned this lesson firsthand. Mr. Jamison, an eighty-two-year-old retired attorney/accountant, had a reputation for planning ahead. He developed a sudden bowel obstruction that required emergency surgery. Fortunately, he not only had Medicare Parts A, B, and D and a supplemental policy with United Healthcare, but also an additional policy that paid the hospital $400 per day in addition to what his other policies paid. He developed a post-surgery complication that extended his hospitalization an additional week. He waited until he regained his strength and could think more clearly before he and his wife scrutinized and corrected some hospital and doctor billing errors. They made certain that all his insurance policies paid the full amount they were responsible for before they paid their portion. The final amount he owed came to only $102.50. Being a curious fellow, he asked the manager of the hospital's finance office what he would have owed if he'd had only Medicare Parts A, B and D. The amount would have been $55,000! It's advisable for those of us in our thirties, forties, and fifties to consider a supplemental policy and to put money into a special saving account, such as health or flexible saving account, for unexpected medical expenses.

What We as Patients Need to Know About Medical Bills

What most of us don't know is that medical bills are negotiable before and even after they are incurred. Also, medical bills are fraught with errors. There is a whole industry of experts trained to spot these errors and negotiate medical bills down to reasonable levels. They are called medical billing advocates.[4] Some work for free or charge reasonable fees. Of course, we can successfully negotiate on our own behalf. So why don't we?

Why We Don't Negotiate Medical Bills

Why don't we think of negotiating our medical bills? Do we think it's impolite to question our doctor or hospital about anticipated medical expenses before we actually receive medical care? Many people think it's offensive, disrespectful, or even rude to discuss such matters. And many of us don't have experience in broaching these issues with healthcare providers.

---

4   http://www.needhelppayingbills.com

When you are ill, your main focus is on getting medical help, whatever the cost. You may feel vulnerable and less sure of yourself and view your doctor as a healer who has the answers to get you well. You put great trust, hope, and faith in your healer and comparatively less in yourself. Doctors don't want to spend their valuable time talking about money issues with their patients. They delegate this to their office billing manager. So, you are actually doing yourself and your doctor or hospital a favor by openly discussing billing matters before actually getting medical care because this conveys to them that you are a thoughtful, reliable, responsible person who wants to know what your expenses are likely to be and that you intend to meet your financial responsibilities. If you are acutely ill and not feeling up to discussing financial matters, you can enlist the help of your patient advocate or a trusted family member to assist you in understanding the approximate cost you'll be responsible for after your insurance has paid.

Think of it this way: When you buy a new car, do you assume that the sticker price on the window is what you are going to pay? Probably not. You're likely to check prices at other dealers or Internet sites to see where you can get the best deal. This takes time and negotiating skills, but it's time well spent. So, consider looking at doctor and hospital fees in a similar light. There is no need to be shy about asking!

How Medical Billing Really Works

Your doctor and hospital have contracts with many insurance companies. Insurance companies have agreements to pay doctors and hospitals a certain amount for particular medical exams, tests, and procedures. No matter how much money the doctor or hospital bills, the insurance company pays based on the amount negotiated beforehand, often referred to as the "approved" amount. For example, a doctor may bill your insurance company $500 for an initial one-hour comprehensive medical examination. Your insurance company, because of the previously negotiated agreed-upon amount, may "approve" $300, which is the maximum the doctor can collect. Insurance pays the doctor (depending on your particular insurance policy) 80 percent ($240) of the approved amount. You may be responsible for the co-payment (or the balance) of $60, if you have already met your yearly deductible. A co-payment is usually a fixed amount for a particular service, such as the above $60 for an initial comprehensive exam. If you have a supplemental insurance policy, it may pay your doctor part or all of the $60. If your doctor is an in-network contracted physician with your insurance, he/she is not permitted to collect more than $300.

Your yearly insurance deductible is another important issue. If your policy (like most) has a yearly deductible (which often begins on January 1 of every year) of, let's say, $2,000 and you have not yet paid out-of-pocket the $2,000 for medical, medication, hospital, and other expenses, you are responsible, using the above example, for paying your doctor the $300 of your $2,000 deductible. You will still be responsible for paying the remaining $1,700 for other medical costs out-of-pocket until you've met the $2,000 deductible.

Once you've met your deductible, your insurance company will begin paying (depending on your particular policy) about 80 percent of the approved amount of subsequent medical bills. This is analogous to the $500 deductible for automobile collision insurance you pay out-of-pocket before your insurance company begins to pay.

You or your doctor's billing manager could contact your insurance company to find out – before you incur any medical bills – the following: (1) What is your yearly deductible, and how much has been met? (2) Does your insurance cover the proposed test, procedure, or surgery? (3) Is the doctor, hospital, and specialist you may need in-network? (4) What is the approved amount for the procedure? (5) What portion of the approved amount (the co-pay) will be your responsibility? (6) What is the approximate cost if an out-of-network physician specialist needs to be involved in your care? (7) Will your insurance cover any of the costs if an out-of-network specialist is needed?

Returning to Carol's plight with her husband's medical bills from his ski accident, she did not know that her husband's two specialists (the radiologist and anesthesiologist) were out-of-network. We'll soon learn how she dealt with her financial dilemma.

There are also free Internet sites, such as Healthcare Blue Book[5] and Fair Health, Inc.,[6] where you can find out what your insurer actually pays the doctor or hospital for a particular procedure near where you live (sometimes 80 percent of the approved amount). New Choice Health lets you compare fair prices with the list prices for particular procedures. For example, the "fair price" (or the approximate approved amount) for knee arthroscopy in 2014 in Brentwood, Tennessee was $9,200 in an outpatient surgery center (surgicenter) compared to the list price of $20,200. Using this example, the surgicenter may be paid 80 percent of the approved amount ($7,360), and the patient's responsibility may be 20 percent ($1,840). The above costs are just approximations depending on your insurance and other factors. It's certainly helpful to have all this information before surgery.

Before deciding to have an expensive procedure such as surgery, make sure your hospital, physician, and specialists you may be seeing, are contracted providers (in-network) with your health insurance plan. If they are out-of-network (not contracted with your insurance plan), your insurance may pay little to nothing of the bill, and your financial responsibility will be high. So, you need to know all these details beforehand. Also, your doctor's office manager and hospital may need to obtain prior approval *before* an expensive procedure (such as surgery) even if the doctor is in-network, but especially if he/she is out-of-network. Having all this information helps you avoid "surprise bills". Don't assume that the hospital and doctors have all the correct answers. You may want to call your insurance company to substantiate these important issues.

If your financial situation permits, try not to let cost considerations supersede the quality of healthcare, especially if you have a serious health problem. You can research comparative information about patient outcomes and quality of care for different procedures at hospitals that you are considering for your own care.[7]

---

5   www.healthcarebluebook.com.
6   www.fairhealthconsumer.org.
7   www.hospitalcompare.hhs.gov

If you do not have insurance, the doctor or hospital is not bound by any "approved" amount, so you may be billed the full ("list") price for the doctor's and hospital's services, which is usually much higher than the negotiated "approved" amount if you had insurance. So, whether or not you have insurance, it's wise to know beforehand not only the list price but also the approved amount for a procedure, such as surgery. You can find this out beforehand by learning what the CPT (current procedural terminology) code is for a particular medical test or procedure. The CPT code is a long numerical code (there are hundreds of different ones) used by commercial and government insurance carriers such as Medicare. Your doctor's or hospital's billing manager may be able to tell you the CPT code and the approximate approved amount for a particular procedure that your insurance company would pay a portion of. By having this information, you will know beforehand what your approximate financial responsibility will be (sometimes it's 20 percent of the approved amount).

If you are fortunate enough to have the assistance of your doctor's or hospital's experienced billing manager, he/she may be willing to gather all this information from your insurance company. If the billing manager doesn't know, you can go to the American Medical Association website[8] and find out the CPT code for the procedure you are having. Then contact your insurance company to find out the approximate dollar amount of the approved amount the insurance company will pay and the amount that is your responsibility.

If your procedure, for example knee surgery, is only partially covered by your insurance and your portion of the cost is high, you can use your knowledge of the approved amount to negotiate close to that amount. You can say to the doctor's office manager, "My insurance only partially covers this procedure, and I'll be paying a lot of money for out-of-pocket costs (the co-pay). Could you lower my portion of the approved amount?"

If you are having financial problems, don't feel ashamed or embarrassed about mentioning this because doctors and their staff are understanding, especially during rough economic times. Billing managers, after discussion with your doctor or hospital's financial officer, may lower your portion or suggest a payment plan.

If you have been a longtime reliable patient and no longer have insurance, ask if the doctor or hospital would consider accepting from you as full payment what an insurance company's approved fee would be. You may be pleasantly surprised to not have to pay the much higher list price.

It doesn't hurt to try any of the above strategies.[9] This worked for one of the author's patients who lost her insurance along with her job. The doctor agreed to continue treatment at a discount of 50 percent of her previous insurance's approved fee until she obtained another job that paid for her health insurance. She gradually paid the doctor what was owed.

If all this does not seem daunting and time-consuming enough, what if you need a complicated procedure, such as heart surgery, that requires not only a surgeon but also an anesthesiologist, consultation with one or more specialists, and post-operative physical and occupational therapy? Before starting this whole complicated process, we suggest meeting with the hospital's and doctors' business managers. Ask their assistance in figuring out – as best they can and given unpredictable complications – what your insurance

8   ama-assn.org.
9   Lacie Glover. 5 Expert tips for negotiating your medical bills. http://health.usnews.com/health-news/patient-advice/articles/2014/10/16/5-expert-tips-for.

is likely to pay and what will be your responsibility. Bring along a family member and/or your patient advocate to be your second set of eyes and ears. Be sure to verify what medical care will be in-network, what may be out-of-network, and how that will affect your financial responsibility.

When Carol learned that two of her husband's specialists were out-of-network she made appointments with their billing managers, who understood her financial hardship. After discussions with the out-of-network specialists, they agreed not only to reduce their bill to what an insurance company would consider the approved amount, but further reduced their bill by another 20 percent.

Balance Billing

Balance billing can happen after your insurance company has paid everything that it's obligated to pay toward your medical bill and you've paid your deductible, co-insurance, or co-payment. In other words, your bill has been completely paid. If there is still a *balance owed* that you're expected to pay, it's likely that you're being balance-billed [1]. An illustration helps. Say your in-network doctor sent your insurance company a bill for $100 for medical services, and the agreed upon "approved" amount was $80. Your insurance company has paid its share (80 percent, or $64), and you paid your doctor (20 percent, or $16). The payments total $80, which is the approved amount. If the medical provider expects you to pay the remaining balance of $20, this may be an instance of balance billing. It's usually best to give your provider the benefit of the doubt. Call his/her billing manager and try to resolve the problem locally. It may be a simple billing error. Sometimes this is legal, but often it is not and should not be paid. A recent newspaper article indicates that 30 percent of adults with private health insurance fall victim to balance billing, known also as "surprise bills" [5]. For additional information and resources on this topic, please go to our website.

Scrutinize and Pay Bills Promptly

Be sure to request an itemized bill so each charge can be scrutinized (billing errors are very common). Make certain that your insurance company has paid the maximum amount that it is responsible for *before* you pay what's required of you. If you have secondary or perhaps even tertiary insurance, make sure they've met their full responsibility. The hospital's and doctor's billing departments may be less aggressive in pursuing the maximum amount from your insurance company if you prematurely make payments.

Once you're satisfied that the remaining amount you owe is correct, try to pay it as soon as possible or arrange a payment plan because you don't want your bill to go to a collection agency, which can tarnish your credit rating. It is much easier to resolve a billing problem or negotiate a discount before your bill goes to collections. Once in collections, that company has taken over your debt, and the doctor and/or hospital is no longer obliged to negotiate with you.

Billing Errors

Billing errors are common. Diagnoses, medical procedures, and tests have specific codes sent on bills from your doctor's and hospital's billing offices to your insurance company. A simple clerical coding error such as an incorrect letter or number can result in insufficient payment or denial by the insurance company. If your provider's billing staff does not catch the errors and re-submit the bill, the bill can then become your financial burden. You may need to contact the doctor's or hospital's billing manager about these and other suspected errors.

So, it's important to keep copies of all your bills and to ask for an itemized statement. Many doctors and hospitals may send you a summary bill with a single "amount due". Instead, you want an itemized statement that has every single charge on it so you, your advocate, or a professional billing advocate can scrutinize the bill for charges you did not incur or for incorrect coding – both are common occurrences.

In addition, keep a record of all phone calls, emails, and written correspondence with your insurance company and your doctor's and hospital's billing offices. Ask for that person's name, location, and call reference number, and write down exactly what was discussed. If answers to your questions are pending, tell the person that you will follow up with another call or email in two to three weeks. Be sure to follow through, which demonstrates your reliability and resolve.

Consider Payment Options

If you have put away money in a health or flexible savings plan, consider using these funds to pay off your medical bills. The doctor's and hospital's billing departments want to get monies owed off their books as soon as possible, so if you are able to pay promptly, they may even consider a discount. You have nothing to lose by inquiring. If you are not financially able to pay right away, arrange a payment plan that is realistically within your financial means. All your previous discussions with your providers about billing issues have substantiated your reliability. Doctors and hospitals will want to work with you.

Avoid Paying by Credit Card

If you pay all your remaining bills with a credit card, your debt has been paid and you weaken your ability to negotiate the remainder of your hospital's and doctor's bills. And if you don't pay your credit card bill in a timely manner, you'll be subjected to high interest rates.

You Can Still Negotiate Later On

If you have huge bills, even after your insurer has paid its maximum, you can still ask your doctor's and hospital's billing departments for a discount. You have nothing to lose by offering to pay 30 to 40 percent of the remaining bill right now as payment in full. Even if your initial offer is not accepted, it may by countered with a reasonable discount. Hospitals and doctors want to avoid a lengthy collection process and paying the collection company a high percentage of what is collected. If you have been paying reliably on a monthly payment plan, have been a longtime patient, and encounter rough economic times, you can request that part or all of your remaining balance be waived. You can also ask if your payment plan can be extended or changed to an interest-free plan.

If you can't negotiate a reduction yourself, consider enlisting the help of a non-profit, professional billing advocate such as the Access Project.[10] It provides free one-on-one coaching, including negotiating on your behalf your remaining bill with your hospital and doctors. You can fill out an online form, and an Access Project staff member will call you. Other options include Medical Billing Advocates of America, which keeps a percentage (about a third) of the reduction negotiated for you. Two others are Morgans and also Lambs.

Reducing the High Cost of Medications

Generic medications are much less expensive than brand-name medications. Your physician usually doesn't know your insurance's particular drug benefits, so before your doctor writes a prescription, ask if a generic is available. Even before a visit to your doctor, review the brand-name medications you routinely use and call the pharmacy department of your insurance company (the telephone number is sometimes on

---

10   https://www.rwjf.org/en/library/research/2007/03/the-access-project.html

the back of your insurance card) or your neighborhood pharmacy and ask the cost of a one-month supply of your brand-name medication. Ask if an equally effective generic medication is available and if so, what is the difference in cost. Your insurance card or information booklet may provide a website that lists prices for generic, brand-name, and alternative but less expensive drugs used to treat the same medical condition that have been on the market a long time. You can also compare retail pharmacy prices for specific drugs on the Internet. Many discount stores, such as Walmart and Costco, offer hundreds of commonly used generic medications for $10 to $20 a month.

If your physician thinks it's important for you to take a specific brand-name medication that is not covered by your insurance, your doctor can submit an authorization request explaining the reasons why the brand-name drug is much preferred and why it should be approved. In addition, ask your doctor if he/she has free samples of the brand-name medication available in the office, but the supply may be limited. Also, pharmaceutical companies offer free supplies of specific brand-name medications for patients whose yearly income is below a certain amount, so the doctor's staff or you can check the pharmaceutical company's website for details. (*See Chapter 10 for additional ways to reduce medication costs*).

Ask Your Doctor for a Discount

If you have become uninsured or your insurance has a high yearly deductible or co-payment and you've had a longtime good working relationship with your physician, you have nothing to lose by asking the office manager to consider a discount or a payment plan. If you need an expensive procedure, such as surgery, ask your PCPhys. to recommend a surgeon and hospital that he/she would consider given your financial constraints.

Put Money into a Health or Flexible Savings Account

Most large-company employers allow you to set aside part of your paycheck with pre-tax dollars in some type of savings account to pay for healthcare expenses. If you are self-employed, you can set up one of these accounts. This money can be used to cover deductibles, co-pays, medications and other out-of-pocket medical costs not totally paid for by your insurance. There are two major types of medical savings accounts: a health savings account and a flexible savings account.

Health Savings Account

A health savings account (HSA) is a tax-advantaged medical savings account that you can contribute to with pre-tax dollars and withdraw money from tax-free if used for out-of-pocket medical, dental, and eye care expenses. If you use an HSA for other than health-related expenses, you'll pay taxes on the money withdrawn and the interest earned.

To qualify for an HSA, your insurance policy has to have an annual deductible over $1,300 for individual coverage or over $2,600 for family coverage. As long as you hold an "HSA eligible" high-deductible insurance policy, you can contribute tax-free dollars up to the annual limit every year.[11]

An HSA can't be used to pay for health insurance premiums, but it has tax and other benefits. The money you put into an HSA is tax deductible, and you can invest the money in various ways. The money remaining in the HSA can eventually be rolled over into a retirement account when you are eligible for Medicare.

For 2016, HSA's annual contribution limit was $3,350 for an individual and $6,750 for a family of four. For 2018, an individual can contribute a maximum of $3,450 and $6,900 for a family. If you are fifty-five or older you can contribute an extra $1,000 a year.

Because HSA contributions are tax deductible, contributions may reduce your modified adjusted gross income (MAGI) and thereby reduce your taxes as well as increase your chance, if it lowers your MAGI, of being eligible for an insurance subsidy.[12] If you fund an HSA, be sure to file tax form 8889 so you'll deduct the correct amount from your taxable income. You can compare different HSA terms at different financial institutions, such as the HSA Bank.

It's usually advisable to invest the HSA in a safe investment, such as a bank savings account, so the money is readily available in emergency situations for out-of-pocket medical expenses. But if you and your family are young and healthy, have the financial means and want to take advantage of the savings component of an HSA, you could consider some variation of the following.

For a family of four, if you invest $5,000 at the beginning of every year for ten years in a bank or similar savings account paying, say, 2 percent interest per year, it would be worth approximately $68,528 – minus any withdrawals to pay out-of-pocket medical expenses. But if you invested the $5,000 each year in good, safe mutual funds or exchange traded funds (ETFs) that have minimal management fees, and the fund appreciated 7 percent per year (considering stock market downturns), and there were no withdrawals for medical expenses, after ten years it could be worth over $73,417. The money, which may appreciate more in subsequent years, could later be rolled over into a retirement account when you reach the age for Medicare. Granted, most of us need our salaries just to make ends meet, but if you want to plan for an early retirement and are an astute saver, you may want to talk with your financial or tax advisor, especially because of the complexity and potential yearly changes of how an HSA works.

11   http://obamacarefacts.com/health-insurance/health-savings-account-hsa/.
12   http://obamacarefacts.com/modified-adjusted-gross-income-magi/ http://obamacarefacts.com/obamacare-subsidies/.

Returning to Carol's financial predicament, she and her husband had contributed $2,000 at the beginning of each of the last ten years into an HSA. The monies were invested in an exchange traded fund (ETF) that tracked the S&P 500. Fortunately, the fund appreciated about eight percent a year and after ten years was worth approximately $32,500, which was enough to pay off the remainder of her husband's bills.

Flexible Savings Account (FSA)

A flexible savings account (FSA) allows employees of companies that offer this account to contribute pre-tax dollars to pay out-of-pocket healthcare expenses not covered by medical insurance. If your company doesn't offer an FSA or you are self-employed, an FSA can be obtained on your own.

Before you put money into an FSA, estimate your out-of-pocket expenses for the coming year. To do this, figure out your annual out-of-pocket expenses for the past few years to arrive at an estimate of your next year's medical expenses and then add in any anticipated extra medical expenses.

For 2017, the FSA contribution limit was $2,600 and for 2018 it was $2,650, under the rules of the ACA. If you fund an FSA, you can't also fund an HSA that same year. You can always use your HSA, even if you can't fund it that year.[13]

You can sign up for an FSA with your company during open enrollment or after a "life change" (for example, marriage or the birth of a child). The human resources department of your company can assist you in estimating the amount to put into your FSA. FSAs are very popular; an estimated 35 million Americans used them in 2015.

Other Ways to Reduce Medical Expenses

Consider Surgery in a Surgicenter Rather Than a Hospital

Some types of surgery, such as knee surgery, can be performed in an outpatient surgery center (surgicenter) at a much lower cost than in the hospital, which may require an expensive overnight stay. Mrs. Jones needed a left knee replacement. She read the Healthcare Blue Book[14] about the benefits of having it done in a surgicenter and suggested this to her surgeon, who readily agreed. If she had surgery in the hospital rather than the surgicenter, the cost to her would have been $12,000 more. Also, outpatient surgery reduces the risk of a hospital-acquired infection and other hospital-related complications. Many other types of surgery can now be carried out in a surgicenter, so it's worthwhile to inquire.

13   http://obamacarefacts.com/health-insurance/health-savings-account-hsa/.
14   www.healthcarebluebook.com.

Alternatives to an Expensive Emergency Department (ED) Visit

Emergency departments are noisy, brightly lit, and filled with sick patients (and their families or friends) waiting impatiently to be seen. The staff prioritizes who needs to be seen right away, but you can wait a long time before receiving care.

If you have a minor illness, such as a head cold, sprained ankle, or the ubiquitous low back pain, rather than an expensive visit to an ED, it's much less costly, less stressful, and more time efficient (whether or not you have health insurance) to consider one of the following:

- Appointment with your PCPhys. or PCP.

- Workplace clinic – Many large companies have inexpensive or no-cost clinics staffed by a nurse practitioner or other health professional who can handle minor ailments. (*See Chapter 4*).

- Large retail chain drugstores – An increasing number of chain drugstores have clinics managed by nurse practitioners. Whether or not you have insurance, they are much less costly than an ED.

- Urgent care clinics – As the name implies, these clinics are for problems more serious than minor ailments. Staffed by physicians and nurse practitioners, they are much less costly than an ED.

When to Consider the Emergency Department (ED)

Hospital emergency departments are appropriate for serious medical problems, such as signs of heart attack, stroke, or kidney stones. If possible, you or your patient advocate should notify both the ED and your insurance company in advance about your symptoms so the ED can be better prepared when you arrive. Some insurance companies may be reluctant to pay if they are not notified in advance or if they subsequently determine that your symptoms or diagnosis were not serious enough to warrant the ED. (*See Chapter 4*). If you are seriously ill, have a family member or your patient advocate make the calls.

The cost for a simple ED visit for an uninsured person can be well over $3,000 depending on the nature of your problem and where you live. Ambulance service is also very expensive. If your health problem is severe, have a responsible family member drive you to the ED. If no one is available, call for an ambulance for your and other's safety and to reduce your stress.

Bring with you to the ED your personal health record (PHR), your insurance card(s), and an overnight suitcase with clothing and toiletries in case you are admitted to the hospital. If you don't have a PHR, bring a list of all your current medications, dosages, and the medications themselves; a list of past and current medical problems; and all legal documents including your living will, patient advocate agreement and healthcare and financial proxy should you become incapacitated. If you have your PHR in your smartphone bring it to the ED. If your PHR is not available, the person who has a copy should bring it to the ED.

Continuing Your Insurance with COBRA

If you have the financial means, set aside money you can afford into an emergency fund for six months' worth of household, medical, and other expenses in case you or your spouse becomes unemployed or ill. That fund can provide you with peace of mind if your insurance ends along with unemployment or if you incur unexpected expenses. If your insurance ends along with your job, be sure to discuss with your employer's human resources department the option of continuing your insurance under COBRA (Consolidated Omnibus Budget Reconciliation Act).

If your employer has twenty or more employees and you lose your insurance, you may have the option of extending your health insurance under COBRA for up to eighteen months, and under certain qualifying events, for an additional eleven or eighteen months.

COBRA requires that insurance coverage be offered to employees of private sector jobs, state or local government employees, their spouses, and dependent children when group insurance coverage is lost due to qualifying events, such as termination of employment, reduction of number of hours of employment, divorce or legal separation from the spouse who has group insurance from the employer, and other life events.

Individual health insurance under COBRA is more expensive for you than group insurance was when you were employed because the employer usually pays a substantial portion of the employed employees' coverage. However, COBRA insurance is usually less costly than purchasing a new individual policy with similar coverage and benefits on one's own because the employer pays a portion of the cost. But continuing insurance under COBRA can be very expensive for former employees, especially those who are financially strapped. Continuing insurance under COBRA may not apply to some insurance plans sponsored by the federal government (for example, Medicare) or certain church-related organizations.

Try your best to purchase insurance via COBRA, especially if you or a family member has serious health problems, because one recurrence of a serious illness that occurs when uninsured can lead to bankruptcy and accompanying emotional stress.

There is a thirty-day grace period after employment ends during which you can sign up for COBRA with no interruption in insurance coverage. It's essential to pay your monthly premium on time and pay attention to any increase in your monthly premium, especially at the beginning of a new year, because some insurance companies will drop your coverage for one late or insufficient payment. If you lose your insurance, it can be difficult to get reinstated.

If your eighteen months of COBRA insurance is soon to expire, consider whether you have a second qualifying event, such as a disability, that may enable you to continue COBRA for an additional eleven or eighteen months.

Before deciding on COBRA, consider other options that may be more affordable, such as getting insurance coverage under your spouse's plan, the health insurance exchange (see *Chapter 3 on the ACA*), Medicaid, or medical care at a local Veteran's Administration clinic or hospital (if you served in the military).

Because of the ACA, if you've lost your insurance, you can purchase insurance any time of year so you don't have to wait for the next enrollment period. If you can't afford insurance, you can obtain healthcare from a neighborhood, city, state, or federally supported non-profit healthcare center or from a university medical center. As we have emphasized throughout this book, don't give up your pursuit of quality medical care. Your persistence and determination will be rewarded.

Why Patients, Doctors, and the Healthcare System May Over-Test and Over-Treat

Modern medicine has miraculously extended life, saved lives, and helped patients regain productive lives. Unfortunately, there are medical illnesses for which there are no cures. And there are periods at the end of life when lack of pleasure, social interactions, and physical and emotional pain and suffering make one question the purpose of living [3].

It's astonishing that about 25 percent of the billions of dollars that Medicare spends every year on medical costs are spent on patients in their last weeks of life. Many terminally ill patients undergo tests, procedures, and surgeries and spend time in expensive intensive care units with little to no prospect of returning to any meaningful quality of life. Why does this happen?

The problem can be looked at from three perspectives – the point of view of patients, doctors, and America's complicated healthcare system.

Patient's Viewpoint

Americans believe that life is precious and everything should be done to preserve it even when it may not be worth the pain, suffering, stress, and financial burden on ourselves and distraught family members. It's certainly not easy, and many of us have probably never had the "tough talk" with our family members to make clear how we would want to be cared for should we have a terminal incurable illness. We have not prepared for the inevitability of our aging and eventual death. Most families avoid using the words "cancer" and "dying" or speak them only in hushed voices.

Many of us have never filled out a healthcare directive (living will), which spells out what we want done and not done if faced with a terminal illness. It's normal and natural to deal emotionally with all these issues by putting off thoughts about one's mortality to "another day." We don't think about the inevitable, especially when we are young and healthy. When Woody Allen entered his geriatric years, he was asked how he felt about growing old and dying. In typical Woody fashion, he replied, "That's been done!" implying that the whole issue is an old and bad joke.

Some of us have unrealistic expectations of our doctors and life-saving advances of modern medicine, such as organ transplants and kidney dialysis. If we become sick, it's natural to bestow upon our doctor our belief in his/her superhuman healing powers. At times, we suspend our own discriminating judgment with the hope that if we follow the doctor's advice, we will be cured. But end-of-life preferences should be discussed well before our lives are ending. In the rare occasion the topic comes up, it may happen in a brief office visit with your overworked new doctor, who you've just met because of your change to new health insurance.

A Wise Elderly Lady Asserts Herself

Elizabeth Sanders, an elegant ninety-two-year-old woman from an old New England family, living independently at home, fell and was taken to a nearby hospital. An enthusiastic orthopedic surgeon, who looked younger than her grandson, mistakenly called her by her first name (not respectful to an elderly woman). He said authoritatively, "Your hip is broken, and you need immediate surgery." He asked her to sign the consent form.

"Not so quick, young man," she retorted. "Let's see the X-ray together, and then I'll decide." Taken aback by her forthright manner, the surgeon acquiesced. Although having no medical training, Mrs. Sanders had been an interior designer known for her attention to detail. She perceived a delicate, thin-line fracture at the head of her thigh bone and politely asked the surgeon if, rather than surgery, "a few weeks of bed rest would suffice?" She quickly followed with: "If I were your beloved grandmother, what would you recommend?" Needless to say, she was discharged home the same day and recovered uneventfully.

Doctor's Viewpoint

Doctors are trained to heal and cure. Older doctors may not have received much training in the benefits of hospice and palliative care for terminally ill patients. Physicians are inclined to follow the wishes of their patients and their patients' families, even when overtreatment can be fraught with pain and suffering that is worse than the underlying illness. Doctors are also concerned about litigation should they fail to carry out what they perceive are their patients' and families' wishes. Communication problems and brief office visits can interfere with doctors' abilities to truly understand their patients' wishes, especially regarding sensitive end-of-life preferences [2].

Healthcare System Viewpoint

From the perspective of our complicated, sometimes poorly coordinated healthcare system, patients, especially the elderly, often see specialists, social workers, and other health professionals in addition to their PCP. Multiple physicians seeing the same patient often don't have time to talk with one another to facilitate a coordinated treatment plan. It isn't always clear which doctor is the "captain" of the healthcare team responsible for coordinating treatment with other health professionals and for clarifying the patient's end-of-life wishes. Who takes responsibility and the time to help patients complete important legal documents such as a living will and healthcare proxy? Is it the PCP, the physician specialist, or an attorney? These important life decisions can be overlooked [6] [7].

Some hospitals, because of religious or other reasons, practice the philosophy that life should be preserved at all costs. Sometimes financial considerations, whether conscious or unconscious, can lead to overzealous treatment to preserve life even when there is little hope of restoring a patient to a meaningful quality of life.

A striking example of how the patient-doctor-healthcare system interface can unknowingly over-treat, with dire consequences, is epitomized by Dr. Murray's seventy-six-year-old longtime patient, Joseph, who had a history of multiple surgeries and chronic illnesses.[15] Joseph had repeatedly told Dr. Murray and his family, substantiated with legal documents, that if he became terminally ill, he never wanted to be resuscitated and kept alive on life support equipment. Then he had a massive stroke and was unconscious when brought by ambulance to the nearest ED, where no one knew him. He was unaccompanied by any family members and didn't have his smart phone, which had his living will, healthcare proxy, and his PHR. Not knowing his wishes, the ED staff resuscitated him and admitted him to the intensive care unit under the care of a hospitalist who didn't know him. Fortunately, Dr. Murray returned home a few days later, took over Joseph's care, brought to the hospital his patient's living will, and talked over the situation with the family. Surrounded and comforted by his family and doctor, the patient's true wishes were respected. The life-support machines were turned off, and he died peacefully.

Another example is that of a ninety-five-year-old comatose woman with advanced dementia and many chronic illnesses who was brought to an ED. The physician did not know the patient or her family. Language barriers interfered with communication. When the doctor explained several times the patient's dire situation and asked what the family wanted, like a choir they said, "We want everything done to save her life!" The doctor patiently asked what the family meant by "everything." To make matters worse, the elderly woman had never communicated to her family what her end-of-life wishes were; nor had she completed a living will. Much to the detriment of the patient, she was resuscitated and spent a week in the intensive care unit experiencing pain and discomfort before she died. The final bill was $38,500, which neither the patient nor family could afford.

Author's Aunt Knew What She Wanted

A former off-Broadway actress, art lover, and subsequent museum docent lived an exciting life until age eighty-two, when she suffered from mild Alzheimer's disease and depression. She had previously filled out a living will indicating that she did not wish any heroic measure to stay alive if she were to become severely incapacitated and totally dependent on others. She then had a massive stroke that paralyzed the left side of her body. Her family knew she did not want to live her last months or years in a wheelchair in a nursing home. When her family visited, she repeatedly and slowly moved the index finger of her right hand across her throat, signaling she had "had it." She readily agreed to move into the nursing home's hospice program, where she received excellent, compassionate care. She was comforted with visits, calls, and cards from family members and died peacefully a week later.

---

15   Murray, Ken. How doctors die; It's not like the rest of us but it should be. http://www.zocalopublicsquare.org/2015/11/30/how-doctors-die/ideas/nexus/.

What Can We Learn from How Doctors Deal with End-of-Life Issues

———————————

Doctors die, just like all people, but most physicians have a different perspective about life and death. Doctors know the limits of modern medicine. They know that people, especially the elderly, fear dying alone and in pain more than they fear death itself. Doctors have witnessed firsthand when fruitless, heroic efforts are made to keep people alive without any prospect of recovery to a meaningful quality of life.

That is why most doctors have a living will that indicates they choose not to be resuscitated if terminally ill with little chance of recovery and have appointed a trustworthy healthcare proxy and an alternate. Their doctors, attorney, hospital administrator, and close family members have copies of these documents. Doctors have explained to their family members what their end-of-life wishes are to protect family from feelings of guilt and to avoid family quarreling when the time comes for the family to support and respect their wish to "go quietly into the night." Their doctors and family can then act as a united team to carry out their end-of- life wishes. Doctors don't want tens of thousands of dollars spent fruitlessly for days of suffering in an intensive care unit if there is no hope of recovery.

Many doctors keep all these legal documents and PHR on their smartphone or other electronic device and carry it with them should they end up in an emergency department where no one knows them. Some elderly health professionals with chronic illnesses even wear a medallion around their neck stamped "DO NOT RESUSCITATE." Doctors know what they want and don't want when their life is ending. With some realistic planning, discussion with family, and completion of necessary legal documents, your wishes will be respected and tended to just as doctors expect for themselves. Dr. Atul Gwande, in his eloquent *New Yorker* article "Overkill." emphasizes that there is an "avalanche of unnecessary medical care that is harming patients physically and financially." [4]

We hope that you can benefit from how doctors cope with end-of-life issues and be empowered to make your wishes known and respected. Most people can find a way to die in peace at home without much pain and discomfort. Hospice and palliative care provide terminally ill patients with comfort and dignity as an alternative to fruitless invasive tests and desperate treatments. Some studies have found that people receiving hospice care often live longer than those with the same disease who are subjected to last ditch attempts at cures.

Chapter 2 Key Points

Key Points: Why We Are Burdened by Medical Debt

- Medical costs continue to escalate.
- Employers have shifted costs onto employees.
- Medicare alone can't be relied upon during post-retirement years.
- We are reluctant to discuss costs before incurring them.
- Medical bills are negotiable!

Key Points: Negotiating Medical Bills

- It's not rude to discuss medical costs with doctors/hospitals.
- By discussing costs early on, you demonstrate that you are reliable and responsible.
- Consider enlisting the help of your patient advocate, family member, or professional billing company.

Key Points: Scrutinize Bills for Errors: Try to Pay Promptly

- Billing errors are very common. Request an itemized statement.
- Review your bill for tests/procedures that you never had.
- Avoid bills going to collections. Negotiate a payment plan.

Key Points: Reduce High Cost of Medications

- Consider generic rather than expensive brand-name medications.
- Compare prices at different pharmacies – www.drx.com.
- Pharmaceutical companies offer free brand medications for those with a low yearly income.
- Discount stores (K-Mart, Walmart, or Costco) offer hundreds of generic medications for $10 to $20 per month.
- Use discount drug cards.
- Ask your doctor for samples.

Key Points: Why Patients, Doctors, and the Healthcare System Over-test and Over-treat

Patient's Viewpoint:

- Patients or their family tend to tell the doctor to "do everything" to save a life.
- We all tend to avoid dealing with end-of-life issues.
- Brief doctor visits are not conducive to address end-of-life wishes.
- Many patients have not completed documents expressing end-of-life wishes.

Doctor's Viewpoint:

- Many doctors have insufficient knowledge of the advantages of hospice and palliative care.
- Doctors are concerned about litigation if they fail to abide by unrealistic patient/family wishes.
- Miscommunication between the patient and the doctor.

Healthcare System Viewpoint:

- Patients' true wishes sometimes go unknown.
- Often unclear who takes the responsibility and time to discuss end-of-life wishes.
- Philosophical and religious beliefs may lead to overzealous treatment.

References

1. Davis, E. *Balance billing—what it is & how it works.* August 18, 2015 [cited October 20, 2018].

2. Gordon, Michael, MD, MSc, FRCPC and Giulia-Anna Perri, MD, CCFP. *Conflicting demands of family at the end of life and challenges for the palliative care team.* Annals of Long-Term Care, January 2015, P. 25-26.

3. Gwande, A. Being Mortal. New York: Metropolitan Books, 2015, p. 149-190.

4. Gwande, A. Overkill: America's epidemic of unnecessary care, in The New Yorker, New York, 5/11/15 p. 42-53.

5. Hoadley, J., S. Ahn, and K. Lucia. *Balance Billing: How are states protecting consumers from unexpected charges?* 2015 [cited October 30, 2018].

6. Michelson, L.D., The Patient's Playbook, Alfred A. Knopf, New York, 2015, p. 238-241.

7. Press, M.F., Instant replay: A quarterback's view of care coordination. New England Journal of Medicine, 371:489-497, 2014.

CHAPTER 3

Taking Advantage of the Affordable Care Act (ACA) and Other Insurance Options

Joseph Simmons is a forty-two-year-old married father of two daughters, ages ten and twelve; he is a self-employed housing contractor living in a small Midwest city. Before the Affordable Care Act (ACA) was fully implemented in 2014, the only health insurance he could find excluded coverage of his wife, Clara's difficult to control juvenile onset diabetes mellitus because it was a pre-existing condition. He had heard that in 2014 such exclusions were no longer legal, but he didn't know if this was true. He'd heard of "insurance exchanges" in 2015, but they seemed too complicated. He needed to focus all his attention on his business, which was failing.

Joseph consulted an insurance agent, who helped him get a high-deductible family policy that met ACA standards and covered Clara's diabetes. However, in late 2015 he found out that the insurance company stopped offering his plan as of January 1, 2016. His insurance agent found his family a new policy, but it had even higher premiums and deductibles.

Clara highly valued her longtime internist, Dr. Jones, the only expert on juvenile onset diabetes within 200 miles of their home. She reminded her husband to make certain that Dr. Jones was in-network with the new insurer before purchasing the new insurance. Joseph checked the insurance company's website, which listed Dr. Jones was in-network. But when Clara called Dr. Jones for an appointment, she was shocked to learn that he had dropped out of her new insurance four months ago. The insurance company had not updated its website; a common problem. Because no other nearby doctor had the special expertise to treat her, Clara was determined to keep Dr. Jones. We'll find out later how she accomplished this.

Have you or a family member had the disheartening task of finding a new doctor because your employer changed to a different insurer, your long-term doctor you trusted retired early, or your doctor terminated his/her contract with your insurance company?

Read on for how you can handle this and many other obstacles to getting the best healthcare possible. We show you the benefits of comparing insurance policies, whether you're employed by a large or small company or self-employed, with those available through government and private health insurance exchanges. Policies are also available from independent insurance agents so you can compare what's available and select the best, most cost-effective and affordable policy for you and your family. Then we help you determine if you qualify for a federal tax credit or subsidy that may greatly reduce your cost for insurance. If you have insurance with a high deductible, you may be able to contribute tax deductible money into a health savings account (HSA) that may lower your tax bracket.

We explain the ACA's positive impact on Medicare, such as reducing your cost of medications, providing a free yearly doctor checkup, and free screening tests. We discuss how to take advantage of the not widely known, "Jimmo Agreement" and the government's recent removal of the financial cap for rehabilitative services if it's determined that you or a family member with Medicare can benefit from additional rehabilitation services. We explain what recourse you have if Medicare denies payment for these additional services.

We discuss the importance of finding a good primary care physician (PCPhys.) or provider (PCP) now, if you don't already have one, because of the worsening doctor shortage. We then explain how the expansion of Medicaid has enabled millions of low-income Americans to obtain health insurance, often for the first time in their lives. We assess the accomplishments and shortcomings of the ACA from its implementation in January 2014 to January 2018 and additional strategies to reduce your cost for insurance and medical care.

Armed with inside knowledge from two seasoned doctors, with more years of experience than we'd like to admit, of how American's changing healthcare system really works, you will be better equipped to tackle its complexities to make it work the best way possible for you and your family.

We are the first to admit that this chapter is detailed and challenging. But, so is our changing healthcare system! So, we suggest reading sections most pertinent to your personal situation. If you are employed by a large or small business and figuring out what insurance to select for the forthcoming year, read the section: *If You are Employed by a Large or Small Company*.

If you have, or are about to begin Medicare, we suggest reading the ACA's impact on Medicare to learn about improved benefits and about selecting or changing to different plans to save money as you get older (and wiser!)

You may want to read the key points section at the end of the chapter. Additional key points and appendices can be found on our website. Good luck with your selections.

Deficiencies of America's Healthcare System Before the ACA

In 2011, the percentage of Americans without health insurance reached a staggering high of 15.7 percent (48.6 million Americans). Three groups made up the bulk of the uninsured: young adults (age nineteen to twenty-five), low-income families with annual incomes of less than $25,000, and foreign-born residents without U.S. citizenship.

Before the ACA began in earnest in 2014, even those who had health insurance found it too limited, expensive, and riddled with exclusions. It did not cover persons with certain pre-existing illnesses, like

Clara's juvenile onset diabetes discussed at the beginning of this chapter. Insurance policies had yearly and lifetime maximum limits on the amount of money they would pay out for medical treatments. And insurance company payouts were often insufficient to cover a catastrophic illness. A serious medical problem often led to bankruptcy. Unpaid medical and hospital bills were, and still are, the number-one cause of personal bankruptcy in America. So even people with health insurance, especially those with high deductible plans, as well as the uninsured, put off seeking medical care until their illness became more serious. Delaying treatment lessened chances for recovery, lead to an expensive emergency department visit, and often a hospitalization.

Another shortcoming before the ACA was that doctors and hospitals were financially rewarded for the number of tests, procedures, and hospitalizations they prescribed. The more tests and services, the greater the profit. So, there was less incentive for controlling costs and rewarding good, cost-efficient patient outcomes [1] [2] [3].

The United States spent about 17.4 percent of its gross domestic product (GDP) on healthcare (about $9,255 per person) in 2013 and 2014, and 23 percent of its GDP in 2018 (the highest of any industrialized nation). Given this high expenditure for medical care, it's astonishing that treatment outcomes for various illnesses and life expectancy in the United States still lags behind those of other industrialized nations.

Healthcare experts believed that the above deficiencies of America's healthcare system would improve if more Americans had health insurance; if insurance covered pre-existing illnesses and preventative care; if it emphasized early medical intervention, and greater integration and coordination of healthcare services.

Enter the Patient Protection and Affordable Care Act (PPACA) or simply Obamacare or the Affordable Care Act (ACA). For simplicity, we'll use the terms ACA or Obamacare throughout this book. The ACA's goal was to remedy many of the inefficiencies and shortcomings of America's healthcare system. The ultimate success of the ACA would depend partly on whether it could transform an industry that rewarded excessive tests and procedures into an efficient healthcare system that rewarded excellent patient care, coordinated services, and cost efficiency.

The Affordable Care Act (ACA)

The ACA was passed by Congress and signed by President Barack Obama on March 23, 2010. The U.S. Supreme Court affirmed the constitutionality of most provisions of the ACA on June 28, 2012. The Court's decision permitted the ACA's provisions and improvements to America's healthcare system to proceed. It provided clarity to states, employers, and the public about what changes would begin in 2014. Since 2014, America's healthcare insurance and delivery systems changed dramatically.

How important is the ACA? "Historians will compare Obama's Health Care Reform to F.D.R.'s Social Security and Lyndon Johnson's Medicare." Robert Dallek made this comment in the *New York Times* on June 29, 2012.

Main Features of the ACA

One of the major goals of the ACA was to provide health insurance for the majority of the 48.6 million (15.7 percent) Americans without insurance in 2011 [5]. This was attempted in two major ways: by requiring all Americans to purchase health insurance or pay a tax penalty. A second way was to encourage all states to expand their existing Medicaid program by making eligibility less restrictive.

Beginning in 2014, almost every American was expected to have health insurance. Those who did not would pay a federal tax penalty on their yearly income tax. The penalty in 2017 for an adult, was $695 or 2.5 percent of the adjusted gross yearly income (AGI) above $10,150, whichever was higher; the flat amount of $695 was adjusted for inflation. The penalty for each child under age eighteen was $347.50. The maximum penalty per family was $2,085. There was no tax penalty if you (1) were unable to find insurance that costs less than 8 percent of your annual income, (2) earned below the amount required to file a tax return, (3) were a member of an Indian tribe, or (4) were a member of a religious group that opposed health insurance [7]. The penalty for going without health insurance ended in 2019.

The federal government, under President Obama, encouraged all states to expand their existing Medicaid program. Medicaid is a federal and state-financed insurance program for citizens with low income and the disabled. Since the ACA began, newly insured Medicaid recipients have accounted for more than half the increase in the number of insured Americans. As of January 2018, thirty-two states and the District of Columbia have expanded Medicaid, partly by making requirements for enrollment less restrictive. For a list of states that expanded, or are considering expanding Medicaid, see footnote[16].

A second major provision of the ACA is that Americans can no longer be denied health insurance because of pre-existing medical conditions (so pre-existing medical illnesses are covered). This greatly benefitted Clara, whose medical needs for her juvenile onset diabetes were now covered. And, you can't be charged higher rates because of poor health, although insurance rates are higher for older people because of their higher risks.

A third major provision allows adults under the age of twenty-six to be covered by their parents' insurance. This benefited Clara's two young daughters. Some states had this provision before 2014. Adults twenty-six and older were required to buy their own insurance if it was not provided by their employer or a government insurer. But the cost of insurance for those between age twenty-six and sixty-four has become more expensive, depending on the type of insurance purchased and other factors, and has become increasingly more expensive from 2017-2019. The cost will likely be even higher in subsequent years.

A large number of young, healthy Americans dropped their insurance in 2019 after the tax penalty ended unless they realized the benefits of having insurance or could find affordable policies. The penalty was a very important part of the ACA because it insured a large pool of young, healthy people whose medical

---

16   See www.kff.org.

needs were comparatively low. This offset the large pool of chronically ill elderly patients whose healthcare costs were much higher.

A fourth provision prevents insurance companies from limiting the yearly amount of money they pay for essential health benefits on claims (the yearly limit) while you're enrolled in that plan. Also, insurers cannot restrict how much they spend on essential health benefits during the entire time you're enrolled in that plan (the lifetime limit). Ending the restrictions greatly benefited patients like Clara who need long-term healthcare for a chronic illness. Before the ACA, many health insurance policies set lifetime limits of $100,000 to $500,000 – usually insufficient to cover a catastrophic illness [5].

Health Insurance Exchanges

Health insurance exchanges are electronic marketplaces operated by a network of specialized computers and software. The exchanges were set up in 2013 and 2014 by individual states that chose to develop their own exchange and/or by the federal government (healthcare.gov) for states that decided not to establish their own exchange. Subsequently, many commercial insurance companies have established their own exchanges. If you consider a policy through a private commercial insurance exchange, you'll want to make certain the policy offered meets ACA mandated standards, such as covering pre-existing illnesses and essential health benefits.

Americans who purchase insurance through these government or private insurance exchanges are the self-employed, employees without, or dissatisfied with, insurance from their employers, and others wanting a good policy whose benefits meet ACA standards. Also, U.S. citizens with low income or a disability who believe that they may qualify, can apply for Medicaid insurance through these government exchanges any time of the year. The window of time to enroll is not limited by official enrollment time periods.

You do not need to purchase insurance through these exchanges if you already have government insurance such as Medicare and the Children's Health Insurance Program (CHIP); you're satisfied with the insurance provided by your employer, or if you are under age twenty-six and insured under your parents' policy.

Whatever insurance you currently have, it's wise to have a yearly "insurance checkup." Find out which insurance companies continue to offer policies on the exchanges in your state; see what's available from your employer; when eligible, enroll or consider making changes in your Medicare policy, and also learn from an independent insurance agent what other options are available.

Because your insurance needs may change over time, or the policy you presently have may change or no longer be available, it's important to carefully compare what policies are available from the sources mentioned above during each year's open enrollment period. So, check out the exchange website for your state (if your state has its own website) or the federal exchange (healthcare.gov), enter the required information about your income, number of family members, where you live, et cetera, and then click on the different insurance plans that are available.

The insurance exchanges initially offered different health insurance policies with competitive rates that included ACA-established essential health benefits. As we painfully know, insurance choices in many states have become much more limited because many insurers have left the exchanges and no longer offer policies. The government expected that many insurance companies would compete for Americans wanting a good policy, thereby keeping costs reasonable. Unfortunately, that has not been the case, as we'll learn more about later.

The cost of policies offered through the exchanges varies widely depending on the annual deductible, where you live, your age, and other factors. Policies offered on the federal and state insurance exchanges are graded beginning with the lowest-cost bronze, then silver, gold, and the most expensive platinum. It's no surprise that the better policies cost more.

Suppose you need assistance in studying different policies offered through the exchanges. You can get personal assistance with the insurance exchange applications from specially trained staff working in private, public and university medical clinics and hospitals. They usually go by the title "Patient Advocate". Some PCPhys. and PCP's office staff and insurance agents can provide assistance. Unfortunately, the Trump administration drastically reduced the number of government-funded facilitators in 2017 and 2018, but they are still available. Call ahead for an appointment and find out what information to bring to your face-to-face meeting. You can also learn about 2019 premium rates, insurance benefits, and cost for health insurance purchased through the government exchanges by going to your state's website (if your state established one) or the Federal Exchange (healthcare.gov).

Take advantage of each year's open enrollment period, which usually runs for about three months starting November 1. Many states have different enrollment time periods. Fully understand the pros and cons of different policies. This is especially important if your life situation has changed (such as the birth of a child) to make certain that the policy has the benefits you need. Keep in mind that plans available on the insurance exchanges in 2019, 2020 and subsequent years may not be from the same insurers because many, due to financial and other reasons, have dropped out of, or plan to leave the exchanges.

If you want to keep your PCPhys. or PCP and specialist doctor(s), make sure they are still contracted with your current insurer or the new insurance company you are considering. Call your doctor's office to make certain rather than relying on outdated information on the insurance company's website. You don't want to be disappointed, as Clara was, to learn that your trusted, long-term doctor is no longer a contracted provider (in-network) with your insurer. Clara found an innovative way to maintain her relationship with her specialist, Dr. Jones. We'll soon learn how Clara was able to continue under his care for her diabetes even though he was now "out-of-network".

Most of us unpleasantly know, insurance premiums in 2019 for some <u>individuals</u> and especially for the self-employed, but less so for employer-provided <u>group</u> plans, increased by double-digit percentages. Additional increases are expected in 2020. But federal tax credits or subsidies for those who qualify on the basis of low income may significantly reduce the cost of insurance.

Your premium for an individual plan will vary widely depending on where you live, past medical costs for persons living in your region, number of your family members, and a myriad of other factors. It makes good sense, if you can afford it, to set aside some money each year in a savings plan, such as a health or flexible savings account (*See Chapter 2*), for future out-of-pocket medical expenses and costs, such as out-of-pocket payments to reach your yearly deductible. Later in this chapter we'll discuss effective strategies for lowering your cost for insurance and out-of-pocket medical expenses.

You May Be Eligible for a Federal Tax Credit or Subsidy

The ACA was designed to help people with low income pay for costly health insurance by providing federal tax credits or cost-sharing subsidies. For tax year 2016 (this may change based on inflation in future years), you may have been eligible for a federal tax credit to help pay part of the cost of your insurance if you purchased insurance through a government exchange or a government-approved private insurance exchange and met certain requirements. *See our website for details.*

Immediate and Long-Term Effects of the December 2017 Tax Law on the Health of Americans

Healthcare consequences of the December 2017 major tax bill passed by Congress and White House received very little debate and attention. David Blumenthal, founder of the Commonwealth Fund, and other health experts believe the law has huge implications for the health and welfare of Americans and the economy. Blumenthal summed up these implications in two words: <u>Less</u> and <u>De-Stimulus</u>.

Why Less?

The Obamacare mandate that all Americans (with some exceptions) obtain insurance or pay a tax penalty, expected that the young and healthy would join the pool of insured older, sicker Americans and thus keep insurance premiums reasonable. However, the tax penalty ends in 2019.

The Congressional Budget Office (CBO) estimated that in 2019 four million Americans (mostly the young and healthy) will elect to go without insurance. By 2027, thirteen million more will join the ranks of the uninsured.

Among those especially affected will be low-income workers, Americans between ages 50-64 (not yet eligible for Medicare and more vulnerable than younger people to illnesses), and the self-employed whose individual health policies will be increasingly more expensive. Even employees of companies that provide the major share of the cost of insurance may see a slow but steady rise in their portion of the cost of insurance and out-of-pocket medical expenses.

For the average middle class 60-year-old who doesn't qualify for a federal tax credit or subsidy to lower the cost of insurance, it's projected that monthly insurance premiums will increase substantially.

With fewer insured Americans, it's projected that there will be greater demands on public healthcare clinics and hospitals provided by city, state, and the federal government. This safety net may not be prepared to provide the healthcare needs of the increased number of uninsured. Those without insurance may delay getting medical care, which means fewer doctor visits, fewer hospitalizations, and less sale of medications and medical devices.

Why De-Stimulus?

Blumenthal believes the cutbacks in the overall use of medical services and facilities may ripple through the economy. Healthcare companies will be employing fewer workers who will buy fewer cars, home furnishings, and take fewer vacations. Unemployed healthcare employees will lose their health insurance and will join the ranks of the uninsured.

That's unfortunate! Studies have already demonstrated improved health-status among low-income Americans who became insured for the first time through the ACA's expansion of Medicaid. And there's a strong relationship between having health insurance and improved overall health and work productivity. So, also at risk is a decline in the overall health of Americans in general and on the health of America's workforce. If the December 2017 tax law, which was meant to stimulate the economy by reducing corporate taxes from 35 to 21 percent, increases the federal deficit as we've already witnessed in 2018, then expect discussion in Congress to cut back government spending for Medicare and Medicaid. Cutbacks in Medicare, Medicaid, and other government medical and social programs will add insult to an already injured healthcare system. Hopefully, as lawmakers in Washington, D.C. become aware of how the new tax law adversely affects the health of Americans, legislation will be proposed to remedy these deficiencies.

Our apologies for painting an overly pessimistic view of the long-term effects of the new tax law on America's healthcare system and the economy. But, if some of these dire predictions come true, the following strategies may protect you and your family's accessibility to good healthcare services. Any redundancies in what you've already read are meant to emphasize what action you can take now to protect you and your family's access to quality healthcare.

- Maintain quality health insurance that provides the essential healthcare benefits mandated by the ACA.

- Find out if you qualify for a tax subsidy or credit to reduce your cost for insurance.

- Consider the many benefits of a high deductible insurance policy. It's less costly and you may qualify for an HSA.

- If you qualify for a Health Savings Account (HSA), try to make contributions, even if only small amounts. Money in an HSA can be withdrawn yearly, tax-free if used to pay out-of-pocket medical costs. Or, consider a Flexible Savings Account. Your employers' human services department can provide advice. If your employer can't help you establish an HSA or FSA, or if you are self-employed, look into setting up your own plan at any number of financial institutions, such as the HSA Bank.

- If your current employer pays a good portion of your (and your family's) health insurance, factor in those benefits before changing to a job whose insurance benefits are inferior and/or don't meet the needs of your family.

- If you don't have insurance, become enrolled in your neighborhood government-supported free or low-cost clinic <u>now</u> before greater numbers of uninsured apply. University medical centers also provide quality care for the uninsured.

- If you served in the military, you may qualify for care at a Veteran's Administration facility.

- See *Chapter 2, Strategies for Keeping Costs Down* and *Chapter 10, Medications: What You Need to Know* for many other strategies to reduce your cost of medical care.

ACA's Impact on Medicare

During the yearly Medicare open enrollment period, usually from October 15, to December 7, those already on Medicare can consider switching from a traditional Medicare plan to a Medicare Advantage (MA) plan (or vice versa) and make changes to other parts of Medicare, such as changing to a different Part D (drug) plan. For those newly eligible for Medicare, you can begin enrolling in Medicare three months before you turn age sixty-five, the month of your birthdate, and for three months after. So, you have a total of seven months to enroll. If you enroll later, you'll be penalized by having to pay higher premiums thereafter.

Medicare Advantage plans (also known as Medicare HMOs, PPOs, and PFFS), are for-profit insurance plans that are an alternative to a traditional Medicare plan. The government pays these private insurance companies on a yearly basis depending on the amount of medical care expected to be provided per person enrolled in Medicare Parts A (hospital) and B (doctor visits) in different regions of the country. Most Advantage plans offer drug coverage, so a separate Part D plan does not need to be purchased. Some advantage plans provide extra benefits such as eyeglasses and hearing aids.

If you select an advantage plan rather than regular (traditional) Medicare, the benefits and medical services in Part A and B are packaged together, and medical services are paid for by the insurer you select rather than directly by the federal government. If you choose an advantage plan with an insurance company located only in the state where you live, let's say Colorado, rather than a nationally known company like Blue Cross, and you become ill in another state, your local insurer may not be easily recognized by the health providers you see. So, payment for medical services may be delayed.

Most seniors eligible for Medicare, select traditional Medicare A, B, and D and don't add a supplemental plan. But, it's advisable to purchase a supplemental plan if you can afford it, to cover expenses not covered by your Plan A, B, and D. There are a great variety of supplemental plans, designated from Plan A through N. Cost of the premium varies with the extensiveness of the benefits. Some plans cover medical services if you become ill in other countries. Uncertainty about the future of our healthcare system under the current administration in Washington is another reason to choose the best plan you can afford while additional changes to our healthcare system are debated in 2019 - 2020, and thereafter.

We strongly encourage getting expert advice from Medicare (1-800-Medicare), an independent insurance agent, a knowledgeable family member or friend, or your doctor's office manager before deciding on traditional Medicare or a Medicare Advantage plan. Some advantage plans have disadvantages, such as a smaller network of physicians to choose from, higher out-of-pocket costs, and difficulty getting approval to see an out-of-network specialist who's not contracted with your supplemental plan. A main advantage of Medicare Advantage is lower cost.[17]

Premiums for Medicare in 2019 rose modestly, and are projected to rise modestly in subsequent years, as in the past, but these increases reflect existing law; the ACA was not responsible for the increases. Premiums will rise more for individuals who earn over $85,000 a year and for couples with annual incomes over $170,000.

The ACA is responsible for some improvements in Part D (drug benefit) coverage. Consider making a change in your drug plan (Part D) every year, especially if you are taking several expensive medications. Different Part D drug plans make changes every year in the medications they will pay for. And, the price for the same drug you've been using for years may jump two or three-fold beginning in January 2019 and subsequent years. So, in mid-October of 2018 and again in October 2019, make a list of all your prescribed medications. Call your local pharmacist or Medicare (1-800-Medicare) and ask which Part D is economically the best for you to choose for 2019 before you request a change to your Medicare Part D plan. Do this in October every year to keep your prescription costs reasonable. This may save you hundreds, even thousands of dollars over time. For more details about Part D, go to our *Chapter 3 Appendix: Details About Medicare Part D (Drug) Coverage.* You may need to read it several times to understand all the particulars.[18]

Beginning in 2012, the ACA made other improvements to Medicare. Improvements include a free annual medical checkup and free preventive and screening tests such as a mammogram and colorectal-cancer screening if your doctor believes they are warranted. Beginning in 2014, Medicare entitled you to an additional free annual wellness visit[19] to talk with your doctor in more detail about your medical concerns.

A longstanding Medicare program worth mentioning is the Eldercare locator. A public service of the U.S. Administration on Aging, it finds local agencies that assist community dwelling elderly with information about Medicare-supported home and community-based services, such as assistance with transportation, home-delivered meals, and caregiver support services.[20] These services assist elderly people who want to remain in the familiar setting of their own home as long as possible, to avoid going into an institutional setting such as a nursing home.

Important Medicare Development: Jimmo Settlement Agreement

There has been a long-standing erroneous belief that for Medicare to continue to pay over a certain dollar cap for rehabilitative services, such as physical, occupational, and speech therapy, in a patient's home, rehabilitation facility, nursing home, or outpatient clinic, a patient had to demonstrate "improvement." The

---

17   www.senior65.com.
18   www.medicare.gov or call 1-800-Medicare.
19   http://obamacarefacts.com.
20   www.eldercare.gov or call 1-800-677-1116.

Jimmo agreement, which was settled in January 2013, clarified that Medicare would also pay for these medically necessary rehabilitative services if the services are needed to "maintain" an individual's condition or "to prevent or slow deterioration."[21]

The agreement is not limited to patients with particular diseases or conditions. And it applies to patients who have a traditional or a Medicare Advantage plan. If you or a loved one have been notified that rehabilitative services have, or are about to be discontinued, you, a family member, or your patient advocate may want to show a copy of the Jimmo Agreement[22] to your doctor. Your physician may not be fully aware of the Jimmo agreement and he/she can assist you in challenging the discontinuation of therapy.

Let's use as an example, at-home physical therapy. If your doctor believes that continued therapy is warranted, he/she needs to write a letter to Medicare. It must explain exactly how your unique medical condition(s) will benefit from continued physical therapy at home from a qualified physical therapist in order for you to make "further progress," "maintain your present level of functioning," or "prevent or slow deterioration." Using the above example, if your doctor's request for continued at-home physical therapy is denied, or Medicare denies payment for therapy that you've already had, detailed information about how to appeal the denial is available from the Medicare Center's self-help packet.[23] It is important to appeal a denial!

If your medical problems interfere with your ability to take up the challenge of appealing, enlist the assistance of your patient advocate or a family member. Otherwise, the hard-earned monies you paid into Medicare over many decades will not be used to pay for continued rehabilitative services. If you don't appeal Medicare's denial, you may be responsible for the cost of services after Medicare's cutoff.

There continue to be challenges about the legality and enforcement of the Jimmo Agreement, so be assertive and remain steadfast. Consider enlisting the help of a lawyer specializing in healthcare and Medicare law or the patient advocate foundation[24] to help you appeal a Medicare denial. This is yet another example where your determination and resourcefulness will be rewarded. Since the vast majority of Americans don't pursue the challenge, those that do are taken seriously by officials at Medicare.

In February, 2018 the long-standing payment caps for out-patient physical, speech, and occupational therapy were permanently repealed as part of the federal budget deal signed into law.[25] For example, the top limit that Medicare previously paid for occupational therapy was $2,010. Now that this arbitrary limit has been lifted, Medicare beneficiaries will be able, if medically warranted, to receive extended services, enabling many elderly people to maintain their independence at home rather than having to enter a nursing home. Because the devil is often in the details, time will tell how beneficial this repeal will be for those that have Medicare. As this change filters down to rehabilitation settings, it may be helpful to have a copy of the Jimmo agreement and the article about the repeal in hand.

---

21   http://www.medicareadvocacy.org/jimmo-v-sebelius.
22   agreement available at www.medicareadvocacy.org.
23   www.medicareadvocacy.org "issue brief in the therapy cap exemptions process". http://www.medicareadvocacy.org/jimmo-v-sebelius-the-improve-mtne-standard-case-faqs/.
24   www.patientadvocate.org tel. 800-532-5274
25   AARP (www.aarp.org) Feb. 9, 2018.

How Improved Medicare Benefits Will Be Paid For

To pay for these additional Medicare benefits, the federal government continues efforts to eliminate waste and fraud. Medicare payroll taxes have been increased for the wealthy. It's expected that improved, more efficient, and coordinated patient care will reduce hospital and physician errors, lessen rates of re-hospitalization, and eliminate unnecessary duplication of tests, resulting in reduced Medicare costs.

Medicare and ACA-Supported Pilot Projects

Many Medicare and ACA-supported pilot projects were launched since 2012 to study whether new, innovative payment and healthcare delivery models could improve patient outcomes while reducing medical costs.

One study sought to determine whether paying one agreed-upon total fee for a heart operation, such as cardiac bypass surgery, rather than separate payments to various members of the surgery team and the hospital, would result in shorter hospital stays, fewer complications and reduced need for re-hospitalization. It was hypothesized that this method of payment would encourage greater collaboration amongst team members and improve patient outcomes. Results thus far have been positive.

Other ongoing pilot projects expect to determine whether innovative ways of rewarding doctors and hospitals based on efficiency and *quality* of care rather than *quantity* of care will improve patient outcomes while reducing costs. Results of these studies may determine which practice models may eventually be adopted nationwide. But, it may take many years for the positive results of these studies to be implemented as new standards of medical care. Currently, every part of our healthcare system is moving to value-based methods of financially rewarding components of the healthcare system that demonstrate better quality of care while containing costs. See our *website Chapter 3: Appendix: Accountable Care Organizations Study (ACO)* about another pilot project.

ACA's Impact on Patients with Mental and Substance Use Disorders

---

Higher standards established by the ACA require insurance companies to provide benefits and payments for mental health and substance use treatment at parity (equal coverage) with other types of medical disorders. Citizens living in states where insurance policies formerly provided limited or no coverage for these conditions are now assured that insurance policies meeting ACA standards include these benefits.

Because the devil is too often in the details, there have been barriers to full implementation of the principle of parity. Some insurance companies and states were initially slow to implement parity for treatment of these disorders. Also, hundreds of thousands of Americans with these medical conditions, who may qualify for Medicaid and other types of insurance, are still without insurance because of lack of knowledge of, and motivation to obtain insurance, limitations imposed by their illness, or unwillingness to obtain government insurance because of stigma and shame.

Another roadblock for patients with Medicaid to get treatment for substance use disorders in a hospital inpatient or residential treatment program is an obscure fifty-year-old federal law that pays for this treatment only for programs having sixteen or fewer beds.[26] As of 2014, the majority of inpatient facilities across the country had programs with thirty to forty beds. Because of this old federal law, treatment programs could not be reimbursed by Medicaid. To remedy this problem, many states have downsized their inpatient programs to sixteen or fewer beds and many have obtained special waivers from the federal government.

It was long ago in the 1950s, when medical experts concluded that drug and alcohol use disorders were diseases that were treatable like other medical diseases rather than a sign of a character flaw or moral weakness. It's difficult to believe that sixty years later, in 2013, only 10 percent of the 23 million Americans with substance use disorders received treatment either because of lack of insurance, the scarcity of treatment centers and specialized health professionals, and social stigma associated with these illnesses. In 2013, those without insurance and wanting treatment were limited to publicly funded programs that had long waiting lists and insufficient health professionals specially trained in addiction medicine.

By 2014, because of the ACA, several million Americans with substance use disorders now had commercial insurance or Medicaid that paid for treatment. The number of Americans seeking treatment doubled from 2013 to 2014, as did the need for specialized health professionals.

Having insurance can mean the difference between getting quickly into a medically-oriented treatment program or a long wait to get into a publicly subsidized program, as the following real-life story demonstrates. Mrs. Ellis' nineteen-year-old son, John, became part of a disturbing trend of suburban teenagers hooked on heroin. Because he was uninsured, he was put on a three-month waiting list for a state-supported hospital program. The family couldn't afford the $28,000 cost of private residential treatment or the $2,000 per month cost for injections of medicine (Naloxone) to block heroin's high. Fortunately, because of an early benefit of the ACA that provided insurance under his parent's policy (for those under age twenty-six), John was able to quickly obtain counseling from a private specialist. After slowly being tapered off buprenorphine, a synthetic opioid used in treatment, he then received the monthly injections of Naloxone to discourage relapse. Because he now had insurance, the family's out-of-pocket cost of Naloxone injections was $40 per month. He's now back in school full time and has a job. Families struggling to help a family member or friend with substance abuse should take advantage of the opportunities now available under the ACA that have opened new avenues for help and hope. *See Chapter 10 – Medications: What You Need to Know.*

---

26   http://www.nytimes.com/2014/07/11/health/obamacare-substance-abuse-treatment-hurdles.html/.

Expansion of the Medicaid Program

Medicaid is a joint federal and state-funded program that began in the 1960s to provide health insurance to low-income persons and the disabled. Depending on the particular state where one lives, Medicaid often pays the total cost for medical care, including medications. To encourage more low-income Americans to obtain Medicaid, the ACA hoped that all states would expand their existing Medicaid program by lowering eligibility requirements. But it was left to each state whether or not to expand their program.

Healthcare experts believed that expanding Medicaid would not only provide health insurance to a larger segment of a state's residents, but would enable the newly insured to seek medical care at early signs of illness rather than delaying help until an illness had worsened or become chronic. Increasing Medicaid enrollment would enable patients to see their doctors sooner, thus reducing the burden and cost of frequent, often unnecessary and expensive emergency department visits and hospitalizations. Health experts believed that improved overall health of a state's citizens would also increase their work productivity, reduce emotional stress, improve mental functioning, life satisfaction and parental care of young family members.

To encourage more states to expand their existing Medicaid programs, in the initial years from 2014 through 2016, the federal government paid 100 percent of the cost of the Medicaid expansion. But beginning in 2017, states were expected to shoulder a portion of the cost. Some states believed that the eventual cost to them would be substantial. This is one of several reasons why some state legislatures and governors chose not to expand Medicaid.

The Obama administration had hoped that all states would expand Medicaid so that by year 2020, between 17 million and 33 million low-income uninsured Americans (the number of people if all states participated in the expansion) would be covered by Medicaid. Since the ACA began, the expansion of Medicaid, as of 2018, has accounted for a little more than half of all newly insured Americans.

As of January 2018, thirty-three states and the District of Columbia expanded Medicaid. The seventeen states not currently participating in the expansion still receive their current Medicaid funding from the federal and state government to continue their existing program. Since 2018, some states began applying for federal waivers to have their citizens on Medicaid shoulder some of the medical costs. For information about who is eligible for Medicaid, go to our *website Chapter 3 Appendix: Who Is Eligible for Medicaid?*

Change from Written to Electronic Medical Records

The ACA incentivized all medical facilities, doctors, and other health professionals to change from hand-written record keeping to electronic medical records to facilitate faster communication. To learn more about the transition to electronic medical records and how you can benefit, go to our *website Chapter 3 Appendix: How You Can Benefit from Electronic Medical Records*

Finding a Doctor Now Despite the Worsening Shortage

———————————

The current shortage of physicians and PCPs is expected to worsen in 2019 and subsequent years when more Americans have insurance because of the ACA, even if it's estimated that five million Americans are expected to drop their insurance. In 2019 many more baby boomers will qualify for Medicare. If you do not presently have a PCPhys. or a PCP, secure one now even if only to have an initial medical exam. More and more doctors have full practices and are not accepting new patients.

If you currently have, or anticipate having, government insurance such as Medicare or Medicaid or CHIP for your children, it's even more imperative to find a PCPhys. or PCP now who is contracted with these government plans because doctors and PCPs are limiting the number of patients with government insurance, especially as their practice becomes full. Consider the strategies discussed in *Chapter 5 – Finding the Best Primary Care and Medical Specialists* – which provides creative, little known strategies to become a patient of your preferred physician.

If you can't engage a PCPhys. or PCP in private practice, consider enrolling now in one of your community's public outpatient medical clinics, one affiliated with a nearby university medical center [6] or, if you qualify as a Veteran, at a V.A. Medical Center. Having insurance makes it easier to find a healthcare provider.

If you are young and healthy and believe you don't need or can't afford insurance, you may be able to purchase an affordable ACA-approved plan, perhaps with a higher deductible. You may even qualify for a federal tax credit or subsidy to substantially reduce the cost of insurance premiums. Having insurance may relieve your family's worry should fate deal you a bad hand.

Be very wary of low-cost policies that are inferior to ACA-approved plans from insurance companies you've never heard of that are being allowed to re-enter the marketplace in 2019-2020. If they seem too good to be true, it's probably not good.

A 28-year-old unemployed college graduate suffered from social phobia. He consistently found excuses for not applying for Medicaid insurance. Every time he set up an appointment at a local clinic to obtain assistance with the application process, he was stricken with overwhelming anxiety and feelings of shame about needing help from government insurance. After a year of counselling sessions, plus an additional dose of anti-anxiety medication hours before his appointment to get enrolled, he overcame his anxiety and obtained Medicaid. Two years later, he broke several bones in a ski accident and was hospitalized for two weeks. He and his family were relieved that he had insurance.

What to Do Now About the ACA and Your Insurance

It is an understatement to say that the many changes to our healthcare system brought about by the ACA are complicated. It's extremely worthwhile to keep abreast of current and future changes in the ACA and other insurance options that pertain to you and your family, especially because of the major impact on health insurance and the healthcare system with the passage of the December 2017 tax bill. Find out all your insurance options from the human resource department at your workplace, your doctor's office manager, an independent insurance agent, government healthcare websites, and others who are knowledgeable about our rapidly changing healthcare system.

Purchasers of our book and others are encouraged to visit our monthly medical forum on our website www.qualityaffordablehealthcare.net where we suggest strategies to take advantage of current and future changes in America's healthcare system. Please share your experiences and also ask us questions; our answers may benefit others and will be posted on the following month's website or emailed to you.

We hope the following suggestions will specifically address your life situation and particular healthcare concerns.

If You Are Employed by a Large Company

Even before the ACA, most large companies with more than 200 employees, accounting for over 16 million American workers, provided health insurance for their employees. Under the ACA, all businesses (including the fast food industry which previously didn't provide insurance) with fifty or more full-time employees (FTE) are required to provide health insurance to at least 95 percent of their full-time employees and their dependents under twenty-six years of age or pay a fine. This mandate doesn't apply to employers with forty-nine or fewer full-time employees. Details are available about the ACA's insurance mandates for different size companies[27] and insurance requirements for small businesses in your state.[28]

Employers of large companies choose the insurance policies for their employees. Insurance plans are required to meet ACA-mandated standards. Find out about plans offered by your employer so you can choose one that is best for you and your family. If your employer offers plans that you find inadequate, you can look into policies on government and private insurance exchanges and with an insurance agent. But find out from your employer's human services department what the financial and other consequences would be if you purchase health insurance on your own. There are obvious advantages of buying a policy that meets ACA standards.

If your share of the health insurance premiums through your employer is more than 9.5 percent of your income, you can consider health insurance through the government's insurance exchange. If you do, you may be eligible for a tax credit or subsidy to help pay the cost. But you can't claim the tax credit if your

---

27   www.obamacarefacts.com-ObamaCare Employer Mandate. You can also speak to an insurance agent: 1-800-508-6754.
28   http://www.ncsl.org/research/health/small-business-health-insurance.aspx.

employer offers health insurance equal to or less than 9.5 percent of your income and you buy insurance through the government exchange.

You may feel discouraged that your employer has, in recent years, chosen insurance plans that place more of the healthcare costs onto you in the form of higher yearly deductibles, co-pays, and other out-of-pocket expenses. The following suggestions may help you deal with these increasing out-of-pocket costs.

If you are single and healthy and have a high-deductible insurance plan from your employer but just need an annual medical checkup, consider reducing your portion of the monthly premium by choosing, if it's available, a plan with an even higher deductible. This type of policy may be similar, in some ways, to a catastrophic coverage plan. Make certain that the high-deductible policy meets ACA standards so it provides adequate medical benefits were you to become seriously ill.

Take Advantage of a High Deductible Plan

Let's suppose that you, like many of us, are saddled with a high yearly deductible of $4,000 or more. If you know that you and family members will need expensive medical and/or surgical care, find out from your physician(s) if the expensive procedure(s) can be postponed to the following January. If so, try to group all the expenses at the beginning of the year to satisfy the deductible. You know you'll have to pay out-of-pocket for all the family's medical expenses until you've met your deductible. But after the deductible has been met, you'll only be responsible for about twenty percent (depending on your policy) of the insurance company's approved amount for subsequent medical and surgical costs, assuming all your doctors and facilities are in-network. Also, once you've reached the maximum (the limit) of your yearly out-of-pocket costs, some policies then pay 100 percent of subsequent medical expenses. Also, with some high deductible insurance plans you may be eligible to put tax-deductible money into a Health Savings Account. Or, consider a Flexible Savings Account. See *Chapter 2* for information about these two types of savings accounts and additional ways to reduce your medical costs.

If You Are an Employee or Owner of a Small Business

Small businesses are generally defined as having a hundred or fewer employees. Because of their smaller size, they've usually had to pay 8 to 18 percent more than large companies to insure their employees. To level the playing field, beginning in 2014, small businesses could join a Small Business Health Option Program (called SHOP) where, because of a larger pool of employees, the cost for insuring employees was less. SHOP exchanges usually offer more insurance choices, and enrollment is available throughout the year. Small business owners who purchase insurance through SHOP may also be eligible for tax credits.

As of May 2015, about 85,000 employees of small businesses had insurance through the SHOP program. Although that number is low, SHOP programs are growing, making it easier for small business owners to provide less expensive policies. Small business owners can also find insurance for their employees through the Federal Health Exchange,[29] where employers can compare different plans. Employers can also find insurance plans from independent insurance agents or commercial insurance companies.

As of September 2015, companies with fewer than fifty full-time employees were not required to provide insurance. But the government encourages owners of smaller businesses to provide insurance by offering financial incentives such as tax credits.

The good news for small business employees is that employers with fifty to ninety-nine fulltime employees were required to provide insurance for their employees by 2016. This applies to about 7 percent of the U.S. private workforce.

If You Are Self-Employed and Need Insurance

The federal and most state and private insurance exchanges offer insurance plans for the self-employed that meet ACA standards. Premiums were fairly reasonable in 2014 when major parts of the ACA became effective, but premiums have increased substantially each year from 2015 through 2019, with yet higher premiums projected for 2020 and subsequent years. Find out if you qualify for a federal tax credit or subsidy.

Check the insurance exchanges, and talk with an independent insurance agent to see what policies are available. Make certain that the plan you purchase meets ACA standards.

Be careful of purchasing insurance from a questionable commercial or other insurance company over the Internet or telephone. As an exercise, the friend of one of the authors used the Internet in February 2015 to request an insurance plan for a forty-year-old single, self-employed, healthy man living in New Mexico earning $40,000 a year. The good news – the cost of available plans varied from $51 to $400 per month. The bad news – it was term health insurance (good for a maximum of eleven months) with a $2,500 deductible and a yearly maximum payout limit of $100,000, insufficient to cover a serious illness. The insurance plans didn't meet ACA-mandated standards. The policy would be in effect only the remaining ten months (from March – December) of 2015 and had to be renewed in January 2016 – if the insurance company was still in business. If he developed a serious medical problem during that ten-month period, there was no assurance he could renew the policy for 2016. The adage "Look before you leap!" applies here.

It's worth repeating that the federal government may be allowing out-of-state insurance companies to re-enter the marketplace. Many may offer low cost policies that are substandard and seem "too good to be true."

Obtaining Insurance Outside the Open Enrollment Period

Open enrollment through the insurance exchanges for most people not insured by their employer or a government plan, usually begins every November 1, (varies in different states). But, you can apply for insurance anytime throughout the year if you have recently experienced, or expect to experience, one of the following events: (1) become a U.S. citizen, (2) lost or will be losing your existing health insurance, (3)

---

29   www.healthcare.gov— go to HHS Premium Estimation Tool.

marriage or divorce, or (4) moved permanently to a new county or state. More details about qualifying events can be found on the Internet.

Assessment of the ACA: January 2014 to January 2018
(The Good, the Bad, and the Ugly)

The Good

There are 10 major features of the ACA that are very positive. First and foremost, as of May 2016, more than 20 million previously uninsured Americans gained the security of health insurance. So, more parents can now afford to take their children to the doctor, and more families have a lower risk of losing their homes or savings due to medical bills. Since the ACA became implemented in 2014, the number of the uninsured Americans has been cut by about a third. By 2016, about 90 percent of Americans had health insurance. Three years previously, in 2013, only 72 percent had insurance. Because of the ACA, more than 3 million previously uninsured Americans under the age of twenty-six have gained insurance under their parents' policies.

Prior to the federal tax law in December 2017, the Congressional Budget Office (CBO) estimated that by year 2020, about 27 million Americans, an additional 7 million, will have obtained insurance because of the ACA. This estimate will be substantially less because the December 2017 tax law ended, as of 2019, the mandate that everyone have insurance or pay a tax penalty.

When the three-month open-enrollment period ended in February 2015, about 12 million Americans chose an insurance plan through the health insurance exchanges. In keeping with the ACA's goal to make insurance affordable, 87 percent of the 12 million insurance marketplace customers qualified for a federal tax credit or subsidy to help pay for their insurance.

This significant improvement in the number of insured Americans is mostly attributable to those signing up on government exchanges, the expansion of Medicaid, healthcare marketplaces for small businesses, and the increasing use of private company insurance exchanges. Because most big companies already provided insurance for their employees before the ACA, the percentage of large companies' employees with insurance hasn't substantially changed.

Second, there has been a significant increase (to twenty-nine percent of all covered employees in large companies) in enrollment in high deductible consumer-directed health plans (CDHPs). Paycheck deductions from employee salaries are less for CDHPs than for low deductible insurance plans. Being insured in a CDHP costs about 22 percent less than coverage in a large company traditional PPO plan. The trend for large employers to offer CDHPs is likely to continue because they cost considerably less for both the employer and employee. Many employers have also reduced employees' out-of-pocket healthcare costs by making telemedicine and urgent care center visits, that are less costly than office visits with a PCPhys., more available to employees.[30]

Third, the ACA's mandate that insurance policies provide improved benefits, including coverage for preexisting illnesses, mental and substance abuse disorders, and preventative care has improved the overall health status of millions of Americans. By having insurance, people are more motivated to see a health professional at early signs of an illness when improvement or cure is more likely.

Fourth, of the 20 million newly insured Americans, a little more than half had signed up through their state's expanded Medicaid program for those with low-income and/or disabilities. As of the end of 2017, thirty-three states and the District of Columbia have expanded their Medicaid program. States that expanded Medicaid saw their Medicaid enrollment grow by 26 percent from 2013 to April 2015, whereas states that did not expand saw only an 8 percent increase. The 8 percent increase in states not expanding Medicaid is partly because some persons seeking insurance through the ACA marketplace discovered that they were, in fact, eligible for Medicaid under the pre-ACA law. As of May 2018, several additional states were considering the expansion.

Groups that have historically been at the greatest risk for lacking insurance – young adults, Hispanics, blacks, and those with low incomes – have made the greatest coverage gains. These improvements are meaningful and unprecedented in the United States healthcare system.

Fifth, many hospitals' financial problems have improved in the states that expanded Medicaid, especially those who had previously treated a high proportion of uninsured patients. People without any insurance and those unable to afford their deductibles and co-payments make up the majority of hospitals' unpaid bills. Nonprofit hospitals, which make up the majority of hospitals in the United States, are required to treat everyone, regardless of ability to pay, who comes to their emergency departments. States that expanded Medicaid saw their hospitals benefit financially because more patients now had Medicaid that paid at least a portion of the costs. Hospitals in states that expanded Medicaid have had about twice the reduction in uncompensated bills compared with states that did not expand Medicaid. This has particularly benefited smaller, financially stressed hospitals, such as those in rural areas with a high proportion of Medicaid patients, which often had struggled, and continue to have difficulty to remain open.

Sixth, healthcare centers, non-profit advocacy groups, and offices of some PCPhys. and PCPs have continued to provide assistance to those applying for insurance through the exchanges. Because of major funding cutbacks for these facilitators by the federal government the number of Patient Advocate helpers has been significantly reduced.

Seventh, the nation's healthcare spending has slowed since the ACA was started in 2010. In the seven years before the ACA, the nation's overall spending for healthcare increased by 5.7 percent/year. But, from 2010 to 2016, it slowed to 4.3% (adjusting for low inflation, healthcare spending actually decreased to 2.7%/year.)

---

30   Mercer survey: Health benefit cost growth slows to 2.4% in www.mercer.com/content/mercer/global/all/en/newsroom/national-survey-of-employer-sponsored-health-plans-2016.html .

Hospitals and Accountable Care Organizations (ACO) were financially rewarded by Medicare if they became more efficient by reducing hospital-and-physician-related medical complications and reducing re-admissions to the hospital. Doctors and hospitals in the ACOs worked in a more coordinated, efficient manner and modestly achieved these objectives. Hospitals with high rates of readmission whose patients developed complications, such as a hospital-acquired infection, were financially penalized.[31]

Eighth, the ACA mandated that patients with mental and/or substance-abuse disorders had insurance benefits comparable (at parity with) patients with other medical problems. This parity rule was strengthened in April 2015 when the Center for Medicare and Medicaid (CMS) ruled that the provisions of the Mental Health Parity Act and Addiction Act (MHPAEA) of 2008, which mandated parity, should apply to insurance plans meeting ACA standards and to the majority of ACA's Medicaid and Children's Health Insurance Program (CHIP) plans.

Ninth, the percentage of hospitals that reported using certified electronic health records in 2017 reached an all-time high of over 95 percent.

Tenth, the ACA appears here to stay. Congress has tried unsuccessfully innumerable times to repeal or dismantle the ACA without a viable plan to replace it. Failing the repeal, the President issued the following executive orders during 2017 – 2018 to undermine the ACA in the hope that it would weaken and slowly die:

- In 2019, there will no longer be a tax penalty for going without insurance.

- Funding for helpers ("navigators") to assist Americans to choose an insurance plan using health insurance exchanges was reduced substantially.

- Reduced the number of open enrollment days for citizens to obtain insurance from the exchanges. Many states, though, extended the enrollment period.

- Threatened, but was unable to cut off federal money to provide subsidies to lower the cost of insurance for low income Americans. In 2017, the government provided $7 billion in subsidies.

- Considering state requests to have Medicaid recipients pay monthly premiums or require them to find a job.

Despite Congressional efforts to undermine the ACA:

- During the enrollment period that ended December 2017, the number of Americans who signed up for 2018 Obamacare insurance policies was just shy of the previous year's enrollment.

- Despite threats to end government subsidies to help low income people pay for insurance, about 57 percent of those who bought insurance through the Obamacare exchanges qualified for the subsidies, according to the Kaiser Family Foundation.

- Public support for Obamacare has grown. A Gallup Poll in the summer of 2017 found that 52 percent of Americans support the ACA. Another poll found that just 13 percent wanted it repealed.

---

31 Antos, J.R., Lapretta, J.C. "ObamaCare's Failed Cost Controls. The Wall Street Journal, 12/21/17 p. A17.

- Americans have grown accustomed to, and appreciative of, popular parts of the ACA, such as coverage for pre-existing illnesses and keeping adult children on their parents' policy until age twenty-six.

The Bad

As we know, conservative politicians and advocacy groups have tried repeatedly, since the ACA became law in 2010, to have parts or all of the ACA repealed. They ideologically perceive the ACA as an expansion of big government into the personal decision making of individuals and a harbinger of higher taxes and increased government deficits.

Although the ACA has had many successes, it has its deficiencies. It is projected that by 2020 there will be 30 million people in the United States without health insurance. The number of uninsured will probably be higher because of the increasing cost of insurance and because there is no longer a tax penalty for going without insurance. Those without insurance will be people in the U.S. illegally; young healthy adults twenty-six and older who believe that they don't need insurance or can't afford it; those with religious beliefs that oppose medical care; and those who are so impaired by medical, mental, and/or substance use disorders and other isolating factors that they have difficulty applying for insurance. Many disadvantaged citizens living in the states that have not expanded Medicaid will also remain uninsured which makes access to medical care difficult. Hopefully, once it's apparent that the number of uninsured has escalated, Congress and the White House will consider legislation to remedy this problem. Who is going to pay for all the substantial benefits mandated by the ACA?

One group paying much more for these improved insurance benefits are Americans with their own individual – as opposed to group –insurance policy, such as middle-class, self-employed individuals not covered by an employer, a group, or a government plan. Individual policies are much more expensive than group policies, such as employees of a big corporation, because the latter with a large pool of insured, poses less risk for the insurer. Some self-employed people with individual plans saw their yearly insurance premiums increase in 2018 and again in 2019, by 15 and as much as 50 percent (although some qualified for a federal tax credit or subsidy).

Another parcel of bad news is that in 2018, premiums for the lowest cost insurance plan on the government exchanges – the bronze plans with high deductibles – increased an average of seventeen percent nationwide (depending on where one lives), according to Kaiser. The second lowest-cost silver plan increased an average of thirty percent while the cost of the second highest gold plans increased about eighteen percent.

But, to soften this bad news, the silver plans are used by the United States Government as the benchmark to determine the number of subsidies to those qualified low-and middle-income people who purchase insurance from the government exchange. So, for those who qualified for the tax credit or subsidy, the cost of a bronze plan (after the subsidy was applied) was, for some people, less in 2018 than in 2017.[32]

---

32   www.usnews.com/topics/author/susan-milligan.

The percent of adults without health insurance rose in the first quarter of 2017 to 11.3 percent compared to 10.9 percent in the third and fourth quarters of 2016 and will increase more in 2019 when the mandate to have insurance ends. This also has been attributed to the rising cost of insurance and the uncertainty about the ACA's long-term future. Despite this increase to 11.3 percent, this remains well below the peak of the 18 percent who lacked insurance before the ACA Exchanges were opened in 2013, according to a Gallup Poll.[33]

Those unable to afford these increasingly more expensive policies, even with the benefit of tax credits or subsidies, had to shop around in 2017 and 2018 to find an affordable policy, often with higher deductibles, co-pays, and other out-of-pocket costs. Others, unable to afford the increased cost, decided to go without insurance, pay the tax penalty for year 2018, and hope they didn't become seriously ill.

The Ugly

The ACA provided financial support for low-cost, consumer-governed health insurance plans, known as healthcare co-ops, to spur competition with large insurance companies in order to keep the cost of insurance reasonable. These healthcare co-ops sold some of the lowest-cost plans through government healthcare exchanges. But limitations of government subsidies to these startups, along with their low-priced policies (hence lower profits), contributed to their financial difficulties. About eight insurance co-ops, or about a third nationwide, were shut down in 2015, leaving a half million Americans covered by these plans scrambling to find coverage for 2016.[34] Some of the remaining co-ops may share a similar fate in 2019, especially because of the current Administration's attempts to dismantle many beneficial aspects of Obamacare.

Another problem, not necessarily a failing of the ACA, has seriously affected those with individual, as opposed to group, preferred provider organization (PPO) plans. Those with PPO plans could see any in-network physician and specialist they choose, even in another state, without the need for referral by their PCPhys. Some big insurance companies in six states, (California, Florida, Illinois, New Mexico, Texas, and New York), as of October 2016 stopped offering individual PPO plans[35] through insurance exchanges. These insurers claim they've lost considerable money providing individual PPO plans in past years because patients with these plans tend to have chronic, more costly illnesses and search for expensive in-network doctors and specialists in other cities and states.

In contrast, group PPO plans that insure big businesses have a large pool of patients, thereby reducing the insurers' risk. So, group PPO insurance premiums are less than individual plans. Many insurers have continued offering group PPO plans.

Some insurers are offering HMO plans to those who previously had an individual PPO plan. HMO plans require patients to obtain a referral from their PCPhys. or PCP (who serves as gatekeeper and coordinator) in order to be referred to an in-network physician specialist. HMOs are less expensive than PPOs because they control costs more tightly, but they often have fewer in-network PCPhys., PCPs, and specialists to choose from. For an example of how a patient was adversely affected when his PPO plan ended, *see our website Chapter 3 Appendix: How People Were Affected When Their Individual PPO Plans were Terminated.*

---

33   Lauren Thomas. The number of Americans without insurance rose in first quarter 2017, Health Insurance, April 11, 2017.
34   The New Mexican. October 14, 2015.1,2. Closure of healthcare co-ops cuts consumer choices.
35   The New Mexican. October 18, 2015. A1, A4.

Another ugly development is that even insured Americans can't afford their medical bills, especially if they unknowingly go to out-of-network physicians and health facilities. Just because you are insured doesn't mean you can actually afford your doctor, hospital, medication, and other medical bills. High deductibles and copays often discourage patients from seeing their doctor, even when it's a necessity.

Out-of-pocket spending by Americans with employer-provided health insurance increased by more than 50 percent from 2010 to 2016. The yearly deductible for 36 percent of employees of small companies in 2015 was over $2,000. A 2015 poll discovered that 26 percent of Americans surveyed claimed medical bills caused severe damage to their family's finances. Another poll in early 2017 found that 55 percent of those surveyed claimed that during a one-year period they had received at least one medical bill they could not afford.

Another problem, years before the ACA began, is the steady increase in out-of-pocket costs for employees of big and small businesses and the self-employed in the form of higher premiums, deductibles, and co-payments. For example, premiums for employer-sponsored group health plans increased 4.2 percent from 2014 to 2015. But more striking is that deductibles increased proportionately more than premiums and wages.[36] The annual deductible for coverage of an employee at a large company in 2006 averaged $584. In year 2015, it was $1,318, according to the Kaiser Family Foundation.

The appeal to businesses and insurers to shift more out-of-pocket costs onto employees is to deter employees from excessively using healthcare services, thereby reducing healthcare costs and increasing the company's profits. But this is detrimental for those needing medical care, especially for serious illnesses. A November 2014 Gallup poll [37] revealed that one in three people said they had put off medical treatment because of high out-of-pocket costs, and two-thirds acknowledged that the treatment they needed was for a serious condition.

Another unintended consequence of the ACA, often not written or talked about, has been the disruption of many patients' relationships with their longstanding PCPhys. or PCP. If a company employer changes to a different insurance company for its employees, and the employee's current PCPhys. or PCP is not a provider (is out-of-network) with the new insurer, the employee has to find another provider who is in-network. Compounding this problem, many doctors, for various reasons, have discontinued being providers for certain, and sometimes all insurers, so most of their patients have also had to search for a new doctor who accepts their insurance.

The consequence for millions of patients has been a disruption of a very important longstanding doctor-patient relationship. Some patients experienced this disruption as a very significant, disheartening loss. It's difficult to measure the emotional and medical consequences of these disruptions and transitions. Returning to Clara whose juvenile onset diabetes we learned about at the beginning of this chapter, she was determined and cleverly succeeded in keeping the doctor she so highly valued. You may want to consider some strategy discussed in the next section for keeping your doctor even though he/she may now no longer be a provider with your insurer.

---

36   The *New York Times*, September 23, 2015/ Health Insurance deductibles rising faster than wages, a study finds.
37   According to a Gallup Heathway's poll.

Another ugly development is that some major insurance companies, such as Aetna, Humana, and United Health Care,[38] decided in August 2016 to stop offering individual health insurance plans through the health insurance exchanges in 2017. Aetna, for example, ceased offering health insurance to its customers in eleven of fifteen states, which affected 80 percent of those insured with Aetna. These insurers explained that they have been losing significant amounts of money because premiums, although increasing, couldn't keep up with medical costs and because those signing up on the exchanges tended to have more medical problems. The trend of insurance companies pulling out from the exchanges continued in 2018-2019, resulting in less competition for the remaining companies and still higher premiums for Americans.

To help fill the void, in November 2017 Obamacare began offering a new plan called "Simple Choice"[39], which is generally exempt from a yearly deductible when patients see their PCPhys., PCP, or specialist, receive outpatient mental health services, and prescription drugs. Such standardized health plans offer a uniform set of features for each plan level – bronze, silver, and gold. For example, for 2017, all gold-level standardized plans will have a deductible of $1,250 but you can see your primary care doctor for $20 per visit at any time, even if you haven't met your deductible[40]. In other words, those purchasing "Simple Choice" may have co-payments but will not have to meet a deductible for certain services before their insurance kicks in. Nevertheless, these plans may be costly because in most cases premiums are regulated by state insurance organizations.[41]

Looking into the future can be disheartening, especially for those with individual health insurance plans, such as the self-employed, compared to those with group, employer, or government insurance. A pessimistic outlook is presented by Dr. Stephen Parents,[42] professor of health finance, who predicts that the cost of individual (and family) insurance plans will rise about 6 percent per year over the next decade, even when factoring in federal tax credits and subsidies. So, by year 2025, the yearly premium for an individual plan may cost $5,500/year and $23,500 for a family. Dr. Parents also predicts a steady increase in out-of-pocket costs. As all these costs rise, more Americans may be discouraged from purchasing increasingly more expensive insurance, opting instead to go without insurance and overwhelming the public, not-for-profit healthcare system, and hoping they won't become ill.

Additional Constructive Strategies to Consider

We would like you to consider other strategies you can implement now to reduce the cost of medical care and medications and take advantage of ACA plans, which have maintained high standards and benefits.

---

38   By pulling out, Aetna highlights "Obamacare" weaknesses. The New Mexican 8/17/16.
39   www.nytimes.com/2016/10/18/us/affordable-care-act-health-insurance-simple-choice-plan.html
40   www.legalconsumer.com/obamacare/topic.php?TopicID=100&ST=NY
41   *The New Mexican*, Oct. 18, 2016.
42   Dr. Stephen T. Parents, "New Mexico's affordable care act future." *The New Mexican,* January 19, 2016.

- It goes without saying that you may be more likely to avoid expensive doctor, hospital, and medication bills by adhering to a healthy diet, exercise program, and obtaining good medical attention at early signs of an illness.

- If you have Medicare or other government insurance such as Medicaid, Veterans Administration (VA) insurance, or CHIP, you have good insurance coverage. But it's important to review your insurance plan yearly, especially if there are changes in your life situation, overall health, or the medications you take. If you don't have a personal PCPhys. or PCP, find one <u>now</u> because an increasing number of doctors are limiting the number of patients who have government insurance.

- If you are employed by a large or a small company and they provide you with insurance, review your policy with your employer's human services department every year during open enrollment to learn about available insurance plans, especially if your life situation has changed. Consider the many advantages of a high deductible plan, such as reduced cost, especially if you and your family are relatively healthy.

- If you don't have employer or government insurance and want insurance that meets ACA standards for yourself and your family, see what's available from the government exchanges and ACA-approved private insurance exchanges. Find out if you qualify for a tax credit or subsidy that can substantially lower your premium. Also, seek advice from an independent insurance agent, your doctor's office manager, and knowledgeable friends and relatives. One of the many benefits of health insurance exchanges (both government and private) is the transparency when comparing prices and benefits.[43]

- If your company offers a health savings account, try to invest tax-deductible money into the account (even if it's a small amount) to be used to meet your deductible and other out-of-pocket medical costs. Also, consider a flexible savings account. If your employer doesn't offer these plans, consider establishing your own. See *Chapter 2* for the many benefits of these plans.

- If you want to keep your current long-standing doctor or physician specialist, who is not a provider with your new insurer, find out from your new insurance company if you can be reimbursed for a portion of your full payment to your now out-of-network doctor if you submit his/her detailed, itemized paid bill. Although it's unlikely, it's worthwhile inquiring. Also, you and your doctor can ask your insurer if they would consider a single case contract.

Returning once again to Clara's predicament, Dr. Jones was the only doctor nearby who specialized in juvenile onset diabetes. He wrote a detailed letter to the medical director of Clara's new insurance company explaining why it was essential for Clara to continue under his care. The insurance company requested a copy of Dr. Jones's extensive medical records, which was followed by a telephone discussion between Dr. Jones and the insurance company's medical director who asked additional questions. Finally, Dr. Jones

---

43 *The New Mexican*: October 18, 2015. A-1, A-4. Do your research experts advise.

obtained a "single case contract" with agreed-upon payments from the insurer and modest co-payments from Clara. It's unlikely that this would have been achieved without Dr. Jones' and Clara's determination.

- What if you want to keep your longtime physician who is now out-of-network but a "single case contract" is not an option? If you have the financial means, you could try to negotiate with your doctor's business manager a reasonable fee to continue under his/her care. Some of your out-of-pocket medical expenses may be tax deductible. Find out in advance if your insurer will pay for tests and procedures carried out at an in-network laboratory if they are ordered by your now out-of-network doctor.

- What if you find out beforehand that you're responsible for paying the cost of expensive tests/procedures out-of-pocket because you haven't met your yearly deductible? Ask your doctor if the benefits of proposed tests/procedures outweigh the risks and costs. You might ask, "What would you do if you had the same financial constraints as me?"

- What if your doctor prescribes an expensive brand-name medication that is not covered by your insurance policy, and there is no generic medication available. If your doctor believes that there are justifiable, convincing reasons that the brand-name medication is needed, he/she may be willing to make the argument with your insurer. Keep in mind that the authorization process takes considerable time and persistence.

- The cost of medical care is so high and the personal finances of most Americans are so tight, there is another resource worth exploring. Many charitable organizations provide financial assistance even though the amount of money available is limited.

There are many disease-oriented organizations that have the funds to assist eligible applicants struggling with medical debt. For example, Cancer Care is a nation-wide organization that provides counseling groups for cancer sufferers but also distributes over $4 million a year for assistance with transportation, home and childcare if needed so you can keep your doctor appointments. But the major portion of Cancer Care's aid goes to disease-specific prescription co-pay costs, which sometimes amount to between $4,000 - $15,000 per patient a year to income-eligible patients.

A study in 2016 found that cancer patients who had to declare bankruptcy because of spiraling medical costs were significantly more likely to die than those who didn't need to file for bankruptcy. Increased mortality was attributed to the reduced likelihood of receiving adequate treatment and increased financial and emotional stress.

But, monies available from charitable organizations are severely limited, according to Alan Balch, CEO of the Patient Advocate Foundation that distributed more than $50 million in co-pay medication funds in 2016. There is generally more money available for patients with more well-known diseases, such as breast cancer, than for someone with a rare tumor. The Patient Advocate Foundation's multiple sclerosis funds have been closed to new applicants since 2016.

One way to search for these non-profit charitable organizations is to google the name of the disease, let's say kidney cancer, or google the likely name of a funding source, such as the American Kidney Foundation Fund. If you have a computer savvy teenager at home, ask him/her for assistance in a computer search.

Another resource for assistance with medical bills is non-profit hospitals, which are generally more financially helpful than for-profit hospitals. In an effort to reduce uncollectible bills, a number of hospitals have teamed up with financial service firms like Commercial Bank, to offer patients time-limited interest-free loans.

Other sources of financial assistance occur if a person has medical expenses due to being a victim of acts of international terrorism. Eligible expenses include medical, dental, rehabilitation and mental health care[44]. Sometimes illnesses associated with domestic terrorism or natural disasters can stimulate donors to help the victims. A special donor internet site can be set up and the mechanism is called **Donation-based crowdfunding** [45]. **Crowdfunding** is the practice of funding a project by raising small amounts of money from a large number of people, typically via the Internet. **Charity donation-based crowdfunding** is the collective effort of individuals to help charitable causes. Here donors come together around a common calamity to help fund services and programs for the victims. For example, the Orlando nightclub shootings in 2016 inspired numerous crowd-sharing efforts for everything from survivors' medical bills to help with funeral expenses.

- Learn as much as possible about you and your family members' health problems by using credible healthcare Internet sites, such as Kaiserfoundation.org, Mayoclinic.org and Johnshopkins.org rather than chat rooms and commercial websites, where information can be unreliable [4]. Stay current about changes to America's healthcare system by reading the authors' monthly medical forum at www.qualityaffordablehealthcare.net.

- Be wary of super cheap health insurance policies that do not include the essential health benefits of ACA-approved policies, do not guarantee renewal of your policy should you become ill, and do not provide insurance for pre-existing illnesses.

The more knowledge you have, the more effective and empowered you'll be as one of the most important members of your healthcare team.

---

44   https://www.benefits.gov/benefits/benefit-details/2745
45   https://www.moneyadviceservice.org.uk/en/articles/crowdfunding—what-you-need-to-know#what-are-the-different-types-of-crowdfunding

Chapter 3 Appendix

Details About Medicare Part D (Drug) Coverage

As of 2013, if you had Medicare and purchased one of the many Part D plans (drug coverage), you paid a monthly premium between $0 and $150 and a yearly deductible (about $325 for most plans) before Medicare covered 75 percent of drug costs until the total of what Medicare paid out reached $2,960. You then entered what's termed the "doughnut hole" at which point you then had to pay the entire cost of all prescription drugs until your out-of-pocket expenses totaled $4,750, after which Medicare covered 95 percent of drug costs approved by your particular Part D plan. Because of improvements under the ACA, the doughnut hole has been shrinking. Beginning in 2019, Part D enrollees will pay 25 percent of the cost of prescription drugs from the time they enter the doughnut hole until they reach catastrophic coverage. Before selecting a Part D plan, it's advisable to make a list of all the prescription medications you take regularly and then ask your pharmacist or call Medicare to see which of the many Part D plans covers most, if not all, of your current medications.

Chapter 3 Key Points

Key Points: Deficiencies of Our Healthcare System Before the ACA

- In 2011, 48.6 million Americans (15.7 percent) had no health insurance.
- Medical bills remained the number-one cause of bankruptcy.
- Patient outcomes in the United States were inferior to most industrialized nations.

Key Points: Main Features of the ACA

- Almost every American was expected to have health insurance or pay a tax penalty (penalty ended in 2019).
- The ACA mandated that insurance cover preexisting medical conditions, essential benefits, treatment of drug addiction, and mental illness.
- Citizens under age twenty-six can be covered under their parents' insurance.
- Health insurance exchanges were established in 2013 to purchase ACA policies; enroll in Medicaid.

Key Points: How the Healthcare of Americans May be Impacted by the December 2017 Tax Law

- The Congressional Budget Office estimates that by 2027, 17 million currently insured Americans (a good percentage will be the young and healthy) will join the ranks of the uninsured.

- Most affected will be Americans between ages 50-64 and the self-employed, whose insurance premiums will increase substantially (possibly more than 10 percent/year).

Key Points: Healthcare of Americans May be Impacted by the December 2017 Tax Law

- With less Americans insured there will be greater demands on the unprepared public health sector.
- The uninsured, and even those with insurance, will delay getting medical care, making them more vulnerable to medical illness and resulting in less utilization of medical services.
- If the December 2017 tax law increases the federal deficit, Medicare and Medicaid, may become targets to reduce the deficit.
- Cutbacks in Medicare/Medicaid would add insult to an already injured healthcare system.

Key Points: Strategies to Protect You and Your Family's Health Include:

- Try to continue your high-quality health insurance, which includes essential health benefits mandated by the ACA.
- To reduce your cost of health insurance, consider the benefits of a high deductible plan. You may be eligible for a health savings account (HSA). Consider a flexible savings account (FSA).

Key Points: ACA's Impact on Medicare

- The ACA resulted in improvements in Part D (medication) coverage. The infamous doughnut hole is gradually closing.
- Medicare provides a free annual check-up plus a free annual wellness visit.
- Before changing from regular (traditional) Medicare to an Advantage plan or vice versa, study the advantages and disadvantages of each.

Key Points: Impact of the December 2017 Tax Law – What to Do

- Keep abreast of current and future changes regarding the ACA and other insurance options.
- Before changing to another insurance company if you want to keep your current physician(s), make certain they are in-network.
- Lower-cost individual policies will be available in 2019 but many will be substandard.
- See if your yearly income makes you eligible for a tax credit or subsidy to lower your cost for insurance.

Key Points: Additional Strategies to Reduce Medical Costs

- If you and your family need expensive medical care, ask your doctor if you can postpone care until the following January. If so, you can satisfy your deductible; subsequent care may require a twenty percent copay.

- If you don't have insurance, enroll at a neighborhood free or low-cost clinic or a university medical center. If you served in the military, you may be eligible for care at a V.A. medical center.

Key Points: Assessment of the ACA: January 2014 to January 2018

The Good

- Since the ACA began in earnest in 2014, 20 million previously uninsured Americans have health insurance (about 88 percent of Americans have insurance).

- More than half of the newly insured is the result of the Medicaid Expansion.

- Depending on your income, you may be eligible for a federal tax credit or subsidy to reduce the cost of insurance.

- Medicare benefits have improved.

- The quality, coordination, and cost of healthcare is improving (according to some healthcare experts).

- Payment for treatment of mental health and substance abuse disorders is similar to medical illnesses (parity).

- Obamacare began offering a new plan "Simple Choice" that exempts the deductible for visits with your PCP and certain specialists.

- The ACA is surviving (as of January 2018), despite attempts to dismantle it.

The Bad

- 30 million Americans will still be without health insurance by 2020 but likely more because of the increasing cost of insurance.

- The insufficient number of specialists to meet rising demand for treatment of patients with substance and mental health disorders.

- There will be substantial increases in the cost of insurance, deductibles, and co-payments, especially for the self-employed and those age 55-64.

The Ugly

- Many healthcare co-ops that offered low-cost insurance have gone out of business.

- Many insurers have stopped offering policies on the exchanges, limiting the number of choices and increasing cost.

- Important doctor-patient relationships have been disrupted when employers or those purchasing insurance on the exchanges change to a new insurer and their doctors are not providers with that insurer.

References

1. Brill, P., *America's Bitter Pill: Money, Politics, Backroom Deals and the Fight to Fix our Broken Healthcare System*. 2015, New York: Random House, pgs.1-12.

2. Gawande, A., *Being Mortal*. 2014, New York: Metropolitan Books, pgs. 149-190.

3. Gawande, A., *Overkill: America's Epidemic of Unnecessary Care*, in *The New Yorker*. May 11, 2015: New York. p. 42-53.

4. Michelson, L.D., *The Patient's Playbook*. 2015, New York: Alfred A. Knoph, pgs. 175-183.

5. Nather, D., *The New Health Care System-Everything You Need to Know*. 2010, New York: Thomas Dunne Books, pgs. 25-36.

6. Roizen, M.F., Oz, M.C. You the Smart Patient. Free Press, New York, 2006, pgs.63-97.

7. Yagoda, L. Affordable Care Act for Dummies, John Wiley & Sons, Inc., Hoboken, NJ, 2014.

CHAPTER 4

Making the Best Outpatient Care Choices

Consider that you are traveling with your family. It's approaching midnight and your young son, Adam, who had been cranky suddenly vomits and appears ill. There is no fever. You need medical advice. You call your at-home pediatrician who is on-call and she gets back to you. She says to watch your child and if there are any further changes such as more vomiting or fever you should get him assessed ASAP. However, she says it doesn't now seem like an urgent or emergency situation. Two hours later there's more vomiting and now a fever also. It's 2 AM—what to do? You call your insurance company to advise on which of the three Emergency Rooms in town to use and are they all covered by your insurance. You call the designated ER and speak to a nurse. You tell her that your son vomited (3 times), has a fever (low grade) and is easily arousable. The nurse says they would be glad to see your child but they don't usually regard this as an emergency unless it continues or worsens. They would be glad to evaluate the child but are unsure if your insurance will cover a non-emergency visit in an Emergency Room.

Issues of where to go, who to see, insurance coverage, getting middle of the night medical advice, knowing which local health services to use whether at home or traveling are but a few of the topics to be discussed in this chapter. We have already discussed the changing insurance coverage options. That is an important part of the "healthcare ice berg" but only a part. Other basic components of the healthcare system are also changing at a rapid pace There are new mixes and types of healthcare professionals, new outpatient facilities, new service delivery models, new high-tech in-home communication systems, and new payment options.

For example, do you know the differences between the following licensed health providers: MA, RN, NP, PA, MD, DO, MSW, PhD, PsyD? You'll likely meet many of them over the years and it's important to understand their differing skills and training. Do you know when to use each type of outpatient facility: Retail Clinic, Urgent Care Clinic, Workplace on site Clinic, Primary Care offices, Patient-Centered Medical Home, Emergency Room? Are you aware of whether they are accredited and what such certification indicates? Is your computer ready to communicate with the new Patient Portals and Telemedicine services? Have you encountered the growing use of new payment mechanisms such as "concierge services" and "direct primary care"?

All these changes show us that the average reader will benefit from an upgrade in his or her health system knowledge. This will allow you to confidently navigate through this changing "healthscape". This chapter will guide you through each of the areas.

Healthcare Professionals

Often you may be in the doctor's waiting room and suddenly you hear your name being called. You are greeted by a person in a white coat who invites you to come into the treatment rooms—may or may not tell you his/her name—and often doesn't tell you their medical profession. You must become comfortable to politely ask something like "Could you tell me your professional background…" The person will never be offended by the question and will quickly identify their title. Typically, the title will be that of Medical Assistant or Nurse or Nurse Practitioner or Physician Assistant. That's a good start—but do you know what to expect from their title? Let's take a closer look so that when you hear their title you can relax and know their role and what to expect from them. The various types of healthcare providers have a range of skills (sometimes called "competencies"). Distinctions between the professionals include an appreciation of their training pathways and the different or similar skills that they acquire in order to help you when you are ill. Once these are understood it will bolster your respect and confidence in them. Later you may prefer a particular type of provider that best fits your needs.

Registered Nurses (RNs), Nurse Practitioners (NPs) and Clinical Nurse Specialists (CNSs)

Let's start with nurse practitioners (NPs), who are first registered nurses (RNs). An overview of their course work and clinical experiences are given in *Chapter 4 Appendix: Training of Nurses and Nurse Practitioners*. The differences in their training affect the healthcare services they provide, called "scope of practice". The scope of practice of RNs includes:

- Performing physical exams and obtaining health histories

- Administering medications, wound care, and numerous other personal interventions

- Interpreting patient information and making decisions about needed actions

- Directing and supervising care delivered by other healthcare professionals, such as licensed practical nurses (LPNs)[46] and nurse aides

Because NPs are also RNs, they can do all that RNs can do plus provide additional services, which include:

- Ordering, performing, and interpreting diagnostic tests such as lab work and X-rays

- Diagnosing and treating acute and chronic conditions such as diabetes, high blood pressure, infections, and injuries

- Prescribing medications and other treatments

---

46   See www.practicalnursing.org

- Managing patients' overall care (i.e., primary care function)

- Counseling

- Educating patients on disease prevention and positive health and lifestyle choices

Note that NPs frequently work as part of a medical team, but—unlike physician assistants (PAs)—they do not work under the formal legal supervision of a physician and can work independently.

Clinical Nurse Specialists (CNSs) are registered nurses who have graduate level nurse training at the master's or doctoral level. They have expertise in a specialized area of nursing practice (e.g. pediatrics, geriatrics, rehabilitation, psychiatry – to name a few). They practice in a variety of settings depending on their specialty (e.g. pediatric clinics), provide expert consultation and education to nursing staff nurses in training, participate and lead research, and implement improvements in healthcare delivery systems. Some clinical nurse specialists provide direct patient care in hospitals and clinics, but they do not usually act as a patient's primary care provider. On the other hand, this is exactly what Nurse Practitioners can do.

Primary Care Physicians (PCPs) and Physician Assistants (PAs)

A primary health care provider is a professional who acts as the principal point of contact for a patient in the health care system. The term PCP is sometimes used more broadly to indicate "Primary Care *Provider*" where the "provider" could be a physician or an NP or a PA. Here we will use the term "PCP" to indicate Primary Care *Physician*". There are two types of "physicians" and two types of PCPs. Understanding the differences may help you choose your provider. The term "physician" refers to two slightly different medical degrees: MD (doctor of medicine) or DO (doctor of osteopathic medicine). There is no practical difference between these two degrees. DOs made up approximately 6.5% of the total U.S. physician population. Both DOs and MDs can practice in any specialty of medicine—such as pediatrics, family medicine, psychiatry, surgery, or ophthalmology. DOs and MDs must pass comparable examinations to be eligible to obtain state licenses, and both practice in accredited and licensed healthcare facilities. Osteopathic medical schools emphasize training medical students to become **primary care physicians.**

With that awareness, let's unpack the term PCP a bit more. There are two types of PCP—family medicine doctors (family practitioners) and internal medicine doctors (internists). According to the American College of Physicians (ACP)[47], "Internal medicine physicians are specialists who apply scientific knowledge and clinical expertise to the diagnosis, treatment, and compassionate care of adults across the spectrum from health to complex illness." Here a key word is "adult" which significantly distinguishes Internal Medicine doctors from Family Medicine doctors who treat a much broader age range of patients. The American Academy of Family Physicians (AAFP)[48] indicates that "Because of their extensive training, family physicians are the only specialists qualified to treat most ailments and provide comprehensive health care for people of all ages– from newborns to seniors."

---

47   See www.acponline.org
48   See www.aafp.org

Family Medicine physicians receive training in six major medical areas: pediatrics; obstetrics and gynecology; internal medicine; psychiatry and neurology; surgery; and community medicine. Internists do not train in pediatrics or obstetrics and gynecology, although they are familiar with gynecologic diseases in adults. In addition to diagnosing and treating illness, both Internal Medicine physicians and Family Medicine physicians also provide preventive care, including routine checkups, health-risk assessments, immunization and screening tests, and personalized counseling on maintaining a healthy lifestyle.

Here's a rundown on the training and skill-set of Physician Assistants (PAs). Their scope of practice includes:

- Taking your medical history
- Conducting physical exams
- Diagnosing and treating illnesses
- Ordering and interpreting tests
- Developing treatment plans
- Counseling on preventive care
- Assisting in surgery
- Writing prescriptions
- Making rounds in hospitals and nursing homes

You'll note that some of these skills repeat those of NPs and RNs. However, unlike nurse practitioners, physician assistants must work under the supervision of a physician. Supervision does not necessarily require the physical presence of a physician at the place where services are rendered although it is imperative that the PA and a supervising physician are or can be in contact with each other by telecommunication.

Social Worker

You may meet Social Workers in private practice or in health care settings. It is important to understand their broad scope of practice. According to the National Association of Social Workers (NASW), in the health care setting their roles and responsibilities include[49]:

- Understanding of common ethical and legal issues in social work practice in health care settings
- Biopsychosocial–spiritual assessment
- Client and family engagement in all aspects of social work intervention
- Case management/care management/care coordination/health care navigation

---

49   https://www.socialworkers.org/Practice

- Discharge and transition planning

- Client concordance with and adherence to the plan of care

- Advance care planning

- Palliative care, including pain and symptom management

- Hospice and end-of-life care

- Identification of child/elder/vulnerable adult abuse, trauma, neglect, and exploitation

- Crisis intervention

- Facilitation of benefits and resource acquisition to assist clients and families, including an understanding of related policies, eligibility requirements, and financial and legal issues

- Advocacy with other members of the interdisciplinary team and within the health care institution to promote clients' and families' decision making and quality of life

- Client, family, interdisciplinary, and community education

- Family systems issues, including the impact of health care concerns, illness, and disease on family relationships; life cycles; and caregiving roles and support needs

Medical Assistant

There is another medical position that should not be confused with Physician Assistant. That is the title of Medical Assistant. Their level of training and clinical skills is much less than that of a PA. However, their skill set is in strong demand in medical settings and it is good to take a moment to be familiar with their role and competencies as you are likely to meet them. Medical assistants are cross-trained to perform administrative and clinical duties. The typical range of clinical duties include:

- Taking medical histories

- Explaining treatment procedures to patients

- Preparing patients for examination

- Assisting the physician during exams

- Collecting and preparing laboratory specimens

- Performing basic laboratory tests

- Instructing patients about medication and special diets

- Preparing and administering medications as directed by a physician

- Authorizing prescription refills as directed

- Drawing blood

- Taking electrocardiograms

- Removing sutures and changing dressings

See details of their training in Chapter 4 Appendix: Skills and Training of Medical Assistants

Your Preference for an NP Versus a PA Versus a PCP

Although there is great overlap in the respective services of an NP, a PA, and a PCP, there are some distinctions. For example, NPs can work independently. PAs must work under the supervision of a physician—either in the physical presence of a physician at the place where services are rendered or able to be in contact with each other by telecommunication. Family Medicine doctors can see a broader age range than internal medicine doctors; the range includes pediatric and obstetric cases. If all these providers are available in your community, you may prefer services from one or the other depending on your circumstances.

New Facilities and Levels of Care

Traditionally, care has been given by either solo practitioners or group practices [either single specialty (such as cardiology, urology, gastroenterology) or multispecialty]. Solo practices are generally in decline and group practices are increasingly common. Some advantages of group practices include: a common medical record used by all practitioners; seeing different providers under one roof; your familiarity with supporter staff and the office facility; good coverage by other providers if yours is unavailable; convenient on-site laboratory services and various diagnostic equipment [1].

Not so long ago there were only *two* basic choices. You could get outpatient care at either: (1) a physician medical office located in the community or hospital clinic; or (2) a hospital emergency room. These *two* choices have now expanded to *eight*! The six additional options include:

- Retail Clinic

- Urgent Care Center

- Workplace on-site Clinic

- Patient-Centered Medical Home

- Home-based Telemedicine

- Ambulatory Surgery Center

If you have some, most, or even all of these facilities in your community, it is important that you know the differences between them and when to use each one. The sites vary in their hours of operation, range of services, seriousness of illnesses, staffing and equipment, and whether they meet national quality of care standards indicated by having accreditation by a recognized accrediting organization *[see on website Chapter 4 Appendix: Accreditation of Outpatient Facility]*. In this section we will show you the different "profiles" so you can choose the best facility as your circumstances change.

Primary Care Physician Office

This discussion assumes that your PCP is the "gateway" to all appropriate services, among them diagnostic tests such as blood and urine tests, EKGs, radiology, referrals to specialists, referral to an inpatient hospital, and prescription medications. Your PCP is the most comprehensive of your providers since he/she routinely deals with both chronic (long term) and acute (recent onset) conditions whereas the other facilities focus more on acute medical problems that need immediate attention. However, you may not always be able to benefit from your PCP's care if, for instance, he or she is on vacation, or the office schedule is completely filled and you can't wait for the next available appointment, or you're calling after hours when the office is closed, or you are traveling. So, what should you do if your PCP is not available—or you do not have one? Let's get to know the other facilities.

Retail Healthcare Clinics (RHC)

You may want to consider using an RHC for mild to moderate medical problems, easy access when shopping, and less costly compared to seeing your PCP. Currently they are the least comprehensive facility. These are walk-in clinics where an appointment is not needed. A recent survey found there were about 1,760 retail clinics in the country with estimates that this number would soon double [1] . A further indication of the significance of RHCs is found in the recent purchase by CVS Health of all of the pharmacies and RHCs in Target stores in December 2015[50]. CVS Health will add Target's nearly 80 clinic locations which will be rebranded as MinuteClinic with plans to open another 20 clinics in Target stores projected that they would operate 1,500 clinics by 2017.

Retail healthcare clinics are usually headed by a nurse practitioner (NP) or a physician assistant (PA). Staffing usually does not include an on-site physician, although the PA works under physician supervision. RHCs have the least amount of medical equipment of the three types of outpatient facilities. For example, they usually do not have X-ray or ultrasound machines. They are usually open twelve hours a day on weekdays and eight hours a day on weekends. Access to your medical records is limited to information the patient provides and to other RHC sites in the same corporate system. An RHC can send an electronic medical report to your PCP if you request that. We recommend that you routinely request this as well as a copy for your own records, especially if you don't have a PCP.

Although RHCs are currently the least comprehensive of the three types of outpatient facilities, this might be changing. Walmart is testing a new model ("The Walmart Care Clinic") that would offer services expected from a primary care provider with referrals to specialists as needed. As of January 2015, Walmart had opened seventeen of these new model clinics to assess their success before pursuing further expansion plan.

Illnesses and Services.

Typical conditions and services treated at RHCs include: infections of sinuses, ear, throat, or lungs; urinary tract infections; blood pressure checks; vaccinations; and school or camp exams. The quality of care from RHCs appears to be good when treatments of minor, non-life- threatening illnesses are compared with the same conditions treated at urgent care centers (UCCs) and Emergency Rooms. For example, recent studies of RHC quality of care and relative costs for treating middle ear infections, sore throat, and urinary tract infections showed excellent care and lower costs in such comparisons [1] [2]. RHCs accept many health insurance plans and are the lowest cost facility which appeals to patients with high-deductible healthcare insurance or those without any such insurance. An idea of cost differences for the three above conditions finds: RHCs ($110), UCCs ($156), physician offices ($166), and ERs ($570) [2].

Urgent Care Centers

Midway in the outpatient level of care spectrum is the *Urgent Care Center* (UCC). The term "urgent" indicates that a UCC is the right place to go when an illness or injury has the *potential* to result in disability or death if treatment is delayed even when such a threat is not immediate. However, UCCs are also appropriate for milder conditions, as discussed below. UCCs are walk-in facilities where an appointment is not needed.

UCC staffing typically includes an on-site physician as well as medical assistants and nursing staff (often including a Nurse practitioner) and/or Physician Assistants as well as X-ray technicians. Medical equipment is at a medium level and includes X-ray equipment. The hours are similar to those of RHCs—typically 9 a.m. to 9 p.m. on weekdays and somewhat reduced on weekends. Access to your medical records is variable. If the UCC is freestanding, there may be no access to your medical records, so it's best to have your PHR with you. If the UCC is part of your group medical practice, there is likely full access to your records at the group practice. If the UCC is hospital based, there may be access to your hospital records and also to your medical group records if the medical group is part of the hospital. Request that the UCC send a copy of the diagnostic and treatment records to your PCP and also to you for your own records. You will be asked to sign a form authorizing the UCC to send their report to the professionals you want to receive a copy.

Illnesses and Services.

UCCs treat a broader range and severity of illnesses than do RHCs, although they do overlap. UCCs treat infections of sinuses, ear, throat, or lungs; urinary tract infections; allergies and rashes; and various stomach and bowel conditions. They also do vaccinations and various preventive screenings *[See further details on website in Chapter 4 Appendix: Services at Urgent Care Centers]*. The cost of care at UCCs is intermediate between costs at RHCs and at ERs. Not every UCC may provide every service mentioned above, so it is best to ask them directly about whether a certain service is available. UCCs accept most major health insurance plans.

Here's an example of how a UCC can be beneficial. Jack lives in a community of 100,000 people that has several RHCs and UCCs. His physician is part of a medical group that runs an on-site UCC as one of the group's several Departments. Recently Jack had an abrupt total hearing loss in one ear. He called the group's Ear, Nose & Throat Department, but they couldn't see him for two weeks. They told him to go to the UCC. After a fifteen-minute wait, he was examined by a physician, who found that his bad ear was totally clogged with earwax; his good ear was completely clear. The RN put an earwax softener in his ear, waited twenty minutes, and then used special equipment to flush out the material. Now he could hear! The physician re-examined him and found the ear canal now totally free of any blockage. The total wait and treatment time was about one hour! Before you go to a UCC, you might call them in advance to let them know what condition you are suffering from. Further information about UCCs can be found at the website of the American Academy of Urgent Care Medicine.[51]

Workplace On-Site Clinics

Big businesses often sponsor another type of outpatient facility that is reserved for their employees (and often their dependents). The corporations are usually large, from 500 to 5,000-plus employees. These on-site clinics may vary considerably with regard to: hours (full-time or part time), staffing (physician-led or staffed by RNs, PAs, or NPs), and primary care (some emphasize acute care while having a separate community-based PCP; others offer PCP services). About one-third of large employers have a clinic that provides primary care services.

Workplace clinics originally focused on occupational injuries and illnesses, but they currently offer a much broader range of services, including: work-related injuries, vaccinations, screenings, and primary care. See a more complete list in *website Chapter 4 Appendix: Services at Workplace On-Site Clinics*. The trend for workplace clinics moving toward more primary care services has many contributing factors [3] [4].

Patient-Centered Medical Home (PCMH)

Here the term "medical home" is not a literal residence. Rather, it is a centralized coordinating hub for delivering comprehensive healthcare by an integrated team of providers headed by PCPs. Members of the team may include other physician specialists, advanced practice nurses, physician assistants, nurses,

---

51   See www.aaucm.org

pharmacists, nutritionists, mental health workers, social workers and others. A brief description of the concept of PCMH is helpful from the American Academy of Family Physicians[52] :

"The patient-centered medical home is a transition away from a model of symptom and illness based episodic care to a system of comprehensive coordinated primary care for children, youth and adults. Patient centeredness refers to an ongoing, active partnership with a personal primary care physician who leads a team of professionals dedicated to providing proactive, preventive and chronic care management through all stages of life. These personal physicians are responsible for the patient's coordination of care across all health care systems…"

The PCMH uses advanced information technology to implement the patient care model. The term "clinical decision support tools" (CDS) refers to the integration of sophisticated computer programs that aid the clinicians and improve patient care and outcomes. See further details on our website in *Chapter 4 Appendix: Patient Centered Medical Home—Clinical Decision Support (CDS) Software.*

Actual measurements of PCMH activities have shown promising results that the intended goals are being realized [5] [6]. The concept of PCMH has many supporting healthcare organizations. These include the American Academy of Pediatrics (AAP), the American Academy of Family Physicians (AAFP), the American College of Physicians (ACP) and the American Osteopathic Association (AOA). A history of the evolution of PCMHs is available [see our website *Chapter 4 Appendix: Patient Centered Medical Home—History and Evolution*].

Telemedicine

Telemedicine is perhaps the fastest-growing new "tree" in the changing healthcare landscape with "roots" extending nationally. When news coverage of this change makes the front page of The *New York Times* [7] regarding electronic "doctor house calls," it's time to be aware of what this is all about.

Telemedicine refers to clinical services where the provider and patient are physically separated and are communicating by online video or telephone or email. Telemedicine is particularly helpful for persons living in more rural areas where comprehensive services may not be fully available and travel distances are a significant obstacle for receiving quality healthcare.

But telemedicine is increasingly available even in major urban areas. The service may fill a void when you are traveling or it is after-hours when medical offices are closed and only the ER is open. It may also fill a need during regular hours for people who do not have a PCP or may not have any (or only high-deductible) healthcare insurance. Here is an example of telepsychiatry services. A psychiatric colleague provided telepsychiatry services to a rural clinic and nursing home where it was difficult to recruit psychiatry specialists to provide services on site. If he was asked in advance whether he felt that telepsychiatry could "work," he would have said: "No way. You must have the patient in person in the same office with you to give good care."

---

52   See https://www.aafp.org/practice-management/transformation/pcmh.html

He later said that he would have been wrong. Telepsychiatry works fairly well in the mental health field. Psychiatrists don't usually do a physical exam of the patient, so the inability to physically touch the patient is not a big problem. Psychiatrists do a "mental status exam" instead of a "physical exam" by asking the patient to answer certain questions in order to check memory and cognition, which can easily be done over the video setup. If there is a need to take a blood pressure, he can ask the nurse to obtain it. If he needs to examine for neurologic side-effects of some medications, the nurse at the other site can be asked to assist as he observes and the nurse indicates whether there are abnormal muscle movements that could be felt but not seen. Notice that without a nurse available (for example, if the TV is in a patient's home instead of in a medical facility), doctors are clearly more limited. Psychiatrists pay great attention to emotional expressions that show in tone of voice, pace of speech, and facial and bodily expressions. They also pay great attention to the content of speech, and how the patient says he or she is feeling and functioning. In some cases, reports from family members or caregivers are obtained on how the patient is doing. All these dimensions work reasonably well in live televised interactions where he can see the patient and caregivers on the screen and they can see the doctor on their screen. He can zoom in or out on the facial nuances; they cannot adjust the camera or microphone.

This is not to say that telepsychiatry is as good as being physically present with the patient. Here are some problems and limitations. The patient—especially an older one—is not used to talking interactively with a TV screen and becomes quite anxious and bewildered. If the patient is sitting but lowers his head or turns away, their facial expressions cannot be seen. If the patient is agitated and paces around the room the doctor cannot follow him or her with the camera or calm him such as by walking with him if necessary. If the screen resolution is not ideal, he cannot see tears forming in his eyes. A rash mentioned by the patient that could be due to a medicine may be hard to evaluate if the TV colors are not accurate. If the audio system and microphone location are not ideal, one cannot always hear his speech clearly. Other limitations concern the fact that you might not get the same physician or health provider next time although the next physician will have your EMR from prior contacts with other providers. Also, Physicians can prescribe medicine in most states if they are licensed there—but typically won't give prescriptions for narcotics or DEA controlled substances.

Despite such problems, the clinical interaction is typically good enough to allow valid assessments. Other medical specialists may need more reliance on a physical examination or other interactions with the patient that are limited by the physical distance of the patient. Despite limitations, telemedicine is growing in importance as an additional modality to deliver health services.

The growth of telemedicine reflects growing acceptance and support in the provider communities [8]. The growth is also fueled by the major commercial health insurance companies including such services as a health coverage benefit. For example, Medicare has geographically limited national coverage while UnitedHealth, Cigna and Aetna are expanding this coverage at a rapid rate. Further details are given in *website Chapter 4 Appendix: Telemedicine—Insurance Coverage of Telemedicine Services.* In addition to telemedicine being promoted to individuals, the modality is also used by entities such as the Veterans Administration healthcare system and also some major universities that sponsor medical training and have their own affiliated healthcare facilities.

Communications with Telemedicine providers often occur via computers or Smartphones with the app for the particular telemedicine provider. Telemedicine services may be available on a 24 x 7 basis. As technology evolves there will likely be changes in the equipment that you the patient will need to communicate with a telehealth company. See *website Chapter 4 Appendix Telemedicine: Computer Requirements and Comparison of leading Telemedicine Providers*

For all of the telemedicine companies, their individual healthcare providers operate in many states and are regulated by each state where services are provided. The physician needs to be licensed by the state Medical Board in the state where the patient resides. Not surprisingly, there is a current plan to speed up the licensing process by state Medical Boards.

Ambulatory Surgery Centers

An Ambulatory Surgery Center (ASC; Surgicenter) is a surgical facility where the center focuses on providing same-day surgical care, including diagnostic procedures such as arteriograms. Surgicenters are very cost effective compared to the same procedure being done as a hospital inpatient. *[See further information in Chapter 9 Preparing for Surgery: Before & After]*

Emergency Rooms

An Emergency Room (ER)—usually part of a hospital or medical center—specializes in the acute care of patients who arrive without an appointment. It operates 24 hours a day, 7 days a week, and 365 days a year and accepts most healthcare insurance. Staffing includes physicians, nurses, mid-level providers, various technicians, and administrative support staff. ERs have broad access to hospital labs, radiology, and other diagnostic equipment. Their costs are the highest in outpatient level of care, due partly to their intensive staffing, diagnostic or therapeutic supplies, and equipment costs. Costs are also high because of a great deal of uncompensated care since ERs are required by federal law to provide care to all patients, regardless of their ability to pay. [See *website Chapter 4 Appendix: Emergency Rooms Must Treat All Patients* for details.] Since they cannot be turned away, patients without health insurance or the ability to pay out-of-pocket costs often use ERs as their main healthcare provider even for non-emergency health conditions. With more Americans having health insurance because of the ACA, the overuse of ERs for non-emergency care may gradually diminish.

An informed healthcare consumer needs to be aware of another issue concerning insurance coverage of ER services. Namely, it is possible that your insurance company may determine that the costly ER services you received were not an actual emergency and deny payment for those services. So it is important to understand current standards for determining what constitutes a plausible medical emergency. Should it be based on the symptoms that brought you to the ER? Or should it be based on the final diagnosis that was made in the ER? A prevailing method of managed care plans had been to go with the final diagnosis. But here we meet the concept of how a "prudent layperson" (not an insurance company) would define an emergency medical condition. A study of "prudent laypersons" [9] cites the following definition: "An emergency condition is any medical condition of recent onset and severity, including but not limited to severe pain, that would lead a prudent layperson, possessing an average knowledge of medicine and health, to believe that his or her condition, sickness, or injury is of such a nature that failure to obtain immediate medical care could result in placing the patient's health in serious jeopardy, serious impairment to bodily functions, or serious dysfunction of bodily organ or part." That study found that the following were often considered by laypeople to be "emergency medical conditions": loss of consciousness, seizure, no recognition of one side of the body, paralysis, shock, gangrene, coughing blood, trouble breathing, chest pain, choking, and severe abdominal urinary tract-related pain (renal colic). There are many other medical conditions that a "prudent layperson" might also consider to be legitimate emergencies, including high fever, abrupt difficulty speaking and understanding language, sudden swelling of leg, abrupt weakness, sudden slowness in heartbeat with dizziness, or physical trauma. This list, however incomplete, coupled with the preceding definition of "emergency condition," should give you a good idea of what specific experiences might lead you to correctly use the ER. The prudent layperson standard was included in national healthcare reform legislation (ACA) [10] and applies to almost all health plans in America. The standard requires insurance companies to cover emergency services if a prudent layperson believes he or she is experiencing a medical emergency. In such cases, prior authorization from the plan is not required.

Where to Go When in Doubt

How do you know what facility to use if an after-hours problem occurs during which the RHCs, UCCs, Workplace On-site Clinic, PCMH and PCP offices are closed and you are not sure if your condition warrants an ER visit and meets the prudent layperson standard of an emergency condition? This was the case with Adam, the young boy we met in the opening paragraph of this chapter. His family called their covering PCP, their insurance company and the ER. They took Adam to the ER where he was found to be seriously ill with a gastroenteritis and was admitted to the inpatient Pediatric unit. He made a good recovery and was discharged 3 days later.

So, what can we learn from this concerning your middle-of-night decision whether to wait until morning when the facilities re-open or go immediately to the ER? We suggest the following.

- If you have a PCP, call that office and ask to speak with your PCP or the on-call doctor who can assess and guide you.

- If you do not have a PCP but do have health insurance, call your insurance company for advice.

o For example, UnitedHealthcare has a phone service called "myNurseLine" (1-800-846-4678), available 24 hours a day, 7 days a week, where a registered nurse will help to "decide if you should see a doctor, go to the ER, or treat yourself at home."

o Some Blue Cross and Blue Shield companies also offer a toll-free 24-hour nurse line, which you can find on the back of your member card. For example, a Massachusetts insurance plan calls their service Blue Care Line [1-888-247-BLUE (2583)], which is staffed by RNs where you "Simply explain the situation, detail your symptoms, and our nurses will tell you whether you should see your doctor, go to the emergency room, or care for yourself at home."

o Your health plan may well have a similar service; it's good to know their phone number in advance.

If you do not have a PCP or healthcare insurance, you or your healthcare advocate might try calling the ER directly and ask whether you should go there. You will probably talk with a triage nurse who will ask about your symptoms and tell you whether you need to come in, whether to call the Emergency Medical Service (EMS) ambulance (which can be reached in most areas by calling 911), what you can do before you arrive, and what information you need to bring with you, such as your health history, current medications, and names of your doctors. However, you get to the ER, it is always helpful if your healthcare advocate can accompany you.

You can also decide in advance—when you are feeling quite well—which type of facility to use when the time comes. If you live in a community with each type of outpatient care described above—PCP, RHC, UCC, PCMH and ER—especially if there is more than one of each type in your community—it makes sense to learn about their services via their website or telephone call or even a personal visit. You should feel free to ask any of the following questions: Exactly what conditions do they treat and what services do they provide? What conditions do they not treat? How they distinguish themselves from their competitors. What is their staffing like? Do they have X-ray or other diagnostic equipment? Can they access your health records? Do they accept your health insurance? What are their fees? What, if any, wellness or preventive services do they provide? What are their hours of operation? Are they accredited? Will they send records to your PCP?

You might also ask your PCP which UCC or RHC they recommend. With this sort of specific information, you can select the facility you will want to use should you or a family member become ill.

New Communication Methods: Patient Portals

You've probably noticed a new way that your physicians can communicate with you. "Patient portal" is one term for electronic availability in which you and your physicians can email back and forth. For example, they send you reports, test results, and appointment reminders, and you can ask them questions. This patient portal software is part of the federal government encouraging providers to transition to electronic health records.[53] It is a secure online website that gives patients twenty-four-hour access to personal health information from anywhere with an Internet connection. Using a secure username and password, patients can view health information such as recent doctor visits, discharge summaries, medications, immunizations, allergies, and lab results. Some patient portals also allow patients to exchange secure email with their healthcare teams, request prescription refills, schedule non-urgent appointments, check benefits and coverage, update contact information, make payments, download and complete forms, and view educational materials.

New Payment Methods: Concierge Services (CS) and Direct Primary Care (DPC)

Physicians have a keen interest in reducing their reliance on medical insurance companies as their main source of income. We will discuss the reasons shortly, but first will focus on two new ways of paying your physician other than through your medical insurance. They are called Concierge Services (CS) and Direct Primary Care (DPC) services. Reading this description will help you decide whether these arrangements would be right for you.

CS and DPC both involve you, the patient, paying a retainer fee to your provider in exchange for enhanced services such as much quicker access to medical care, longer appointments, and enhanced communication with your health professionals—either your primary care physician or sometimes other specialists as well. Both CS and DPC services replace the providers' exclusive reliance on insurance with a direct financial relationship with their patients.

Here are some important similarities and distinctions between both services. Both involve retainer fees paid to the practitioners on an annual, quarterly, or monthly basis. In the CS model, of which there are many varieties, the retainer guarantees direct access to the physician. The physician also bills insurance companies for visits and services. By having these two sources of income, the physician can afford to see fewer patients and devote more time to each one. Some physicians use a variation on the CS model; they have a number of patients in the traditional insurance-based practice along with a smaller number of patients who are under the CS model. With the DPC model, many providers do not take insurance at all but rely solely on the direct-pay retainer fees from their patients.

The DPC model has been approved by the American Academy of Family Physicians (AAFP)[54] and an excerpt from its policy is helpful in understanding benefits to the both the patient and provider.

---

53   See www.healthit.gov/providers-professionals/faqs/what-patient-portal
54   See www.aafp.org/about/policies/all/direct-primary.html

"Typically, these retainer fees guarantee patients enhanced services such as 24/7 access to their personal physician, extended visits, electronic communications, in some cases home-based medical visits, and highly personalized, coordinated, and comprehensive care administration…The DPC contract between a patient and his/her physician provides for regular, recurring monthly revenue to practices which typically replaces traditional fee-for-service billing to third party insurance plan providers. For family physicians, this revenue model can stabilize practice finances, allowing the physician and office staff to focus on the needs of the patient and improving their health outcomes rather than coding and billing. Patients, in turn, benefit from having a DPC practice because the contract fee covers the cost of all primary care services furnished in the DPC practice…"

The AAFP notes that patients who can afford it may also choose to still carry some form of insurance, such as a high-deductible health plan, for coverage of healthcare services that cannot be provided in the primary care practice setting, such as specialty care and hospitalizations.

We think it can be helpful for you to understand the motivation of doctors to reduce their reliance on medical insurance income. Both CS and DPC models apply particularly to primary care providers. PCPs are under great pressure from growing patient panels; time-consuming billing and compliance issues with multiple insurance companies; patient and provider dissatisfactions with brief office visits; sometimes long waits for appointments; and being among the lowest physician income groups [11]. A recent survey documents that: PCPs have among the lowest compensation of all medical specialties; are under pressure to see large numbers of patients spending on average 9-16 minutes with each; typically spend 10 or more hours per week on paperwork and administration; and about 9% participate in either Concierge (4%) or Cash-only practice (5%) which is similar to the general physician population (3% and 5% respectively) [12]. As noted, while these non-insurance income streams provide relief to many of these issues, some practices continue to also see traditional insurance-based fee for service patients.

While only 8% of all physicians currently use such business models, there is potential growth that includes specialists as well as PCPs. An example occurs with some neurologists who are also experimenting with offering direct pay retainer services [13] [14].

Chapter 4 Appendix

Training of Nurses (RN) and Nurse Practitioners (NP)

In these sections on training requirements for healthcare providers, we deliberately give more information than usual for two reasons. First, many people have told us "Gee, I had no idea of their training and find it very interesting and relevant". Second, it will allow more informed confidence in your dealings with all these providers regarding both the differences and overlaps in their professional training and clinical skills. So, let's begin with Nurse Practitioners (NPs) who are first trained as RNs and then do advanced training to become NPs.

A national licensing exam is required to become an RN. There is more than one educational pathway to become eligible to take the exam. At the undergraduate level there is a **Diploma in Nursing**, available through hospital-based schools of nursing. There is also an **Associate Degree in Nursing (ADN)**, which is a two-year degree offered by community colleges and hospital-based schools of nursing. There is also a **Bachelor of Science in Nursing (BS/BSN)**, which is a four-year degree offered at colleges and universities. The first two years concentrates on psychology, human growth and development, biology, microbiology, organic chemistry, nutrition, anatomy, and physiology. The final two years often focus on adult acute and chronic disease, maternal/child health, pediatrics, psychiatric/mental health nursing, and community health nursing. This training offers a deeper understanding of the cultural, political, economic, and social issues that affect patients and influence healthcare delivery. The curriculum includes nursing theory, physical and behavioral sciences, and humanities with additional content in research, leadership, and may include such topics as healthcare economics, health informatics, and health policy.

RN training at the graduate level offers three further levels of degrees and specialization: **Master's Degree (MSN)** programs for Advanced Practice Nurses[55], nurse administrators, and nurse educators; **Doctor of Philosophy (PhD)** programs for teaching and/or conducting research; and **Doctor of Nursing Practice (DNP)** programs for clinical practice or leadership roles.

After completing their nursing curriculum, nurse practitioners take advanced training. The American Association of Nurse Practitioners (AANP)[56] stipulates that NPs must complete a master's or doctoral degree program and have advanced clinical training beyond RN training. Didactic and clinical courses prepare nurses with specialized knowledge and clinical competency to practice in primary care, acute care, and long-term healthcare settings.

Training of Physician Assistants (PAs)

We learn from the American Academy of Physician Assistants (AAPA)[57] that applicants typically need to complete at least two years of college coursework in basic and behavioral sciences before applying to a PA program. The majority of PA programs have the following prerequisites: Chemistry; Physiology; Anatomy; Microbiology;

---

55   The term "advanced practice registered nurse (APRN)" is an umbrella term given to a registered nurse who has at least a master's educational and clinical practice requirements beyond the basic nursing education and licensing required of all RNs and who provides at least some direct care to patients. Under this umbrella fit the principal types of APRNs: nurse practitioner (NP), certified nurse-midwife (CNM), clinical nurse specialist (CNS), and certified registered nurse anesthetists (CRNA).

56   See www.aanp.org

57   See www.aapa.org

Biology. Many PA programs also require prior healthcare experience with hands-on patient care. Most PA programs are approximately twenty-six months (three academic years) and award master's degrees. They include classroom instruction and clinical rotations. Classroom instruction includes: Anatomy; Physiology; Biochemistry; Pharmacology; Physical diagnosis; Pathophysiology; Microbiology; Clinical laboratory science; Behavioral science and Medical ethics. There are more than more than 2,000 hours of clinical rotations, including: family medicine, Internal medicine, Obstetrics and Gynecology, Pediatrics, General Surgery, Emergency Medicine, and Psychiatry.

Skills and Training of Medical Assistants

According to the American Association of Medical Assistants[58], MAs have clinical skills previously outlined and also typical administrative duties such as:

- Using computer applications
- Answering telephones
- Greeting patients
- Updating and filing patient medical records
- Coding and filling out insurance forms
- Scheduling appointments
- Arranging for hospital admissions and laboratory services
- Handling correspondence, billing, and bookkeeping

There are two pathways to becoming a Medical Assistant: either a Certified Medical Assistant (CMA) or a Registered Medical Assistant (RMA). Both must complete a training program that is accredited through either the Accrediting Bureau of Health Education Schools (ABHES) or the Commission on Accreditation of Allied Health Education Programs (CAAHEP). Typically, these programs take around a year to complete and include coursework as well as hands-on practical experience. The education, training, and job responsibilities of CMAs and RMAs are essentially the same[59]. The Registered Medical Assistant credential, or RMA credential is offered through the American Medical Technologists (AMT). The CMA certification, is offered through the American Association of Medical Assistants (AAMA).

---

58   See: http://www.aama-ntl.org/medical-assisting/what-is-a-cma#.V7jhqZgrKUl
59   See: http://www.medicalassistantcoursesonline.net/types/certifiedma/

Chapter 4 Key Points

Key Points: Know Your Healthcare Providers

- Nurse Practitioners (NPs)
    - o   All are Advanced Practice nurses
    - o   All have a master's or doctoral degree and have advanced clinical training beyond their initial professional registered nurse (RN) preparation. They can diagnose, order & interpret tests and can prescribe medicines

- Physician Assistants (PAs)
    - o   PAs Can diagnose, order & interpret tests and prescribe medicines
    - o   They work under the supervision of a physician on site or via telecommunication

- Primary Care Providers (PCPs)
    - o   Physician (internist or family practitioner) or NP or PA
        - ▪   Family Practitioner training includes Pediatrics and Obstetrics & Gynecology

- Licensed Clinical Social Workers (LCSWs)
    - o   Have a Master's Degree
    - o   Can provide mental health services
    - o   Can provide many services in health care setting such as discharge planning, etc.

Key Points: Understanding Levels of Care

- Different facilities treat different levels of seriousness
- Order of severity and complexity (mild to severe)
    - o   RHC→UCC→Workplace On-site Clinic→PCP or PCMH→ER
- RHCs may have NP or PA as main provider
- PCPs treat acute & chronic illness; RHCs & UCCs focus more on acute illness
- Use the "prudent layperson" standard to determine a true emergency condition, where it is appropriate to use the ER
- Make sure that all reports & test results are sent to your PCP so medical care is coordinated
- Consider choosing a facility that has necessary medical equipment

Key Points: Know Where to Get After-Hours Treatment

- Call your PCP office for on-call physician for guidance
- Call your healthcare insurance company 24/7/365 nurse hotline for guidance

- Call the ER directly & speak to the triage nurse for guidance

- Contact a Telemedicine provider for guidance

- Have your healthcare advocate accompany you to treatment

- Make certain your PCP and specialists get all reports

Key Points: Anticipate Healthcare Choices When You Are Well

- Ask your PCP for recommendations regarding after-hours care

- Learn about local RHCs, UCCs, Workplace On-site Clinics, PCMH, Telemedicine providers, & ERs via web sites and/or by in-person visits & reputation from patients

- Check their services, staffing, conditions they do and do not treat, insurance coverage & fees, communication with your PCP, accreditation & hours of operation

- Select an appropriate Telemedicine Provider

    o Register with them & provide on-line medical history

References

1. Shrank, W.H., et al., *Quality of care at retail clinics for 3 common conditions.* American Journal of Managed Care, 2014. **20**(10): p. 794-801.

2. Mehrotra, A., et al., *Comparing costs and quality of care at retail clinics with that of other medical settings for 3 common illnesses.* Annals of Internal Medicine, 2009. **151**(5): p. 321-328.

3. Lee, B.M. *Mercer Newsroom-Mercer's National Survey of Employer-Sponsored Health*

4. Shahly, V., R.C. Kessler, and I. Duncan, *Worksite primary care clinics: a systematic review.* Population Health Management. 2014. **17**(5): p. 306-15.

5. Sandy, L.G., et al., *Measuring physician quality and efficiency in an era of practice transformation: PCMH as a case study.* Annals of Family Medicine, 2015. **13**(3): p. 264-8.

6. Landon, B.E., *Moving ahead with the PCMH: some progress, but more testing needed.* Journal of General Internal Medicine, 2013. **28**(6): p. 753-5.

7. Goodenough, A., *Modern Doctors' House Calls: Skype Chat and Fast Diagnosis*, in *The New York Times*. Sunday, July 12, 2015.

8. Daniel, H., et al., *Policy Recommendations to Guide the Use of Telemedicine in Primary Care Settings: An American College of Physicians Position Paper.* Annals of Internal Medicine, 2015; **163**(10):787-789.

9. Li, J., H.K. Galvin, and S.C. Johnson, *The "prudent layperson" definition of an emergency medical condition.* American Journal of Emergency Medicine, 2002. **20**(1): p. 10-13.

10. Blachly, L. *ACEP initiative supporting "prudent layperson" standard becomes law in Health Care Reform Act.*

ACEP News dated May 2010; [cited 2018 May 20]; Available from: www.acep.org/Clinical—-PracticeManagement/ACEP-Initiative-Supporting—Prudent-Layperson—Standard-Becomes-Law-in-Health-Care-Reform-Act/.

11. Bodenheimer, T., *Primary care—will it survive?* New England Journal of Medicine, 2006. **355**(9): p. 861-4.

12. Peckham, C. *Medscape Physician Compensation Report 2015* dated April 21, 2015; [cited 2018 May 25]; Available from: https://www.medscape.com/slideshow/compensation-2015-overview-6006679

13. Alexander, G.C., J. Kurlander, and M.K. Wynia, *Physicians in retainer ("concierge") practice. A national survey of physician, patient, and practice characteristics.* Journal of General Internal Medicine, 2005. **20**(12): p. 1079-83.

14. Avitzur, O., *More neurologists transition to concierge-type practices-what they're doing to make it work.* Neurology Today, 2015. **15**(7): p. 14-16.

Part 2

Finding the Best Healthcare Providers

Finding the Best Primary Care and Medical Specialists

Finding the best doctors is a challenge. You may have just moved to a new city and need to establish medical care relations and want to find the best new doctors. Or your doctor is retiring and you want to find an excellent replacement. Or you are dissatisfied with the doctor you are using and want to change to a new one. Or you may want to help a friend locate the best professionals. Or you have changed to a new healthcare insurance plan and your current doctor does not participate in it. If any of these circumstances apply, then this chapter will be of great help in systematically locating potential doctors and verifying their credentials both formally and informally.

We begin by distinguishing the **healing side** and **the business side** of choosing your doctors. The **healing side** includes a doctor's professional training and experience; the doctor's reputation among colleagues and patients; any affiliations of the doctor such as what hospitals he or she uses and what academic medical center or medical school faculty appointments he or she may have; and the patient's ability to like and trust the provider and to have an interpersonal "connection" with the provider.

The **business side** concerns the way a doctor is financially compensated by the patients, and the doctor's participation in various health insurance networks, which may include your insurance plan. The business side also relates to the growing trend toward "concierge" and other direct payment models discussed in earlier chapters. Some additional assessment areas include the professionalism and pleasantness of the office staff; the existence of a patient portal for online communications; the ease or difficulty of making timely appointments; no undue waiting when you are on time for appointments; the electronic submission of prescriptions to your pharmacy (both initial and renewal); whether it is a group practice (single or multi-specialty) or solo practice; and communication with other doctors you are seeing.

An important issue we want to emphasize is the *verifiability* of the attributes that you want to find in a candidate doctor. The more verifiability, the better! But keep in mind that some attributes are less verifiable than others. Examples of very verifiable features concern state medical licensure and clinical knowledge and skills. Examples of less objectively verifiable qualities are the personality of the doctor, the demeanor and helpfulness of the office staff, and the professionalism of office operations. Also, keep in mind the role of board certification as an indicator of clinical knowledge and skills. Some doctors are very skilled and very knowledgeable but are not board certified in their specialty, perhaps because they are younger doctors who have not yet taken their board certification exam. Or they may be older practitioners for whom board certifications were not strongly promoted in their early years of practice and they saw no need to undergo the demanding certification process. Because the boards are objective indicators of clinical knowledge and skills, the absence of board certification means it is harder to verify the candidate doctor's knowledge and skills. With this in mind, we look closer at the "architecture" of board certification.

Important Credentials for both PCPhys. and Specialists:
The "Architecture" of Certification of Professional Skills

In this discussion we do not distinguish the "generalist" (primary care physician) from the "specialist." The reason is that primary care physicians also have board certifications (Family Medicine or Internal Medicine or Pediatrics). Thus, they too are "specialists" who choose to treat a wide array of patients and illnesses. With that said, we now approach the **healing side** of choosing a doctor by expanding your understanding of the term "board certified" in regard to verifying the level of skills and knowledge that a candidate doctor objectively has. There are different levels of specialty training. For example, an internist must satisfy *residency training* requirements and pass examinations before receiving specialty certification from the American Board of Internal Medicine (ABIM). If the physician wants to be, for example, a board-certified cardiologist, he/she must take *additional fellowship training* and pass related examinations before receiving certification of having additional qualifications in the various areas of cardiology, such as adult congenital heart disease; advanced heart failure and transplant cardiology; cardiovascular disease; clinical cardiac electrophysiology; and interventional cardiology. There currently are twenty-four recognized board-certified specialties and one hundred recognized subspecialty areas.[60] The American Board of Medical Specialties (ABMS) is the parent organization of these twenty-four specialty boards.

Keep in mind that new specialties formally created as clinical fields evolve and mature. For example, both authors, as geriatric psychiatrists, saw the field of Geriatric Psychiatry become formally recognized as the second subspecialty in Psychiatry (the first was Child and Adolescent Psychiatry). Subsequently there has been the official recognition of the subspecialties of Addiction Psychiatry, Forensic Psychiatry, and Psychosomatic Medicine. Some certifications are lifelong while others are time-limited (such as for ten years) at which time maintenance of the certification is renewed by passing a further examination.

With this overview of training, skills, and certification, you can see that this is an important area to consider in choosing your doctor. Thus, an important source of information is whether the physician is board certified and meeting the requirements of the ABMS program for Maintenance of Certification (ABMS MOC). To find out if your prospective doctor is board certified, you can call the ABMS or visit their online site.[61]

---

60   See full list of medical specialties at www.abms.org/media/84812/guide-to-medicalspecialties_05_2015-2.pdf
61   Call the ABMS Certification Verification Service toll-free at 1-866-ASK-ABMS (275-2267). Operators can assist you in confirming a physician's certification. Alternatively, you can go to www.certificationmatters.org/

Doctor's Reputation

There are two main sources of information that cover a doctor's clinical skills and a doctor's personality. Issues of clinical competence should be addressed by other doctors who might or might not recommend the doctor to his or her patients when they need a referral. A good question to ask the other doctor(s) would be: would you use this doctor for yourself or for your own family? Less reliable but still helpful is asking friends or co-workers who use the doctor about their experience in being helped by the doctor's skills and thoroughness. The issue of personality is a tricky one. As one website notes,[62] word of mouth from friends is one way with two caveats: First, know that a "nice" doctor is not necessarily the most competent. And second, a "competent" doctor isn't always the most pleasant. Draw the line on what you are willing to put up with based on how difficult it is to find another doctor who practices the same specialty or offers the same services. That website notes that another way to get information these days may be to use social media. With the rise in the numbers of doctors who use Facebook, Twitter, or other social networking sites, it's easier than ever to use social media to estimate some aspects of the personality and attitudes of doctors before you ever meet them.

Affiliations

Important affiliations include being on the staff of the best hospitals and being on the faculty of a school of medicine. The credentialing of a doctor at a top hospital is an excellent indicator of very good clinical skills. Having a faculty appointment is a verifying indicator that the doctor has well-regarded clinical skills. It also indicates a good personality since often the faculty is involved in supervising and teaching medical students and residency-training young doctors who routinely rate their teachers.

Other Legal Issues

Two other legal issues to consider include whether the doctor is currently licensed to practice in your state, and whether there are any disciplinary actions or malpractice claims against the doctor. For additional information see chapter *Appendix: Other Legal Issues to Consider.*

Supplementary Credentials

Although the above basic credentials are always important, here are two more "credentials" that may be important to many—but not all—consumers: the *age and experience* of the doctor, and the *non-clinical professional activities* of the doctor. Regarding the first, some prospective patients may prefer a younger doctor because their more recent training may give them an edge on being current in the latest technologies, disease concepts, and advances in disease diagnosis and treatments. Other patients may prefer a somewhat older doctor who has seen more cases and clinical variations in illnesses and patients' response to treatments. These personal preferences depend on what level of clinical experience you value.

---

62   See http://patients.about.com/od/doctorsandproviders/a/How-To-Research-Doctors-Credentials.htm

Beyond direct patient care are professional activities, including publication of medical articles, participation in clinical or basic science research, and involvement in professional organizations such as medical societies, medical boards, and other professional organizations (hospital, state, or national levels). These activities may suggest greater competence based on knowledge and the recognition of peers. However, there is no one-to-one carryover in these areas. That is, other doctors not involved in these activities could be just as good at delivering excellent quality healthcare.

For example, sometimes "politics" also comes into play that can affect a doctor's local reputation either positively or negatively. A senior doctor waiting for a hospital elevator while making rounds on patients had just been elected president of the American Diabetes Association, and congratulations were in order. He laughed, said thanks, and told a brief story of the irony of his ascent to the presidency. He had always had a full-time private practice and never wanted to be on a hospital or medical school payroll. His clinical expertise and qualities had been only reluctantly acknowledged by his department until he was elected to the presidency. Although he was a respected member of his department, he was not an "insider," and the department was focused on promoting "its own" salaried doctors. However, on becoming the president he was suddenly acclaimed as a leading world expert by the Department of Medicine. His attitude? "That's hospital politics for you!" He always delivered the best medical care to his patients. This anecdote shows that participation in these additional activities may not always translate into uniform reliable recognition of clinical excellence.

The Business Side of Choosing a PCPhys. or Specialist

Assuming you have "vetted" the prospective doctor's professional skills, reputation, affiliations, and other legal issues, you can now turn to the business side of the doctor's practice. If you don't have any medical insurance, the first question for you to ask would be what are the typical fees that the doctor would charge for services to you? For this you have to speak directly to the doctor's office staff. However, assuming that you do have medical insurance, the first question is typically whether that doctor participates in your insurance plan (see helpful resources in *Chapter 5 Appendix: Does Your Doctor Participate in Your Insurance Plan?*). If the doctor does participate, does the office accept your plan's reimbursement on an *assigned* [63] basis? Alternatively, are you expected to pay the full fees to the doctor and await insurance reimbursement to you after the office has generated the insurance claim form? A further question may come up concerning whether your doctor (primary care or specialist) has a "concierge" or direct payment component to their practice, as discussed earlier (*see Chapter 4*). If so, then what is the role of your medical insurance under that arrangement? Also, is there a need to establish a health savings account to cover the non-insurance cash payments expected of you? A last question concerns the doctor's policy on late cancellation of an appointment. If the reason for the cancellation is legitimate, are you still charged a fee for the missed appointment?

---

[63] "Assignment" indicates that the insurance payments will be paid directly to the doctor and you pay any applicable co-payment. Conversely, non-assigned payments go directly to the patient.

ABMS Guidance on Selecting and Working With Your PCPhys. or Specialist

The American Board of Medical Specialties (ABMS) has helpful guidance on selecting and working with a doctor of your choice. They fully support our approach thus far and also include additional features to evaluate both the doctor and the medical office. First, they detail three key steps in finding a doctor for yourself or a family member. Then they suggest questions to ask the new doctor. Finally, they describe numerous ways in which you can promote a positive ongoing relationship with the new doctor.

Find a Health Care Partner You Trust [64]

When you choose a doctor, it's important to find someone who will be a valued partner in your care. You want someone you can trust and communicate comfortably with to help you to stay healthy or recover from an illness or injury. Here are three key steps to follow when choosing a doctor for yourself or a family member:

1. Decide what qualities and services matter most to you. These may include having a doctor or surgeon who

   - Is well trained and experienced in the specialty in which you need care

   - Provides clear explanations of conditions and treatments, and welcomes questions

   - Uses technology to improve care and communication

   - Has a convenient office location and office hours

   - Is part of your healthcare plan

   - Has privileges at the hospital of your choice

2. Compile a list of potential choices

   - Ask your current doctors or other health professionals for recommendations

   - Ask family members, co-workers, and friends for recommendations

   - Search[65] to find board-certified doctors by specialty or location

   - Request a list of doctors from your health insurance provider

   - Contact a doctor referral service at your preferred hospital

   - Check with the medical society of the specialty you are looking for

---

64   See http://www.certificationmatters.org/take-charge-of-your-health-care.aspx
65   See www.certificationmatters.org/is-your-doctor-board-certified/search-now.aspx

3. Do your homework

   - Check the doctor's qualifications

   - Use the Web to research the doctor

   - Develop a list of questions on topics and concerns important to you

   - Talk with the office staff and/or the doctor on the phone, or schedule a face-to-face visit (there may be a charge for an in-person visit)

   - Once you've selected a doctor, make the most of your visits by properly preparing and following up

Questions to Ask Your Doctor [66]

Here are some important questions to ask if you're interviewing a doctor or seeing a new doctor for the first time. If you already have an established relationship with a doctor, you may know the answers to most of these questions. If not, take some time during your next visit to learn the answers. Please note that there may not be enough time to pose all these questions, and it is best to prioritize the ones that are most important to you.

   - Are you Board Certified?

   - If you are Board Certified, by which Board? In which specialty?

   - Do you participate in the ABMS Maintenance of Certification® program? What does this involve?

   - Where did you attend medical school? How long have you been in practice?

   - Which hospitals do you use? Are they accredited?

   - What are your office hours?

   - Who covers for you when you are unavailable?

   - How long does it usually take to get a routine appointment?

   - How long is the typical office wait?

   - Will I have to pay if I cancel an appointment?

   - Does the office send reminders about prevention tests?

   - What do I do if I need urgent care or have an emergency?

   - Do you or someone in your office speak the language that I am most comfortable using?

   - Do you (or a nurse or physician's assistant) give advice over the phone for common medical problems?

   - Do you use electronic medical records?

---

66   See http://www.certificationmatters.org/take-charge-of-your-health-care/questions-to-ask-your-doctor.aspx

- Do you perform routine X-rays and laboratory services in your office?

- Do you survey your patients? How do you use the findings?

In addition to these general questions, you may wish to ask questions tailored to doctors in a particular specialty or subspecialty. For example, if you are considering a surgical procedure, you may want to ask how frequently the doctor performs the procedure, what the potential risks are, and what the recovery involves.

Make the Most of Every Visit [67]

Cultivate a good relationship with your doctor by sharing information, asking questions, and listening actively. The more involved you are in your care, the more satisfied you'll be. Here are some suggestions to help you make the most of your doctor's visit:

- Tell your doctor what you think he or she needs to know about your symptoms and health history. Don't neglect family and personal information, even if it makes you feel embarrassed or uncomfortable. Bring a completed health history with you.

- Bring any medicines you are taking, or a list of those medicines (include when and how often you take them). Talk about any allergies or reactions you have had to your medicines.

- Tell your doctor about any natural or alternative medicines or treatments you are undergoing.

- Bring other medical information, such as X-ray film reports, test results, and medical records (if available).

- Ask questions. If you don't, your doctor may think you understand everything that was said.

- Bring someone along to help you ask questions. This person can also help you understand and/or remember the answers.

- Ask your doctor to draw pictures if you think that might help you better understand something.

- Take notes. Some doctors do not mind if you bring a recorder, but always ask first.

- Ask for written instructions, brochures, or videotapes to help you.

- Once you leave the doctor's office, follow up with questions, appointments for lab work or procedures, or additional appointments as needed.

We have covered a lot of information in this discussion. Here are three reputable sources to locate prospective doctors:

1. The American Medical Association's "DoctorFinder" [68] lets you search for doctors by medical specialty or name.

---

67   See http://www.certificationmatters.org/take-charge-of-your-health-care/make-the-most-of-every-visit.aspx
68   See https://apps.ama-assn.org/doctorfinder/recaptcha.jsp

2. MedlinePlus's "Directories" [69] lets you search for doctors (both generalists and specialists), dentists, and hospitals. This is a well recommended and rather unique "directory of directories" to find links to reputable healthcare search engines.

3. Medicare's "Physician Compare" [70] lets you search for providers in a zip code location by specialty (for example, cardiology) or medical condition (for example, diabetes mellitus) or an organ/organ system (for example, the heart).

Further Considerations on Your Expectations of Doctors

Did you notice that in the preceding section, the first ABMS guidance ("Find a Health Care Partner You Trust") uses the words "trust and communicate comfortably with"? This is one of the highly desirable aspects of the doctor-patient relationship that reflects your response to both the professionalism and the humanness of your doctor and the office staff. This is particularly important in your relationship with your doctor over time. Thus, it especially applies to your PCPhys. and any specialist with whom there is an ongoing relationship such as your cardiologist or psychiatrist. If trust and comfortable communication are not (or are no longer) present, it may indicate that this is not the best doctor for you at this time.

Now let's discuss other expectations and issues concerning your doctors.

The Importance of Having a PCP

What to Look for in a PCP

Not surprisingly, doctors are also patients. So this book's authors asked more than a dozen physician colleagues and searched the medical literature to find the main characteristics that doctors look for in choosing their PCPhys.[71] If you currently have a PCP or are in the process of engaging one, we hope you find the following list valuable. Please keep in mind that there is no perfect "10" or perfect PCP. If your PCP or the one you are considering comes close to meeting these characteristics, you'll be in good hands. The following list does not prioritize the order of importance.

- Be the captain of their healthcare team; and be reliable, active, consistent, and skillful in making certain that their overall care is coordinated with their other health professionals and specialists (if needed) [1].

---

69   See https://www.nlm.nih.gov/medlineplus/directories.html sponsored by the National Institutes of Health (NIH) and the U.S. National Library of Medicine
70   See www.medicare.gov/physiciancompare/search.html
71   Consumer Reports (February 2011): "What doctors wished their patients knew: Surprising results from our survey of 660 primary-care physicians"; http://www.consumerreports.org/cro/2012/04/what-doctors-wish-their-patients-knew/index.htm#

- Be invested in your well-being for the long haul. Becomes even more attentive, involved, and reliable if you have a serious illness.

- Takes your physical complaints seriously.

- Returns your call or patient portal system email should you become ill when traveling.

- Carefully weighs the risks and rewards of any test, procedure, and surgery. Makes certain that your questions/concerns are answered [2][3][4].

- Is invested in preventing health problems by encouraging a healthy lifestyle (such as diet, exercise, smoking cessation).

- Tells you and all new patients that they need to play a major role in the physician-patient relationship by asking questions and following treatment recommendations.

- Refers you to the best specialists and makes certain that the specialists' diagnosis and treatment recommendations are fully explained to you.

- If hospitalized and your care is transferred to a "hospitalist" who doesn't know you, makes certain that all your medical information is quickly communicated. The dialogue between your PCPhys. and the hospitalist continues during and after hospitalization.[72]

- Wants you to have the best treatment possible. Will fill out the required authorization forms and, when necessary, call your insurance company to request approval of the best medications and referral to the best (often expensive) specialists.

- Calls or has the assistant call you with test results [5].

- Gives you a follow-up appointment to make certain that you are responding to treatment, and answers additional questions.

- Diligently coordinates your care with other healthcare professionals and (with your permission) keeps your family informed.

- Practices what he or she preaches [for example, stays fit, doesn't smoke, looks professional [6], has no signs of self-abusive behavior (such as alcohol)].

- Makes certain that you have sufficient medication before your next appointment.

- Makes certain you have a designated and alternate healthcare proxy and a living will and they are kept updated.

- Looks comfortable and can be frank and honest with you if you're faced with serious or end-of-life decisions [4].

- Keeps up to date with the latest medical breakthroughs by attending medical conferences. Mentions the latest advances that apply to you.

---

72   J. Gross. New breed of specialist steps in for the family doctor. *New York Times*, 5/26/2010.

When our doctor colleagues were asked who they didn't want as their PCP, they replied they DIDN'T want someone who:

- Says "I'm sorry, I can't do anything more to help you."

- Says "I don't know a specialist who can help us clarify your diagnosis."

- Worsens your problems and finances by needlessly shuffling you from one specialist to another.

- Makes you feel you're taking up too much time. Looks impatient when you ask questions.

- Looks "burned out" and talks about eagerness to retire.[73]

Shortage of Physicians

We strongly encourage you to get a PCPhys. *now* because there is a relative shortage of physicians in the United States. There are now only about 700,000 physicians, whereas there is a current need for well over 800,000 doctors, with an insufficient number graduating from medical and osteopathic schools, and an insufficient number practicing in rural areas. Not enough graduates are going into primary care fields of medicine, such as family practice, internal medicine, general practice, and pediatrics. The current shortage of PCPs will become more acute as increasing numbers of uninsured Americans, under the ACA, become eligible for Medicaid and insurance via exchanges, in addition to the rapidly expanding baby boomer generation eligible for Medicare.

Unfortunately, an increasing number of PCPs are limiting the number of new Medicare and Medicaid patients they admit into their practice, and some have elected to no longer participate as providers for these governmental programs. Yet most insurance plans, especially managed care companies, require patients to have a PCP who serves the important role of coordinating a patient's overall care and making referrals to specialists.

What If a Potential PCPhys. has "Closed" His Practice to New Patients?

If you are determined to enlist the services of a particular physician, here are strategies to achieve your objective. If the office manager tells you that the doctor is not accepting new patients, ask if you could be placed on a waiting list or if you could be seen if a scheduled patient cancels. If relatives or friends are his

---

73   R. C. Rabin, A growing number of primary care doctors are burning out. How does this affect patients? *Washington Post*, 3/31/14.

or her patients, mention their name. Use your interpersonal skills to get to know the office manager. Call a few days later to see if an opening has become available.

Don't be shy about making important inquiries about the doctor you are considering. For example, if you're told that this doctor is the managing physician of a large group practice and sees patients infrequently, you may not want to be under his or her care. If the physician you want is not suitable or available even after trying these strategies, ask the office manager to recommend other physicians.

Out-of-Network Doctors

An increasing number of physicians have not only disenrolled from (or opted out of) Medicare and Medicaid, they have elected, for various reasons, not to be a provider with any insurance company. These physicians are then referred to as "out of network" doctors, and they are sometimes referred to as having a "boutique practice," as described in Chapter 4.

You can ask your insurance company whether or not and to what extent you would be entitled to partial payment from your insurance company if you submit for reimbursement a detailed paid bill from your "out of network" (or "non-participating") physician. You can also ask your insurance company if they would authorize you to see that "out of network" physician as a single-case exemption. The physician and staff would need to be willing to fill out considerable paperwork.

Doctors Who "Opt-Out" of Medicare

Physicians (both PCPs and specialists) and other licensed practitioners can "opt-out" of the Medicare program. This means that neither the physician nor the beneficiary submits the bill to Medicare for services rendered. Instead, the beneficiary pays the physician out-of-pocket and neither party is reimbursed by Medicare. A private contract is signed between the physician and the beneficiary stating that neither one can receive payment from Medicare for the services that were performed.[74]

If you have Medicare *and a secondary insurance* but the physician is not a Medicare provider, neither you nor the physician can send a bill to Medicare. However, some *secondary* insurance companies may provide some reimbursement if your physician's office provides you with a detailed bill and you submit it to your secondary insurer. Find out the details from your secondary insurer beforehand so there are no

---

74   See https://www.cms.gov/Outreach-and-Education/Medicare-Learning-Network-MLN/MLNMattersArticles/downloads/SE1311.pdf

surprises. You may want to ask your secondary insurance company to put its policy in writing to minimize later misunderstandings when you submit the physician's bill.

Finding a Medical Specialist: Overview

Earlier we recommended three online sites to locate PCPs and specialists. The recommendations are worth repeating[75]: The American Medical Association site; the MedlinePlus site; and the Medicare site. You can additionally confirm a potential doctor is Board Certified in a specialty on the American Board of Medical Specialists site. You may want to consider seeing a specialist if your PCP recommends this; or if you are not recovering as quickly as expected from your illness; or if you are not feeling comfortable with your PCP; or if you or a family member intuitively believes its time to get a second opinion (discussed in more detail in Chapter 12).

We recommend that you have a frank discussion with your PCP about seeing a specialist. Your PCP knows and works closely with a number of specialists. With your written permission, the PCP sends copies of your records and/or calls the specialist to discuss your case. The specialist's recommendations are communicated back to your PCP, who integrates the specialist's recommendations into your overall treatment plan.

The role of the PCP is especially important in caring for fragile, elderly patients who often take multiple medications and visit several specialists. It is important that all health professionals know who is "captain of the ship" and who is responsible for which aspects of the elderly patient's treatment, such as who is responsible for adjusting which medications. Otherwise, treatment becomes fragmented and potentially fraught with errors rather than being integrated and coordinated.

You, your PCP, and the specialist can decide if it's best to continue under the specialist's care, continue under the care of your PCP, or utilize the services of both. It's important that all those involved are clear about what role and responsibility each physician will assume.

The following strategies for finding a psychiatrist or therapist are also relevant for finding other specialists.

---

75   See(1) https://apps.ama-assn.org/doctorfinder/recaptcha.jsp; (2) https://www.nlm.nih.gov/medlineplus/directories.html; (3) www.medicare.gov/physician-compare/search.html; and (4) www.certificationmatters.org/is-your-doctor-board-certified/search-now.aspx

Finding a Specialist: Example of Mental Health Professionals

Different Mental Health Professionals

We discuss this example because mental health professionals introduce a new group of licensed non-physician professionals such as clinical psychologists (doctoral level training), psychotherapists (master's level training), and clinical social workers (CSW; master's degree). The main differences between a Psychiatrist, a Therapist, and other mental health professionals can be found on our website. *See further details in Chapter 5 Appendix: Different Mental Health Professionals.*

Making the First Appointment

Making an appointment with a psychiatrist or other mental health professional, such as a psychotherapist or a family counselor, can be a challenging, frustrating experience. This was the case with Julie, an attractive twenty-two-year-old married nurse living in New York City. She had become very depressed after the birth of her first child. Her PCP put her on an antidepressant and told her to call her insurance company to find a psychiatrist. The first few she called were not taking new patients, and the next four no longer were providers with her insurance company and didn't know psychiatrists who were providers. She and her husband considered abandoning the search. Finally, she asked her hospital co-workers for a recommendation. A close friend advised her to call Dr. Clark, who had an excellent reputation but rarely accepted new patients. When Dr. Clark explained that he had no available appointments for several months, Julie became assertive and asked if she could call again in a few days to see if he had a cancellation. She was pleased to be able to see him a week later, felt comforted by his gentle, empathic manner, and was on the road to recovery within a few sessions.

Some psychiatrists have special training and experience in treating children, couples, families, and elderly patients and particular types of problems such as depression, anxiety, or substance abuse. In general, psychiatrists tend to treat patients with major psychiatric problems, and many such patients require a combination of psychotherapy and medication.

Finding a Psychiatrist

If you are looking for a board-certified psychiatrist, you can contact the American Board of Medical Specialties or call the district branch of the American Psychiatric Association (APA) near where you live.[76] If you have an elderly family member suffering from a psychiatric problem, you can contact the American Association for Geriatric Psychiatry to find a geriatric psychiatry specialist.[77]

---

76   To find the district branch, call the APA at 1-888-35-psych or go to www.apa@psych.org.
77   Call the AAGP at 301-654-7850 or go to www.AAGPonline.org.

Another way to find a psychiatrist or a therapist is by calling the psychiatry department of a nearby university medical center. If they have a psychiatric residency training program, there are medical doctors in training you can see who are supervised by experienced psychiatrists. These psychiatric outpatient clinics accept insurance, and fees are usually on a sliding scale commensurate with your financial situation. Additional resources are state- or county-supported community mental health clinics and Veterans Administration hospitals and clinics (for veterans who meet certain criteria).

If you live in a small rural community, you are primarily dependent on your PCP for almost all your healthcare, but your doctor may have access to consultation with a psychiatrist or other specialist in a nearby city. Some rural areas have telepsychiatry programs, where a patient can be interviewed and treatment can be planned via audiovisual equipment connected from the rural physician's office to a psychiatrist's office or the psychiatry department at a university medical center.

Using Your PCPhys. for Mental Health Treatment

Your PCP is usually capable of treating milder depression and anxiety disorders and will refer those with more serious problems to a psychiatrist. For less serious psychological problems, a state-licensed therapist with a background in psychology, social work, or psychiatric nursing is capable of providing psychotherapy, but the majority of psychotherapists are not licensed to prescribe medication.

In group practices of psychiatrists working in collaboration with therapists, therapy is often provided by the latter, and medication along with some psychotherapy is managed by the former. Patients are asked to sign the consent form permitting the psychiatrist, therapist, and PCP to communicate with one another. If your physician or psychiatrist is referring you to a therapist, sign consent forms so clinical records arrive or telephone discussions can take place before your first meeting with the therapist. Communication between psychiatrist and therapist is very important in facilitating a coordinated treatment plan.

Sometimes the psychiatrist and therapist don't know each other and there is a risk that, for various reasons, the psychiatrist and the therapist may work at cross purposes. So, it may be important for you to encourage communication between your two health professionals.

Further Advice in Starting Your Mental Health Treatment

There is a tendency for outpatient providers to be in solo practice rather than in group practices. So don't be surprised if your initial contact is directly with the professional. When making the initial call to a prospective psychiatrist, psychotherapist, or another type of specialist, find out if he or she is accepting new patients and is a provider with your insurance company. Briefly explain your main problem and ask about his/her experience treating patients with similar problems.

If you call a psychiatrist, he or she may ask you to contact your insurance company to find out whether you have a yearly deductible and what portion of it you have met, and what your co-payment is for a typical forty-five-minute session. It's important to understand your coverage and responsibility for the cost before treatment begins to avoid later misunderstandings. Unless the psychiatrist or therapist has office staff to find out these details for you, you may need to assume this responsibility.

The most important take-home message is to decide that you are going to do everything in your power to get the help you need and deserve. Don't allow old-fashioned stereotypical beliefs that it is shameful, a sign of weakness, or an indication of "craziness" to receive help from a psychiatrist or a therapist.

More than half of all psychiatric patients don't complete the first few sessions in most community mental health clinics because of the barriers to engaging with a psychiatrist or psychotherapist. This is often due to discomfort and shame about revealing personal aspects of yourself; cultural biases; ambivalent feelings toward mental health professionals; and transportation and financial limitations. One of the most important determinants of getting well is your willingness to make a commitment to treatment. Studies have shown that patients most likely to benefit from treatment are those who regularly attend their appointments.

Special Problems That May Require Re-evaluating Your Doctors

There are special treatment situations that may unfortunately occur with either a PCP or a specialist that could stress your trust and confidence in your doctor. However, be aware that treatment complications or failures are frequent occurrences in modern medicine, and doctors are ordinarily comfortable discussing them when they occur. Often they will discuss such possibilities in advance and sometimes ask you to sign a consent form verifying that you have been informed of possible unwanted complications. However, even with pre-treatment discussions it feels very different when a complication actually occurs! Let's consider four scenarios concerning non-emergency significant illness and what you might do should such a situation arise.

- Situation 1: Your condition is not getting better despite treatments.
- Situation 2: You're getting some improvement in your condition but experiencing strong adverse side effects of the medications or other interventions.
- Situation 3: The risk-reward balance of the proposed treatment is not good and you are at risk of a poor outcome.
- Situation 4: Your specialists disagree on the most appropriate treatment for your condition.

Here are some approaches that can apply to any of these situations. First, start to become reasonably educated about your condition. This begins with *conversations with your doctor* to explain the treatment problems and the alternatives available.

The process continues with your doing some *online research* on the condition and the currently recommended treatment approaches. The goal here is to acquire enough understanding so you can ask the right questions and understand the answers your doctor may give you. This gives you a chance to have an independent judgment of the information you are getting from your doctor. Is it consistent with what you've been learning? Does it make sense to you? Are there things missing from the explanations and are they provided if you ask about their absence? There are several online sources that can help you in this process. Do a search with the key words "**clinical practice guidelines** for [*insert here your diagnosis or condition*]" to find current recommendations that are intended for health professionals but also can be perused by patients. Such practice guidelines can also be accessed from the **Update** site [78] at a modest cost. An additional useful site is the **Treatment Options** site[79] of the Agency for Healthcare Research & Quality.

Start to build a *list of questions* you want to have answered by your doctor. You might want to use the Agency for Healthcare Research and Quality's "**Question Builder**"[80] to organize and prioritize your questions.

Get a *second opinion* from a specialist in your condition *(see discussion in Chapter 7)*. If your specialists cannot agree, then get a *third opinion* at a reputable comprehensive institution such as the Mayo Clinic in Rochester, Minnesota, or Johns Hopkins Hospital in Baltimore, Maryland or MD Anderson Cancer Center in Houston, Texas, or Dana-Farber Cancer Institute in Boston, Massachusetts. Check with your PCP to refer you to the specialists and check with your insurance carrier that they will respect your PCP's referrals and approve the costs of such further specialist consultations.

---

78   See (1) http://www.uptodate.com/home/about-us;   (2) https://store.uptodate.com/usa/customerinfo/ at a cost of $19.95 for a seven-day subscription.
79   See http://www.ahrq.gov/patients-consumers/treatmentoptions/index.html from the Agency for Healthcare Research & Quality.
80   See http://www.ahrq.gov/apps/qb/

Chapter 5 Appendix

Other Legal Issues to Consider

Because each state licenses its doctors to practice, you can go online to the state medical board in your state[81] and look up the potential doctor. You may also find information concerning any disciplinary issues. The Federation of State Medical Boards itself makes available[82] additional doctor information pertaining to disciplinary sanctions, education, medical specialty, and practice locations. Regarding malpractice claims, the National Practitioner Data Bank is an electronic information repository created by Congress[83] that contains information on medical malpractice payments and certain adverse actions related to healthcare practitioners, entities, providers, and suppliers. Organizations authorized to access these reports use them to make licensing, credentialing, privileging, or employment decisions. However, the reports are *confidential and not available to the public*. Nonetheless, you may see the information reflected in the state medical board record for the doctor. There are additional ways suggested to research malpractice suits and disciplinary actions.[84] For example, do an online search by entering "Dr. Joseph Smith" (be sure to put those quotation marks around the name to keep that phrase intact) and then additional identifiers, such as the words *malpractice* or *lawsuit* or *sanction* or *problem* or whatever you choose.

Does Your Doctor Participate in Your Insurance Plan?

Your doctor's participation can be determined on several websites, often along with other important information. Keep in mind that the lists of doctors and information about them are often outdated so you'll need to call the doctor's office manager to get accurate information.

If you have **Medicare** as your primary insurance and you are looking for a doctor who participates in Medicare, you want to go to a special Medicare site called *"Physician Compare."*[85] All doctors listed on this site are enrolled in Medicare. On this site you can find valuable additional information such as:

- Medicare assignment status (whether accepts or not)
- Office addresses where the professional sees patients
- Primary and secondary specialties including American Board of Medical Specialties (ABMS) board certification
- Medical school education and residency information
- Hospital affiliation
- Whether the individual or group participates in select Centers for Medicare and Medicaid Services (CMS) quality programs
- Gender

---

81   You can find this at the Federation of State Medical Board's "Directory of State Medical and Osteopathic Boards" (www.fsmb.org/state-medical-boards/contacts)
82   See www.docinfo.org
83   See www.npdb.hrsa.gov/
84   See http://patients.about.com/od/doctorinformationwebsites/a/malpracticeinfo.htm
85   See www.medicare.gov/physiciancompare/search.html

If you have **Medicaid**, these are state-run programs so you must go onto your state-specific site to confirm what potential doctors participate in that healthcare coverage.

If you have **UnitedHealthcare**, you can use their "*Find a Doctor*" site[86] to see if your prospective doctor participates in your plan.

If you have **Anthem** as your insurer, you can use their "*Find a Doctor*" site [87] to check if your doctor participates in it.

If your insurance is with **Humana,** you can use their "*Physician Finder*" site[88] to see if your doctor is listed as participating in their networks. You can also check a doctor's specialty, whether the doctor is accepting new patients, and what languages are spoken by his or her office staff.

If your health insurer is **Aetna**, use their "*Find a Doctor, Dentist or Hospital that Accepts Your Plan.*" [89]

If your carrier is **Cigna,** there are at least two sites depending on whether your plan is through employers or school[90] or whether you bought it on your own or through a state or federal insurance marketplace.[91]

The above health insurers are the major ones in the country. However, there are certainly other very reputable plans. Go to their website, look for how to find a doctor, and then see if your prospective doctor participates in your plan.

Different Mental Health Professionals

A psychiatrist is a physician who, after completing four years of medical school, trains for about four additional years at a psychiatric residency training program. The curriculum includes biological, psychological, sociological, and cultural bases for various psychiatric disorders; the theories and practice of different psychotherapies (insight oriented, supportive, cognitive-behavioral, interpersonal, family, and others), and the judicious use of psychiatric medications. Because he or she has a medical background, the psychiatrist is knowledgeable about how a medical illness can present as a psychiatric disorder and contribute to psychiatric symptoms. And because the psychiatrist has specialized training in the use and side effects of psychiatric medications, he or she can prescribe these medications, usually in combination with psychotherapy, to treat various psychiatric illnesses (such as mood and anxiety disorders, schizophrenia, behavioral problems of dementia, and addiction).

Many, but not all, psychiatrists take a special examination under the auspices of the American Board of Psychiatry and Neurology to become board certified in general psychiatry. Some psychiatrists, following successful completion of a four-year residency, elect to train for an additional year or more to become proficient in a formally recognized subspecialty area.

There are other skilled areas that do not have formal ABMS board certification such as expertise in providing psychoanalysis, family therapy, or group therapy. Most specialists take an additional examination, where available, to become board certified in that subspecialty. Board-certified psychiatrists with a subspecialty, and other subspecialty physicians, are expected to become recertified in that subspecialty by passing an examination every ten years or so in order to maintain their board-certified status.

---

86   See www.uhc.com/find-a-physician
87   See https://www.anthem.com/health-insurance/provider-directory/searchcriteria
88   See https://www.hccfl.edu/media/969171/physician%20finder%20english.pdf
89   See https://www.aetna.com/individuals-families/find-a-doctor.html
90   See https://hcpdirectory.cigna.com/web/public/providers
91   See https://ifphcpdir.cigna.com/web/public/ifpproviders?

Concerning clinical psychologists, there are many recognized specialties and proficiencies in professional psychology.[92] Programs and internships are accredited by the American Psychological Association (APA).[93] According to the APA, doctoral graduate programs occur in clinical, counseling, and school psychology. The primary professional degrees offered are the PhD (Doctor of Philosophy) and PsyD (Doctor of Psychology). Most doctoral degrees take five to seven years to complete. In addition, the trainee must pass a comprehensive exam and write and defend a dissertation. In order to practice as a psychologist in clinical, counseling, or school psychology, the trainee will also have to complete a one-year internship as part of the doctoral study in their area of practice. Some universities and professional schools offer a PsyD degree in lieu of the traditional research PhD or EdD degree. PsyD degrees, with their emphasis on clinical psychology, are designed for students who want to do clinical work.[94] An advanced degree in clinical psychology (PsyD) typically includes a Master and Doctoral level program that is completed in four years followed by a one-year approved internship. In contrast to psychiatrists, psychologists are not licensed to prescribe psychiatric medication except in certain states where they undergo special training and need to pass an examination.

With regard to Social Work training, the National Association of Social Workers (NASW) indicates that a social worker must have a degree in social work from a college or university program accredited by the Council on Social Work Education. The undergraduate degree is the bachelor of social work (BSW). Graduate degrees include the master of social work (MSW) and the doctorate in social work (DSW or PhD). Note that an MSW degree is required in order to be able to provide therapy. Degree programs involve classroom study as well as practical field experience. The bachelor's degree prepares graduates for generalist entry-level work, while the master's degree is for more advanced clinical practice. A DSW or PhD is useful for doing research or teaching at the university level.[95] Social workers with MSW credentials work in many areas such as mental health clinics and outpatient facilities as well as in private practice, where their typical services are indicated by the NASW in the previous chapter.

A psychotherapist may have a background in psychology, sociology, nursing, education, or other fields and special training in the theories and practice of various psychotherapies (somewhat like the training of psychiatrists), but they have little to no medical training. To practice psychotherapy, therapists need to be licensed in the state where they practice.

---

92   See http://www.apa.org/ed/graduate/specialize/recognized.aspx
93   See http://www.apa.org/ed/accreditation/about/index.aspx
94   See http://www.apa.org/action/science/clinical/education-training.aspx
95   See http://careers.socialworkers.org/explore/education.asp

Chapter 5 Key Points

Key Points: Verify Potential Doctor's Credentials

- Query professional skills & knowledge
    - Check on specialty board certification
- Verify professional reputation
    - Clinical skills & personality
- Assess professional affiliations
    - Hospital appointments; faculty of a school of medicine
- Confirm there are no legal issues
    - State license is current; no disciplinary actions; no malpractice claims

Key Points: Find Candidate Doctors

- Recommendations from PCP Phys., friends & family, co-workers
- Search specific online sites
    - American Board of Medical Specialties; American Medical Association; MedlinePlus; Medicare *Physician Compare*
- Get a list from your healthcare insurer
- Contact a doctor referral service at a major hospital or school of medicine
- Check with a medical society of the specialty you are looking for

Key Points: Becoming a Patient of a Doctor Who's "Not Taking New Patients"

- Try to get on the waiting list.
- Develop a good rapport with the scheduling secretary.
- Mention the names of relatives and friends under his/her care.
- Call to see if an appointment has become available because of a cancellation.

Key Points: Treatment Complications

- Typical situations are:
    - Not getting better
    - Strong adverse effects of medication or other interventions
    - Specialists disagree on best treatment for your condition
    - Best available treatment is known to have risk of poor outcome
- Have a conversation with your doctor about alternative treatments
- Do online research on your condition
    - See clinical practice guidelines from websites
    - Build a list of questions
- Get a second opinion from a specialist
- If necessary, get a third opinion from a reputable comprehensive institution such as Mayo Clinic, MD Anderson Cancer Center, Johns Hopkins Hospital

References

1. Press, M.J., *Instant replay—a quarterback's view of care coordination.* New England Journal of Medicine, 2014. **371**(6): p. 489-91.

2. Boden, W.E. and e. al., *Optimal medical therapy with and without PCI for stable coronary disease.* New England Journal of Medicine, 2007. **35**: p. 1503-1516.

3. Gawande, A., *Overkill: America's Epidemic of Unnecessary Care*, in *The New Yorker*. May 11, 2015: New York. p. 42-53.

4. Gawande, A., *Being Mortal*. 2014, New York: Metropolitan Books.

5. Casalino, L.P., et al., *Frequency of failure to inform patients of clinically significant outpatient test results.* Archives Internal Medicine, 2009. **169**(12): p. 1123-9.

6. Rehman, S.U., et al., *What to wear today? Effect of Doctor's attire in the trust and confidence of patients.* The American Journal of Medicine, 2005. **118**(11): p. 1279-1286.

Choosing the Best Hospital and Emergency Department (ED)

A Tale of Success

James B is a fifty-four-year-old married engineer with three teenage daughters. The family lives in Westchester County, New York. James was grieving the deaths of his father and older brother, both from heart attacks, six months ago. He was conscientious about all aspects of his life, especially his health and the welfare of his family. He had regular visits with his PCPhys. and cardiologist. He exercised regularly and watched his diet.

Although he always received a clean bill of health from his doctors, he acknowledged his risk of succumbing to a heart attack and was determined to stay healthy for the sake of his wife and his three daughters, who planned to go to college.

James had frank discussions with his cardiologist about risk factors for heart disease and about which nearby hospitals were best equipped to treat heart patients. He and his devoted wife (who was both his patient advocate and proxy) frankly discussed what they would do if he developed heart disease. They each kept a list of all his medications, copies of recent EKGs, and the telephone numbers of the nearby ambulance service and the local Joint Commission-accredited hospital, known for its special cardiology program. He carried with him a medical alert device should he need to contact a local medical emergency team. James periodically confirmed that the nearby hospital and its special cardiac rehabilitative program and their specialty doctors accepted his insurance (were in-network). Otherwise, James and his wife didn't allow their concern about his risk for heart disease to disrupt their normal lives.

Several years later James suffered a heart attack, but because it was mild, and thanks to his advance preparation, he recovered uneventfully after four days in the hospital that he had previously selected. A few years later when his children were in college, he and his wife planned an extended vacation. But throughout their trip, they maintained their preparedness should he experience further heart problems.

A Tale of Woe

Although several older family members had died of a stroke, Mrs. Smith, a fifty-year-old married high school English teacher, always enjoyed good health. She rarely visited her doctor, and she never discussed risk factors for stroke with her husband or physician. She avoided thinking about or getting treatment for her hypertension and her unhealthy, high-fat diet that contributed to high blood lipids – two common risk factors for a stroke. She didn't keep a list of her medications. When the school district where she worked changed to a different health insurance company, which required her to change to a new physician, she put off finding one. She didn't know there were specialized "stroke programs" at designated hospitals where the debilitating effects of an acute stroke could be reversed.

She awoke one morning with weakness on the right side of her body and slurred speech. Her husband called 911 and the EMTs took her to the closest emergency department (ED). Because Mrs. Smith had never found a new primary care physician (PCP), and did not have a personal health record (PHR) or a list of her medications, the ED staff wasted precious time contacting her former physician to learn essential but outdated medical information. Neither she nor her husband notified the emergency room in advance about her new insurance, so they didn't know that her new health plan required her to be transferred, when stabilized, from the ED to another hospital, which further delayed her treatment. The new hospital was not JCAHO-accredited, nor did it have a specialized stroke program. She died seven days later of a hospital-acquired infection.

The moral of these true stories is quite clear: PLAN AHEAD.

Planning in Advance May Save Your and a Loved One's Life

Because it's human nature to not want to think about becoming seriously ill, most of us don't think about preparing for a serious illness or accident. But taking the time to choose the best hospital and emergency department (ED) in your area can have life and death consequences. Some of us spend more time deciding on what new or used car to purchase. When deciding on a car, we do some investigation; we read consumer reports, talk to friends about their cars, test drive some, and look for a good bargain. Why not be as careful about selecting a hospital and ED?

Another factor to consider when choosing a hospital is being aware of who actually decides which ED and hospital to use in an emergency situation. Should you or a loved one have a medical emergency, you likely call 911. Ambulance drivers are usually, but not always, required to take you to the nearest ED, especially if you are critically ill, because getting immediate treatment is paramount. Why is it that we leave the important choice of what ED and hospital up to the ambulance driver we don't even know? However, if you are not too ill, you and a family member or perhaps your advocate could explain and convince the medics to take you to your preferred ED and hospital, even though it may take a little longer to get there. In addition, once you are medically stable, you can request to be transferred to your preferred hospital.

In this chapter, we explain how Medicare and the Affordable Care Act have improved the quality of care and safety of hospitals. We explain the crucial importance for you and your family's health and welfare of proactively assuming responsibility for choosing the best hospital and ED when you are healthy and thinking clearly. Health professionals know that preventable medical errors occurring in hospitals and doctors' offices kill or seriously injure hundreds of thousands of Americans every year. If the U.S. Centers for Disease Control and Prevention (CDC) included "preventable medical errors" as a disease-specific category, it would be the sixth leading cause of death in the United States.[96] We then provide practical advice about what to do before, during, and after a visit to an ED.

Hospitals Have Improved and Are Safer

Even before the ACA (Obamacare) was passed in 2008, Medicare identified preventable medical errors and complications that occurred in hospitals, such as hospital-acquired infections and medication errors. In 2012, Medicare decided not to pay, or to reduce payments, to hospitals and doctors for subsequent care related to hospital errors, such as development of new pressure ulcers, intravenous line-associated infections, and catheter-associated urinary tract infections. The financial viability of hospitals could be jeopardized by frequent occurrences of these avoidable errors. And Medicare gave financial bonuses to hospitals and doctors who had better patient outcomes. Medicare also established a research center to study and improve patient outcome and safety.

Some commercial health insurance companies have followed suit, establishing a similar carrot and stick reward system for reimbursing hospitals and doctors based on good patient outcomes and quality of care.[97] Medicare also required hospitals that receive Medicare funding (most hospitals) to report their medical error and success rate for treating specific conditions, such as heart attack, diabetes, and stroke.

There are two excellent Internet sites to obtain reliable hospital ratings, which can serve as one of a number of guidelines for selecting one of the best available hospitals for you and a loved one. One website is managed by The Joint Commission (JCAHO),[98] the other by Medicare. Regarding Medicare's website, the information comes from hospitals that have agreed to submit their success and error information for review by the public.

Choosing the Best Hospital for You

Before studying the ratings of different hospitals nearby that you are considering, it's most efficient to first find out what hospitals and EDs your health insurance policy has contracts with. This is especially important if you have a Health Maintenance Organization (HMO) insurance policy because these companies may

---

96   http://healthinsurance.about.com/od/reform/a/Medical-Errors-And-Health-Reform.htm?utm_term=Patient%20Safety%20in%20Hospitals&utm_content=p1-mai…
97   http://patients.about.com/od/AffordableCareAct/a/Affordable-Care-Act-And-Patient-Satisfaction-In-Hospitals.htm
98   www.qualitycheck.org

have contracts with a limited number of hospitals near where you live. So first check your insurer's website or, even better, periodically call their customer service department and obtain the names and locations of hospitals and EDs that have contracts/agreements (in other words, are considered in network) with your particular insurance. It's important to periodically check because insurance companies and hospitals change contracts and patients are not immediately informed. This is another example of a transition that can be dangerous to your welfare. Be aware that even though the hospitals you are considering are in network, there may be services such as rehabilitation or groups of doctors such as anesthesiologists who are out of network that your insurance may not pay for, and you will be financially responsible for. An estimated one in three Americans with private health insurance falls victim every two years to what's been called "surprise medical bills." [99] So, when checking out your prospective in-network hospitals, ask what services provided by the hospital are out-of-network just in case you unexpectedly require them so you won't be "surprised." This information may be a major factor in your selection of a hospital and ED.

If you live in an average size city, you probably have several choices of hospitals and EDs, in addition to the one closest to you. If your medical problem is serious – for example, requiring heart surgery – your major decision is what hospital is most capable of treating your condition. There are many different types of hospitals, from small community hospitals to large university-based teaching-research hospitals. Choosing the best hospital can make the difference between a successful recovery without complications, or its opposite.

Finding answers to the following questions ahead of time will help you choose the best hospital [3]. We suggest checking off and prioritizing the items most important to you to assist in selecting the hospital that best meets your or a loved-one's needs.

- Is the hospital and its ED accredited by JCAHO? Accredited facilities are most likely to have the best physicians and state-of-the-art medical equipment. Furthermore, if it is determined in the ED that you require hospitalization, you have a good chance of being admitted to the same hospital. You can check a hospital's accreditation status via www.qualitycheck.org.

- Ask your PCPhys. what hospital he/she would choose for the medical condition you have. Find out if your PCPhys., a hospitalist, or an intensivist (who cares for patients in an Intensive Care Unit (ICU) and often works closely together with the hospitalist) would be in charge of your hospital care. Ask whether or not all the hospitalists are contracted with your insurer (that is, are in-network). Other than in a small hospital in a rural part of the country, you'll most likely be assigned to a hospitalist.

- Does the hospital have board-certified medical specialists who treat your particular medical or surgical condition?

- Will your insurance pay for treatment of your medical condition at the hospital you are considering? Are there some services provided that are out-of-network, such as rehabilitation, in which case you will be financially responsible?

---

99   Edwards, H.S., "You only think you're covered", in Time magazine, New York, 187: 9 3/14/16 p. 45-47.

- If you'll be treated by a hospitalist, how will your PCP convey all your important medical information to the hospitalist and vice versa when you leave the hospital so your care is coordinated?

- Is the hospital a teaching hospital affiliated with a medical school? These hospitals have medical students and residents closely supervised by experienced attending physicians with medical school appointments. On the negative side, teaching hospitals can be more burdensome on you because multiple medical teams are questioning and examining you daily. Medical care in teaching hospitals can be a bit compromised around July of every year when a new crop of less experienced, recent medical school graduates begin their first year of residency and are involved in your care (although they are closely supervised).

- How conveniently located is the hospital for family/friends to visit, and if you will need follow-up visits at the hospital after discharge?

- Does the hospital offer private rooms (if that is important to you)?

- Can a family member or your patient advocate stay near your bedside 24/7?

- For serious conditions, such as those requiring heart bypass surgery, how often is this operation performed in the hospital you are considering? What percentage of patients have "successful" outcomes, and what is the rate of complications? In general, the greater number of such intricate surgeries done at the hospital, the better your chance of a successful outcome.

- If you don't have a patient advocate, can the hospital provide one or suggest an outside agency to contact?

- Consider taking a tour of the prospective hospital; visit someone there and have a meal in their dining room.

- Find out if it's likely you can receive all the care required in the same hospital (for example, rehabilitation or in a skilled nursing unit (if needed). Transferring to a different hospital for rehabilitation or further treatment increases the risk of delay in transferring your records, discontinuity of care, and errors. Recall the high risks associated with transitions!

The Role of the Hospitalist in Caring for Hospitalized Patients

Hospitalists are physicians who dedicate their clinical work to the medical care of hospitalized patients. The majority of hospitalists are board-certified internal medicine specialists, with three years of residency training after graduation from medical school. Some have additional post-residency training, known as a fellowship, such as in pulmonary and critical care medicine. Today, most hospitals with two hundred or more beds have contracts with one or more private practice hospitalist groups to provide services to hospitalized patients. Patients are referred to the hospital by physicians from nearby emergency departments and from PCPhys. and PCPs in the surrounding communities. Once a patient is admitted to the hospital, the hospitalist becomes the captain of the patient's healthcare team, responsible for requesting consultations with subspecialists (for example, in cardiology or infectious diseases when necessary), coordinating patients' care with discharge planners, social workers (who assist with family issues), and, when needed, consultation with palliative care and hospice physicians. Experienced hospitalists are competent in carrying out a variety of procedures, such as lumbar puncture, central venous catheterization, and endotracheal intubation. Their experience in medical procedures has reduced the need for subspecialists to perform such procedures, lowering the cost and number of days patients need to be in the hospital. Shorter hospital stays lessen the risks of hospital-acquired infections, bed sores, and other problems associated with protracted stays. Another benefit is round-the-clock 24/7 in-hospital care by your hospitalist team, as opposed to less attention from your PCPhys. who likely has a busy office practice.

Hospitalists in academic medical settings supervise residents, physicians, and other trainees and are involved in research.

Problems During Transition from Your PCP to a Hospitalist

Potential problems can occur when a patient, who has a long-term, close relationship with his/her PCP, is transferred to a hospitalist whom he/she doesn't know. Confidence and trust developed over years with your PCP is not easily transferred to a new physician (hospitalist). Likewise, your PCP may not know the hospitalist or be familiar with his/her educational and cultural background, including temperament and manner of speech. Your electronic medical records in your PCP's office may be incompatible with your hospitalist's software system, making transmission of your important medical records problematic. This is another example of miscommunication that can occur at crucial periods of transition [2].

What can you do to ensure a smooth transition when your medical care is transferred to a hospitalist or an intensivist?

- Hopefully, you and your patient advocate have maintained your own up-to-date personal health record (PHR), HIPAA, living will, and healthcare proxy that you can hand deliver to your hospitalist or nurse either prior to or upon admission to the hospital. (See *Chapter 1 – Why It's Critical to Assume More Responsibility and Control for Your Healthcare*).

- If you know in advance of your hospitalization, because it is elective (planned in advance) rather than an emergency, encourage your PCP to discuss your medical problems with the hospitalist assigned to you.

- Have a family member or your advocate notify your healthcare proxy and those friends and family members you've selected to be informed of your upcoming hospitalization.

- After admission to the hospital, encourage your hospitalist to keep your PCP informed of your progress and to obtain additional medical information about you that may have been overlooked during the transition to the hospital.

- Don't be hesitant about having your patient advocate or close family member assist you with the above functions. If you lack the capacity to make healthcare decisions, your proxy should know in advance to assume decision-making responsibilities.

- Before discharge home or transfer to another facility, encourage your hospitalist to discuss all your medical information with your PCPhys., PCP, and other health professionals (for example, physician specialists) who will resume responsibility for your post-hospital care. It could take days or longer until the hospitalist dictates your discharge report and even longer until the records reach your doctor's office. So, it is important to obtain your own copy of a summary of your treatment in the hospital. You can add it to your PHR and hand deliver a copy to all your health professionals so everyone is on the same page during this important transition. If you have used the hospital services in the past, you may already have set up a Patient Portal that serves as a communication link with your office physician and other health professionals. In that case you can print out copies of your hospital report from your home.

How the Merger of Hospitals and Healthcare Systems Can Affect You

Hospitals and healthcare systems, like other big industries in the United States, have been merging at a rapid pace. In 2016, there were 102 hospital mergers.[100] How do these mergers affect us as patients wanting high quality healthcare?

A 2017 study supported by the American Hospital Association (AHA) found that mergers decrease costs to patients due to economies of scale, and they have the potential to improve the quality of medical care and expand the scope of services available to patients.

For example, when a smaller hospital merges with a larger, better equipped hospital system, patients at the smaller hospital may benefit from more access to specialists, enhanced communication among health professionals, and greater access to advanced medical technologies, such as high-tech imaging procedures and a more uniform (standardized) electronic medical records system [4].

---

100   http://www.aha.org/presscenter/pressrel/2017/012517-pr-cr.shtml.

On the other hand, some economists believe that the merger of healthcare systems will drive the cost of medical care and insurance premiums higher because of decreasing competition. It could take weeks or months for merging healthcare systems to fully integrate their communication systems and educate the staff about new programs and procedures. If you or a loved one is admitted during the transition, your advocate could be especially helpful in being hyper alert to potential hospital/doctor/nursing errors.

Another potential benefit of consolidation and integration of large healthcare systems is the potential for more science-based studies resulting in more uniform diagnosis and treatment and better outcomes for patients. For example, decades of research have confirmed that patients who undergo complicated surgery have much better outcomes when the surgery is performed by surgeons doing a higher number of such surgeries. (The old adage "practice makes perfect" applies here.) The leading surgeons at Dartmouth-Hitchcock Health System, Johns Hopkins, and the University of Michigan[101] identified ten complex operations (for example, cardiovascular procedures) for which scientific evidence has proven that surgeons who perform a greater number of such surgeries per year have much better patient outcomes. These three institutions have agreed on a "volume pledge," establishing standards for all surgeons at the three institutions. Surgeons who don't perform a minimum number of a specific surgery are now expected to stop performing that surgery and be eligible for advanced training and proctoring before resuming the particular surgery.

The merger of hospital systems has fostered progress in reaching and establishing higher standards of healthcare for many other medical/surgical problems based on scientific evidence and the consensus of medical experts. Patients now and in the future, are very likely to benefit.

Choosing the Best Emergency Department (ED)

Many factors are worth considering *in advance of* deciding what ED is best for you or a loved one. Be prepared for an unexpected emergency by finding the answers to some of these questions that are most relevant to your situation. Talk about it with your spouse, partner, and patient advocate so you are all in agreement [1]. The order of these questions does not imply priority.

- Ask your PCP what ED he/she would choose for a medical emergency.

- What hospitals does the ED have a transfer agreement with should the ED's hospital be filled and you require transfer to another hospital?[102]

- Will your insurance company pay for that particular ED as well as for hospital care if you are admitted? You don't want to waste valuable time being transferred to another hospital that accepts your insurance.

- Is your PCP on staff at that hospital should you need hospitalization, or would a hospitalist take over your care? Today, even in small cities, hospitalists generally assume care.

---

101 http://catalyst.nejm.org/why-health-care-mergers-can-be-good-for-patients/
102 http://health.usnews.com/health-news/articles/2008/09/17/questions-to-ask-before-choosing-an-emergency-room

- Going to the nearest ED may be best if time is essential—for example, if you have a life-threatening event such as a heart attack or stroke.

- What is the closest ED that specializes in trauma? Such EDs have the most expertise and equipment to handle serious accidents and other trauma.[103] If that ED is farther away, it may be worth the longer ambulance ride.

- Are the physicians in the ED board-certified in emergency medicine? If so, that would be a plus in making your decision.

- In some areas of the country, by law, emergency medical technicians (EMTs) in the ambulance may be required to take you to the hospital that they believe is best to treat your particular condition. In other parts of the United States, EMTs are required to take you to the nearest ED. But you and/or your advocate may have a choice, especially if time is not essential. Should the EMTs tell you that a specific hospital's ED is overcrowded, you may ask to go there anyway because of the hospital's reputation.[104]

- For minor medical problems, make an appointment with your PCP or consider a twenty-four-hour-a-day urgent care clinic near you, where getting in and out is faster and far less expensive than a hospital ED. (See *Chapter 4—New Outpatient Choices When Your Doctor is Unavailable.*).

Preparing for Your Visit to the ED

- If you are seriously ill, call or have someone call 911 for an ambulance. Don't drive yourself, for your safety and that of others.

- Ask a family member or your patient advocate to call your PCP to (a) explain your symptoms, (b) ask your PCP to contact the ED to prepare them for your arrival, and (c) ask if he/she can meet you there.

- Ask your family member or advocate to go with you to the ED. Having someone by your side can reduce your stress[105] and be helpful in explaining your condition.

- Ask someone (your advocate or family member) to call your insurance company because some companies prefer advance notification if you use an ambulance and go to an ED.

- Whether or not you expect to be admitted to the hospital, pack a small suitcase with essential clothes, toiletries, your personal healthcare record (PHR), HIPAA, healthcare directive and proxy documents, telephone directory of your important people, a list of all your current medications, pill bottles, insurance cards, and a few family photos.

- Leave jewelry at home.

---

103 http://health.usnews.com/health-news/articles/2008/09/17/questions-to-ask-before-choosing-an-emergency-room

104 http://health.usnews.com/health-news/articles/2008/09/17/questions-to-ask-before-choosing-an-emergency-room

105 http://patients.about.com/od/atthehospital/a/er_tips.htm

After Arriving at the ED

- You, a family member, or your patient advocate should clearly explain to the triage nurse your main symptoms so the nurse can determine the seriousness of your condition. Give the nurse your PHR and a list of current medications. All this information helps the triage nurse expedite the next step in diagnosing and treating your condition.

- If you think you are having a life-threatening event, you or your advocate can tell the nurse you would appreciate seeing the ED's attending physician as soon as possible. (The usual routine is to be first assessed by a nurse or other ED staff before seeing the attending physician.)

- You and/or your advocate should ask questions, which engages you with the staff and provides you with more attention. At important transitions, ask, "What happens next?"[106]

- Remind yourself it is normal to feel scared, not only because of your symptoms but also because most EDs are noisy and brightly lit. You may see patients more critically ill than you. Don't make yourself more upset by taking personally what you may perceive to be some negative remark by a staff member about another patient. Doctors and nurses are under considerable stress and sometimes use humor to cope.

- Despite these stresses, maintain trust and faith in the medical team and be cooperative and appreciative. Think twice about requesting to be discharged against medical advice. Leaving the ED without needed treatment is likely to worsen your medical problem. Your patient advocate should advise you to cooperate and stay the course.

- You and/or your patient advocate should take notes because it's difficult to understand your doctor when you're under stress. If your doctor speaks in medical language you don't understand, ask that he/she explain in plain English.

- Have a family member or your advocate serve as your auxiliary spokesperson to communicate with your doctor(s) and keep family members updated about your progress. This enables you to focus your attention and energy on cooperating and getting well.

- Make certain that your healthcare proxy and alternate are kept updated about your condition in case he/she needs to make healthcare decisions on your behalf should you lose that capacity.

Before Leaving the ED

- Ask for copies of all evaluations and test results to take with you. Emphasize the importance of sending copies ASAP to *all* your doctors and other health professionals so your subsequent care is coordinated. As noted earlier, if you have a Patient Portal established with the hospital, you can print out the ED test results and summaries from your home.

---

106   http://patients.about.com/od/atthehospital/a/er_tips.htm

- Be certain that the ED staff gives you written instructions to follow once you return home. Make sure you know which medications to continue taking before your visit to the ED and new medications prescribed by the ED physician.

- Thank the ED staff for their help and concern. If asked, fill out a questionnaire about your experience so staff can improve services to others.

After returning home, make an appointment with your PCP within a week or sooner for subsequent follow-up care. Bring all the records from the ED visit and all your medications.

Chapter 6 Key Points

Key Points: Choosing the Best Hospital

- Make certain that the hospital accepts your healthcare insurance and that it's in- network for "all" the services you may need.

- Choose a JCAHO-accredited hospital.

- Determine whether your PCPhys., a hospitalist, or an intensivist will be your treating physician.

- Consider how convenient the hospital is for visits from family or friends.

- For complicated procedures, consider a hospital that specializes in your condition.

Key Points: The Role of the Hospitalist

- Hospitalists assume the role of captain of your healthcare team.

- Miscommunication and errors can occur when your care is transferred from your PCPhys. to a hospitalist and vice versa on discharge.

Key Points: Choosing the Best ED

- Ask your PCPhys. what ED he/she would choose for an emergency. In general, the best hospitals usually have top-quality EDs.

- Determine in advance whether the ED, hospital, and its doctors and other services you may need are in-network with your insurance.

Preparing for an ED Visit

- You, your patient advocate, or your PCPhys. should call the ED to prepare them for your arrival.

- Ask a family member or your advocate to accompany you to provide information and reduce your stress.

- Notify your insurance company.

- Pack a small suitcase that includes all health-related legal papers, your PHR, HIPAA, healthcare directive and proxy, list of all current medications, and all insurance cards.

Key Points: After Arriving at the ED

- Provide a concise summary of your main symptoms; ask questions.
- Remind yourself that it is normal to feel nervous. Be cooperative and appreciative.

Key Points: Before Leaving the ED

- Obtain a copy of all evaluations and test results for yourself. Have the staff send copies to all your health professionals ASAP.
- Obtain written instructions to follow after returning home.

References

1. Michelson, L.D., Emergency Room 101, in The Patient's Playbook, Alfred A. Knopf, New York, 139-165, 2015.

2. Press, M.F., Instant replay: A quarterback's view of care coordination. New England Journal of Medicine, 371-497, 2014.

3. Roizson, M.F., Oz, M.C., You – The Smart Patient, Free Press, New York, 2006 p. 169-191.

4. Noether, M., May, S. Hospital merger benefits: views from hospital leaders and econometric analysis. Report by Charles River Associates. 1/25/17, p.1-24.

A Second Opinion Can Save Your Life

Being Steadfast and Assertive Pays Off

Martha Young, a sixty-eight-year-old intelligent, assertive and successful literary agent living in Albuquerque, New Mexico, knew she had an aortic aneurysm (ballooning of a major heart artery) since her early thirties, when it was discovered on a routine chest x-ray. Every five years a CT scan confirmed that the size of the aneurysm was increasing very slightly. Because she was asymptomatic, she was treated with a cardiac medication that improved the functioning of her heart. Her cardiologist cautioned her that she may someday need specialized surgery to repair the aneurysm. It wasn't until Martha reached age sixty-six that she and her cardiologist decided to get an opinion from a cardiac surgeon about repairing the aneurysm. Fortunately, a year earlier she had chosen a Medicare Advantage PPO plan, but the insurance agent did not inform her of important details of the plan, which she soon learned were extremely important.

Her local cardiologist referred her to an in-network nearby heart surgeon. She lacked confidence in the surgeon because he looked younger than her thirty-four-year-old son and he hesitatingly admitted to having performed only two aortic artery surgeries in the past year. Putting her Internet skills to work, she found a heart surgeon with recent publications about aortic aneurysms in prestigious medical journals. He had developed a simpler, safer surgical procedure. In the past year, he had performed over 100 new operations, similar to the one she needed at an acclaimed academic medical center 1,500 miles away. Unfortunately, he was not contracted with her health insurance plan and hence was considered "out-of-network". She could not afford $325,000 out of pocket cost for the surgery, associated tests and cardiac rehabilitation, were she to have the operation by the more experienced surgeon.

She had been erroneously informed by a newly hired representative at her New Mexico Medicare Advantage PPO Plan that her insurance plan would not pay even a small portion of the cost if she had the surgery with an out-of-network surgeon. She decided to get a second opinion about her insurance coverage.

She arranged a three-way telephone conference with her insurance agent and the finance officer at the hospital where the experienced surgeon operated. She was delighted to discover that because she had a New Mexico Medicare-Advantage PPO plan, her insurance would pay almost the entire cost and her maximum out of pocket cost was $10,000. Other states may have different cost sharing rules for patients with Medicare-Advantage PPO plans.

The moral of this true story is that you need to be assertive, have an advocate (in this case, Martha's insurance agent), and obtain a second opinion. For Ms. Young, she not only obtained a second opinion from a renowned surgeon but she also got a second opinion regarding her insurance.

Why Don't More Americans Seek a Second Opinion?

About 30 percent of patients who obtain a second medical opinion discover that the initial diagnosis for their condition was incorrect, or they learn about a better treatment approach.[107] A 2017 study from the Mayo Clinic[108] in Rochester, Minnesota found that as many as 88 percent of medical patients coming to this renowned clinic for a "second opinion" got a new or refined diagnosis – changing their care plan and potentially saving their lives. Autopsy studies have shown that 25 percent of patients had diseases that were never diagnosed when they were alive.

Another argument for obtaining a second opinion emanates from a controversial book, *Demand Better! Revive Our Broken Healthcare System* [1]. They believe that the majority of treatment decisions made by physicians are based on little to no scientific evidence from randomized controlled studies but rather subjective judgment. Even the most experienced physicians make errors in diagnosing patients because of subjective, cognitive biases inherent in human thinking processes. For example, Drs. Kumar and Nash cite studies showing that when a patient goes to his primary care physician with a common problem such as low back pain, the doctor delivers the right treatment with real clinical benefit only about half the time. They believe that a physician's inaccurate decision making is not because doctors lack competence, sincerity, or diligence, but because they often must make decisions about tremendously complex problems with insufficient solid evidence from scientific studies to back them up.

Surprisingly, only 20 percent of patients receiving medical care each year seek a second opinion. The other 80 percent of Americans, according to a Gallup poll, don't think they need a second opinion because they feel confident about their doctor's advice.

Other reasons that account for why we don't seek a second opinion include: fear of acting distrustful of our doctor; concern that our doctor will take it as a personal insult and may be less responsive when called upon in the future; tendency to believe that our doctor is infallible; and inadequate knowledge of how to go about getting a second opinion and insufficient determination. But to paraphrase a longtime survivor of breast cancer: Doctors are not gods. They can do amazing things, and I have the utmost respect for the profession, but they are all human.[109] Don't think that getting a second opinion is an end run around your

---

107   http://www.latimes.com/business/la-fi-healthcare-watch-20150525-story.html

108   http://insider.foxnews.com/2017/04/10/mayo-clinic-study-second-opinion-new-diagnosis-health-wellness?utm_source=share&utm_campaign=share-bu…

109   http://www.latimes.com/business/la-fi-healthcare-watch-20150525-story.html

doctor; think of it as assembling the best team possible to guide you through some critically, potentially life-altering choices.[110]

Some of us may not know that we are entitled to get a second opinion or just how valuable and lifesaving it can be. Obtaining a second medical opinion has become much easier than it used to be. Patient records can be quickly sent electronically or by overnight courier service to a medical expert who specializes in your type of illness. It's easy to find medical experts in various fields of medicine via the Internet. For information about authoritative websites about various illnesses, see *Chapter 7 Appendix: Websites Providing Current Illness-Related Information and Research.* And, second and even third opinions are often covered by your insurance and are usually reasonably priced.

In this chapter, we discuss additional reasons why it's worthwhile to get a second medical opinion, when to consider obtaining one, common diagnoses often missed, important steps in the process of obtaining a second opinion, and strategies to pay the cost.

Why a Second Opinion Is Worthwhile

Although in this chapter we focus on getting a second opinion for a suspected cancer diagnosis, the treatment and diagnostic uncertainties about heart, lung, kidney, and liver and a host of other medical problems also deserve a second opinion. For example, hepatitis C, affecting the liver, has newer medications available without as many side effects as previous medications.

It's important to obtain a second opinion about your diagnosis and treatment because it can save your life, [4] as illustrated by Mary Edwards, a twenty-nine-year-old woman who underwent a breast lumpectomy for suspected cancer. Her oncologist told her that the pathology report indicated she didn't need further surgery or chemotherapy. He added, "You're fine" and "I know what I'm talking about." She was taken aback by his presumptuousness. Her intuition told her that his advice didn't "feel right." She got a second opinion from another oncologist, who re-examined the initial pathology report and biopsy specimen. It showed remaining cancer cells that were not detected by the initial pathologist. She went on to receive the proper treatment and is alive and well twenty years later.

After a biopsy is taken for a suspicious breast mass, a patient usually puts her fate in the hands of an unknown pathologist who may be in a local or faraway pathology laboratory. In that lab, the pathologist decides whether the sliver of tissue is benign or malignant. If the latter, the pathologist judges how aggressive the disease is. All this information crucially influences the subsequent treatment plan.

A study of biopsy slides of over six thousand cancer patients at Johns Hopkins Medical Center found that eighty-six patients (1.4 percent) had significantly incorrect diagnoses that would have led to incorrect or unnecessary treatment. But if it were your or a family member's biopsy specimen that was incorrectly

---

110 http://www.cfah.org/prepared-patient/prepared-patient-articles/seeking-a-secondor-thirdopinion#.WMW8RzvRknQ.email.

diagnosed, it would feel as if the incorrect percentage was 100 percent.

Another Johns Hopkins study reviewed the slides of prostate cancer patients referred for possible prostate surgery. Because errors in the initial pathology report were discovered by a second specialized pathologist, 1.1 percent of the patients did not need to undergo surgery.

Experts attribute the majority of these errors to many benign biopsies mimicking cancer, and to the reverse – malignancies that mimic benign tumors. As options for treating cancer have greatly expanded, it's become even more important to not only make a correct diagnosis but to sub-classify biopsy tissue as more or less aggressive and sometimes to do genetic studies – which greatly influence the choice of treatment options.

To improve accuracy of diagnoses at academic medical centers and at specialized comprehensive cancer centers, when a patient is referred from another hospital where a pathology diagnosis of cancer was made, it's required that an in-house pathologist reexamine the actual slide of the biopsy to verify the diagnosis before deciding on the best treatment approach. In addition, these medical centers have regular conferences to discuss difficult-to-diagnose cases with highly specialized pathologists.

Another advantage is that some academic teaching and research centers offer experimental treatment approaches for treatment-resistant cancers not available at smaller hospitals. For some patients with difficult-to-treat cancers, being part of an innovative, experimental treatment program offers increased hope.

In the past decade, more patients have taken it upon themselves to request a second opinion about their initial diagnosis. Dr. Epstein, an expert oncologist at the Memorial Sloan Kettering Cancer Center, believes that cancer is such a devastating diagnosis with so many implications for treatment that it's perfectly reasonable to obtain a second opinion. And a second opinion for yourself or a loved one can be reassuring if it confirms your doctor's original diagnosis and treatment plan. You then know you've left no stone unturned. A second opinion can sometimes help you avoid being subjected to unnecessary tests, procedures, and even surgery. If the second opinion and treatment plan disagree with the initial ones, it's worthwhile to consider obtaining a third opinion.

It doesn't have to be something as serious as cancer to get a second opinion, and another opinion may be offered when you least expect it. When Mrs. Smith went to her doctor for a dark spot under her toenail, her physician took one look at it and said it was a fungus and prescribed Lamisil, which can have serious side effects. A week later, her pedicurist realized that the dark spot under her toenail was blood from a broken toenail, so medication was discontinued.

It's also worthwhile to obtain a second opinion when an older person is suspected of having Alzheimer's disease. It's important to carry out extensive blood tests and to consider special brain scans because 10-20 percent of older patients with progressive cognitive, intellectual impairment and behavioral changes typical of Alzheimer's disease may have potentially reversible medical problems, such as vitamin B12 or folate deficiency, thyroid disease, depression, autoimmune disorders, heavy metal abnormalities, and other medical problems that may mimic or contribute to what appears to be Alzheimer's disease. If these medical problems can be identified and treated, a patient's apparent cognitive impairment may improve. Although there are medications that can slow the progressive decline characteristic of Alzheimer's disease, there is currently no cure.

A neurologist colleague[111] actually encourages the family of patients with a presumptive diagnosis of Alzheimer's disease to obtain a second opinion to make certain that some potentially reversible and treatable medical problem is not contributing to the signs and symptoms of Alzheimer's disease.

When to Obtain a Second Opinion

The following includes just a few of the many reasons for getting a second opinion.

- You have what is believed to be a serious, life-threatening illness.

Dr. Jones discovered a small black lesion on his lower leg. He consulted his PCP who examined the area and reassured Dr. Jones that there was no cause for concern. No biopsy was performed. A month later, Dr. Jones sought a second opinion from a dermatologist, who recommended a biopsy. The lesion turned out to be a virulent form of melanoma. He had surgery two days later. Five years later there was no recurrence.

- Your illness is not improving.

Mr. Samuels, a seventy-eight-year-old retired construction worker with pain in his right knee, visited his elderly long-term physician. After examining the knee, his physician said, "You're old; it's expected that you'll have aches and pains." Mr. Samuels replied, "My left knee is seventy-eight years old and doesn't hurt. How do you explain that?" They mutually agreed to get a second opinion from an orthopedic surgeon who diagnosed and repaired a torn ligament, resulting in the return of the patient's normal, pain-free gait.

- A diagnosis is not forthcoming.

Mrs. Friedman, a sixty-five-year-old retired New York City journalist, was visiting friends in Florida when she experienced dizzy spells, fainting, and weakness. A physician at the local medical clinic diagnosed anemia and prescribed iron pills, but a simple test for gastrointestinal bleeding was not done. Her two sisters, who were doctors, insisted that Mrs. Friedman return immediately to New York. An emergency colonoscopy discovered an early-stage tumor of the colon, which was successfully surgically removed and alleviated the initial symptoms.

- Unresolvable communication problems exist between you and your doctor. Your doctor doesn't maintain eye contact with you and seems frustrated and distracted as he types your answers to his

111 Personal communication. Dr. Paul Walsky, Santa Fe, New Mexico.

139

questions into his computer during your appointment. Your complaints are not taken seriously. You sense a lack of concern about your welfare.

- Your doctor is not a specialist in the rare illness or condition you have [2].

Consider sarcoma, a rare cancer accounting for only one percent of all cancers affecting connective tissue such as muscle or bone. There are seventy diverse types, so it is essential that a patient see a sarcoma expert, according to Dr. Seth Pollack at the Fred Hutchinson Cancer Research Center, who has treated enough patients to know what works and doesn't work.[112]

- Your doctor tells you "there's nothing more that can be done," but you think otherwise.

Mr. Jones, father of two young children, was diagnosed with a fatal type of leukemia with an expected survival of less than a year. He experienced his doctor as cold and aloof, especially when the doctor suggested he consider donating his body to science so researchers could learn more about his disease. Mr. Samuels and his wife wanted a specialist with a better "personality" who might offer hope and save his life. He finally found a specialist, Dr. Smith, who "looked him in the eyes and whose voice conveyed kindness and hope." Dr. Smith provided treatment that sent Mr. Samuels into a seven-year remission.[113]

- Your intuition and/or your family urges you to seek a second opinion.
- Your doctor wants to refer you to a specialist. This is actually a good indication of your doctor's recognition of the importance of getting a second opinion and efforts to arrange it.
- The recommended treatment is very risky.
- The treatment recommended is experimental, such as a trial of a new drug or surgical technique.

Frequently Missed Illnesses/Conditions Discovered by a Second Opinion

Examples of frequently missed illnesses and conditions include depression, early signs of cognitive impairment (mild cognitive impairment), potentially reversible causes of memory impairment, osteoporosis (the initial sign may be a fracture), hypothyroidism and hyperthyroidism, sexually transmitted diseases (STDs), cancer, and type-2 (adult onset) diabetes.

---

112   https://www.fredhutch.org/en/news/center-news/2015/02/why-second-opinions-critical.html.
113   https://www.fredhutch.org/en/news/center-news/2015/02/why-second-opinions-critical.html.

Process of Obtaining a Second Opinion

Anytime you as a patient raise the issue of a second opinion, your doctor should welcome it, endorse it, and facilitate the process. It's very important to involve your PCPhys. in the process, especially if you want to continue under his/her care.

Everyone involved in the process of obtaining a second opinion needs to cooperate with one another. [3] Ask your doctor who he/she would see for a second opinion for the same problem and symptoms you have. Your PCPhys. can facilitate the referral by making certain that all your medical records, including pathology reports (if relevant) and other test results, are sent electronically or by overnight mail to the consultant. You'll need to sign a form permitting your doctor to release your records. This is yet another example of a transition period we've talked about throughout the book, when errors and omissions occur. Even though you assume that your PCPhys. has sent all your records to the consultant, there may be additional important information that is needed. For example, doctors and specialists you've seen in the past may have important information that your current PCPhys. does not have. So, prepare for your consultation for a second opinion by bringing, or sending in advance of your appointment, your personal health record (PHR), a detailed summary of your illness, the results of treatments tried, and a list of all current and previously tried medications, including over-the-counter medications and nutritional supplements.

Let's assume that your diagnosis is satisfactorily established, and you're interested in alternative treatments. The more knowledge you have about your illness, the more worthwhile a second opinion will be. Use the Internet to learn as much as possible about your medical condition and its treatment. Medical websites can provide the most up-to-date research and the names of researchers carrying out the latest clinical studies that pertain to your diagnosis and treatment. You can find the names of specialists involved in the latest research and the results of their research. The most reliable clinical studies involve large numbers of patients who have participated in well-designed studies carried out at academic medical centers. Research in the United States, Canada, and Western Europe, compared to that in other parts of the world, adhere to stricter, more reliable research standards.

The most useful, reliable Internet sites are those indicated by ".edu" (indicating an educational institution) or by ".gov" (indicating a U.S. government site) and ".org" sites (which are often not-for-profit organizations). But even for these websites, check to see that the information is current and the website identifies the source of the information (for example, studies carried out at acclaimed medical centers such as Johns Hopkins, Harvard, the Mayo Clinic, and Kaiser Permanente), and that the medical articles are published in peer-reviewed journals (submitted studies require approval by experts before acceptance for publication). *Please refer to the list of internet sites in Appendix I.*

Avoid websites with the designation ".com," which indicates a commercial site whose motivation is to sell you something. These companies may be promoting products touted by movie stars or athletes based on hyped-up testimonials claiming 100 percent success rates. Avoid "chat rooms," where laypersons offer strong but unscientific opinions.

Consider getting a second opinion from a specialist at a different institution than the one your PCPhys. is affiliated with. Like other types of institutions, medical centers gradually develop long-standing, accepted diagnostic and treatment approaches. For example, the chairman of a department may be an opinion leader at that institution, influencing other doctors to conform to a particular way of diagnosing and treating certain medical problems. But another institution, in another part of the country, may have a different diagnosis/treatment philosophy that may be more beneficial for you.

Getting a second opinion may not require an expensive cross-country trip to see a specialist because your medical records can be sent electronically to a medical expert. One online resource is Second Opinion Expert,[114]/[115] which enables you to upload your medical records and have them sent for review by a physician specialist. Academic medical centers such as the Cleveland Clinic,[116] the Mayo Clinic[117] and other prestigious centers offer patients online second opinions. For example, although the Cleveland Clinic's *MyConsult* doesn't accept insurance, a second opinion costs about $650, whereas a consultation including a pathology biopsy review costs $800. John Hopkins offers a remote medical opinion program in eleven states, mostly in the eastern part of the United States. Johns Hopkins physicians work directly with your doctor to make recommendations about your diagnosis and treatment options.[118]

If you live in a rural community far from an academic medical center, obtaining a second opinion is now easier using these websites, whereas being able to pay and travel to obtain treatment continues to be a major problem. For example, how does someone living on a farm and needing radiation treatment four times a week get treatment when the nearest radiology treatment facility is a four-hour drive away? Situations such as this require creative planning and determination.

Who Pays for a Second Opinion

Most insurance plans will cover the cost of a second opinion, especially if you see an in-network specialist. So, read your insurance policy or speak with a supervisor at your insurance company. If you obtain a verbal approval for a second opinion, request that the approval be put in writing in case payment is disputed later. Insurers in some states are required to pay for a second opinion. In California, for example, HMOs are required to pay the cost. Some insurers actually require you to get a second opinion before agreeing to pay for very expensive procedures, such as heart bypass surgery or a kidney or liver transplant.

---

114   http://www.latimes.com/business/la-fi-healthcare-watch-20150525-story.html or call 855-573-2663.
115   http://www.secondopinions.com.
116   http://www.clevelandclinic.org.
117   http://www.mayoclinic.org.
118   http://www.hopkinsmedicine.org/second_opinion/contact_us.html or call 410-464-6555.

The consultant you see in person or remotely for a second opinion may want to repeat tests you've already had or order some additional tests. If you don't want to be encumbered with "surprise" bills later on, ask the consultant's business office, and/or take the initiative to make certain that your insurance company will pay for part of the cost, and find out what amount will be your responsibility.

If you want to see an out-of-network expert for a second opinion, you may have to bear the cost. However, there might be circumstances when your insurer may pay – for example, if there are no in-network "experts" within a reasonable distance, or the in-network consultant is not a suitable fit (as was the case with Ms. Young, discussed at the beginning of this chapter). If you think that you have a credible argument to see an out-of-network expert, enlist the support of your PCPhys. to write a strong, convincing authorization request to your insurer that clearly explains the reason(s) for approving a second opinion from an out-of-network expert. If you want to subsequently receive treatment from the "out-of-network" consultant, it can be exceedingly expensive. Strategies to have your insurer pay for an out-of-network consultation and ongoing treatment are discussed in *Chapter 2*.

Should you and your PCPhys. encounter problems obtaining approval from your insurance company for a second opinion, consider enlisting assistance from the Patient Advocate Foundation,[119] a national organization that empowers patients to assume more control over their healthcare. The Foundation can help you with the appeals process if your insurer refuses to pay for a second opinion and associated tests. Since very few patients have the determination and fortitude to challenge their insurer's denial, initiating the appeal process (which includes gathering supportive letters from your specialist and PCPhys.) is taken seriously by your insurer and is often successful. If your insurer won't pay, you may have to bear the costs. But, if it's your life at stake, it's worth the investment.

---

119 www.patientadvocate.org.

Chapter 7 Appendix

Websites Providing Current Illness-Related Information and Research

www.uptodate.com - Up-to-date reference on medical conditions with excellent information from the scientific literature. Scroll to section "Benefits for Patients".

www.cdc.gov/ncidod/diseases - The Centers for Disease Control provide information about various infectious diseases.

www.cancer.gov - The National Cancer Institute provides information about types of cancer, including treatment, coping strategies, and current clinical research trials.

www.nia.nih.gov - The National Institute on Aging (NIA) provides valuable information on health and diseases associated with aging and how to seek enrollment in clinical research trials.

www.psych.org - The American Psychiatric Association (APA) site provides information about psychiatric disorders, district branches where you can obtain a listing of psychiatrists, and related topics.

See also: Mayoclinic.org, Johnshopkins.org, Clevelandclinic.org.

Chapter 7 Key Points

Key Points: The Value of a Second Opinion

- 30 percent of patients who obtain a second opinion discover a different diagnosis or better treatment plan.
- Surprisingly, only 20 percent of patients seek a second opinion

Key Points: Why Second Opinions Are Valuable

- 1-1.5 percent of biopsy reports are incorrect (if it's yours, it feels like 100 percent).
- Incorrect diagnosis can lead to undertreatment or unnecessary treatment.
- A second opinion that confirms the initial diagnosis and treatment plan is very reassuring.

Key Points: When to Consider a Second Opinion

- A diagnosis is not clearly established.
- Your doctor suggests a consultation (second opinion).
- Unresolvable communication problems between you and your doctor.

- The treatment recommended is risky or experimental.

Key Points: Process of Getting a Second Opinion

- Involve your PCPhys. or PCP.
- Prepare like the first visit to a new PCPhys. (bring your PHR, medications, etc.).

Key Points: Finding a Specialist

- Involve your PCPhys. to facilitate the referral.
- Some insurers pay for a second opinion.
- Use the Internet to find physician specialists involved in the latest research.
- Traveling to see a specialist may not be necessary. You can contact acclaimed medical centers to arrange a consultation via Skype or other means of communication.

References

1. Kumar, S., Nash, D. B., Demand Better! Revive Our Broken Healthcare System. Second River Healthcare Press, 2011.

2. Michelson, L.D., "How to find and interview the medical experts you need" in The Patient's Handbook. Alfred A. Knopf, New York, 2015 p. 107-139 and p. 175-197.

3. Nathan, D., The New Health Care System, Thomas Duane Books, 2010.

4. Roizen, M.F., Oz, M.C. You the Smart Patient, Free Press, 2006, pgs. 223-257.

Part 3

Navigating Specific Healthcare Treatments

CHAPTER 8

Strategies for a Successful Hospital Stay

Myrna was born with a defective heart valve. Now in her mid-fifties, she had shortness of breath, extreme fatigue, and heart murmurs due to the faulty valve, and had to avoid strenuous activity. Her symptoms, which mimicked those of congestive heart failure, forced her to face the reality of her own mortality. She scheduled an appointment with her PCPhys. to get his opinion, and then saw her longtime cardiologist. After she described the worsening symptoms, it became clear that it was time to fix or replace the valve. It wasn't difficult to see that the benefits of undergoing open-heart surgery far outweighed the risks, and the procedure was scheduled for the following month. Myrna had ample time to make the necessary preparations to ensure that her hospital stay and return home would go smoothly.

Let's face it. The prospect of being in the hospital for any amount of time is terrifying. We have all heard stories at one time or another of a hospital stay gone terribly wrong, or, at the very least, we've seen it in the movies or on TV. This chapter outlines the steps to take to help ensure a successful, problem-free hospitalization.

A hospital stay can evoke profound, unwelcome feelings of dependency and helplessness. You may be in a weakened, susceptible state to begin with, and your anxiety level may be high. Stripped away is your sense of self—who you are as a person, reinforced by familiarity with your surroundings at home, the comforting security of friends and family, and the sense of having control over your life.

When you enter the hospital, you are expected to conform to a new, strange, and potentially bewildering environment. A hospital gown is substituted for your clothes. You are expected to be passive and compliant with recommended tests and treatments. Meals and the scheduling of tests, procedures, and doctor's appointments are out of your control. Your sense of time becomes distorted as each day blends into the next and even seemingly insignificant events become the major occasions of a day. You may feel dependent on a system that is far from perfect. It's unsettling to know that about 1.7 million Americans become infected in hospitals each year, and about 99,000 of them (close to 6 percent) die from those hospital-acquired infections [1]. What can you do to make your hospital stay safe and successful? Read on for advice on how to prepare before your hospital stay, what actions to take during your stay to secure the best care possible while avoiding hospital risks, and how to prepare for a safe, seamless return home.

Preparing for Your Stay in the Hospital

A week prior to Myrna's surgery, she scheduled a conference call between herself and the key medical personnel who would be involved in her surgery and subsequent care: her PCPhys., cardiologist, and cardiac surgeon. The goal of the call was to have everyone connect and get everyone on the same page. After a bit of discussion, everyone agreed that the cardiac surgeon would be the "captain" of her healthcare team while she was hospitalized since, out of the three of them, he was the only one on staff there. The cardiologist and PCPhys. would be in close contact with the surgeon. Once she was discharged, her PCPhys. would resume the role of lead physician with the cardiologist available for consultation and follow-up appointments. Myrna requested a free exchange of information between her three doctors. They assured her they would be in close contact. They also confirmed that all her medical records had been transferred from her PCPhys. to her cardiologist.

Myrna assembled her own personal team, consisting of her husband, Wayne, their nineteen-year-old son, Corey, and Laura, her best friend. Even though Wayne did not have a medical or nursing background, he was reliable and organized and able to remain calm and rational in a crisis. Myrna designated him as her patient advocate. He had her important medical documents— personal health record (PHR), healthcare advance directive, medical and financial proxy—and her list of medications and insurance cards. He was also appointed the "medical communicator" who would be the one to talk to the doctors and other medical staff on Myrna's behalf, and the main person to ask questions. This was to prevent the doctors from being inundated with questions from multiple people. Laura offered to be the "personal communicator" to keep friends and family informed about her progress and respond to their requests for updates. She planned to use the **Caring Bridge** website (**https://www.caringbridge.org/**) as a convenient and cost-free way to electronically keep everyone posted on Myrna's recovery in the hospital and also her status when she returned home to continue her recuperation. This would allow Myrna to focus her energy on her recovery. Her son would be a permanent fixture by her side at all times and keep a watchful eye on the staff as they came and went, making sure that hands were washed and medical instruments, such as stethoscopes, were cleaned prior to touching his mother. The family also devised a contingency plan should the unlikely event occur that one of them became unavailable. The roles of "medical communicator" and "personal communicator" would be exchanged between Wayne and Laura, and Corey would assume the role of "personal communicator." They would enlist the help of their family friend Sylvia to step in and fill Corey's position as the watchdog.

The evening before being admitted to the hospital, Myrna removed her jewelry, selected a framed photo for her hospital room bedside, and packed a small suitcase with some toiletries, cell phone and charger, reading material, and a change of clothes.

As emphasized in the previous chapter, it's important to choose the hospital that is best for you, and accredited by the JCAHO (Joint Commission on the Accreditation of Healthcare Organizations). It's important to determine who will be the captain of your healthcare team while you're in the hospital—whether it will be your PCPhys., a specialist (for example, a surgeon as in Myrna's case), or a hospital-employed physician (hospitalist). In medium to large cities, the trend is to have hospitalists oversee a patient's care while in the hospital. Hospitalists are physicians, most often internists, specializing in the field of hospital medicine. They have expertise in handling the acute clinical and complicated medical problems associated with hospitalized patients. In any case, during a hospital stay, it is more likely than not that the doctor with whom you are most familiar, your PCPhys., will not be overseeing your care.

Your close family members, patient advocate, and all the healthcare professionals involved in your care should be on the same page. Do not assume that your hospital "captain" will automatically be in contact with your PCPhys. It is important to convey that you would like communication to be open between the key members of your medical team and to give your permission for your medical information to be shared among them. You can reinforce this by periodically asking "How will you communicate this with my PCPhys.?" It is particularly critical for the hospitalist to keep your PCPhys. informed, before discharge from the hospital.

There are several other preparatory steps to take. Make sure to find out if you will require post-hospital rehabilitation or a stay at a skilled nursing facility, and make certain that all facilities and services are in network so they will be covered by your insurance. It is also important to find out if the health providers (such as the radiologist) at the facility are in network. Just because a facility is covered does not guarantee that those working there are too. Figuring out these details ahead of time will help you avoid large, unexpected medical bills. If you have not already, choose your patient advocate prior to being admitted. This person does not necessarily have to have a medical background but rather, like Myrna's husband, be reliable, organized, and able to remain calm in a crisis.

Take some time to decide who, out of your circle of family and friends, you would like to tell about your upcoming hospitalization and how detailed you want to be about your medical problem. Everyone differs in how they feel about sharing personal information—in particular that of a medical nature. So, take some time to consider who you want to tell. Also take into account the possible aftermath from not telling certain individuals were they to find out after the fact. It is also important to consider if anybody *should* be informed irrespective of whether they would be on your "want to tell" list, such as your employer, co-workers, or business associates.

Once you've made those decisions, notify people on your **Caring Bridge** website list as to where you are going and when, and if you will be accepting visitors. People will want to help and will ask what they can do. You can respond by asking that they show their appreciation to the medical staff for the care they are providing you. It is important to request that anyone who is sick, or even slightly "under the weather," refrain from visiting, and try to limit the number of daily visitors to a minimum so you can focus your energy on getting well. You may want to appoint someone to act as your "personal communicator" who will keep family and friends informed of your progress and field their questions, as Myrna did by appointing her friend Laura to fill this role. Let others know who the designated communicator is, how to reach that person for updates, or how to be added to an email list to stay informed of your progress. While you are trying to recuperate, responding to people's inquiries can quickly become an overwhelming and exhausting task.

Paths to the Best Care Possible

Immediately following her open-heart surgery, Myrna was taken to the intensive care unit (ICU), as is customary. Her son and husband were by her side anytime they were permitted. Her husband assumed the role as "medical communicator" and spoke with the surgeon, cardiologist, and other staff, asking questions and taking notes. Meanwhile, her son, Corey remained at her side, keeping a watchful eye on the staff as they came and went, making sure they washed their hands and changed his mother's sheets and pillowcases. Corey and his father covered for each other whenever one of them went outside to make a call or left to use the restroom.

After two days in ICU, she was transferred to the cardiac unit within the main hospital. One day later, she was transferred to a regular hospital room. During each transition, both her son and husband were hypervigilant, making sure they knew what was happening at every step along the way. They heard that errors frequently occur during periods of transition.

Once in her regular hospital room, Myrna placed the framed family photograph next to her bedside along with a bottle of hand sanitizer. She introduced herself and her husband and son by name to all the staff and made sure to ask their names in return so she could address them with a certain familiarity when she saw them next. As friends and family started to contact Laura requesting updates, she assumed her responsibility as "personal communicator." Even to Laura, who was not recovering from surgery, it soon became overwhelming and tiresome answering the same questions over and over and providing progress updates. She wanted to see if emailing an update via the **Caring Bridge** website periodically to a group of friends and family would relieve her, and it did. From then on, she sent two updates a day summarizing Myrna's progress.

Do whatever you can to have your healthcare providers see you as a real person rather than a diagnosis. Follow Myrna's lead and have a picture of you and your loved ones by your bedside. You also need to strike a fine balance between being the consummate diplomat and a hypervigilant sleuth by avoiding being perceived by hospital staff members—who are dedicated to helping you—as cantankerous, mistrustful, and irritable.

Early in your hospital stay, introduce your patient advocate as an active member of your medical team, and explain the role he/she will assume. Doing this may improve the care you receive and result in a shorter, safer stay in the hospital [2]. Since your advocate will likely be your choice to be the "medical communicator," it is especially important that introductions are made early on and communication channels are open so that the staff feels comfortable speaking with your appointed medical communicator/advocate and vice versa.

Early after admission, try to identify and forge a relationship with a hospital "troubleshooter" whom you and your advocate can turn to when something is confusing or just simply not going right. It can be the supervising nurse or even a friendly, experienced nurse's aide who knows the complex inner workings of the hospital system [3].

Diplomacy is the better part of valor. Most complaints stem from misunderstandings or miscommunications and can be resolved simply and directly with the particular staff member before taking up the issue with someone at a higher level, such as the head nurse or your doctor. It would be reasonable to complain if the nurse doesn't respond within a reasonable time if your intravenous line, which provides you with fluids and sometimes medication, becomes infiltrated, causing swelling and discomfort in your arm. Another cause for complaint would be if staff members, after being asked repeatedly, do not wash their hands.

Consider directing nursing complaints to the senior "charge" nurse on your unit. If your complaints are about your clinical care from medical staff, such as an intern or a resident, speak with your lead doctor. If your complaints concern treatment plans or complications, and your principal doctor has not addressed them satisfactorily, ask the doctor if it would be okay to get a second opinion and even who he might recommend. While you don't need his "permission" to get a second opinion, this approach conveys respect and emphasizes the seriousness of the issues and/or questions you have.

If your complaint is not tended to at these levels and you are in a JCAHO-accredited hospital, you can call at 630-792-5800 or file a complaint online at https://www.jointcommission.org. Note that the Joint Commission cannot help you if you have a billing or an insurance dispute or an interpersonal complaint about a particular staff member. This is a sort of "nuclear option" and should be carefully considered after all other avenues have proven unsuccessful.

Your hospital doctor and assistants will have brief visits with you, so it is important to be prepared in advance to make the visit as productive for you as possible. Keeping an ongoing list of questions that arise between visits will not only make efficient use of the time and engage the doctor, but will also demonstrate that you are an inquisitive, knowledgeable, and active member of the team. If your doctor seems overly occupied with inputting information into a handheld computer, or seems otherwise rushed, invite him or her to sit down and have a conversation. If that is not possible, an assistant will likely take the time to sit with you. If you don't understand the rapid-fire delivery of medical jargon, politely ask him/her to slow down and explain things more simply while your advocate is taking notes.

If your principal hospital doctor (hospitalist) is a locum tenens (temporary, often from another city) physician nearing the end of his/her contract, you and your advocate should become as knowledgeable as possible about your current medical status. Even though the departing hospitalist will communicate all pertinent information to the new one, it never hurts to ask directly that this be done.

Avoiding the Risks of Hospitalization

As people started to stop by to visit Myrna, Laura made a point to greet everyone at the door and politely asked how they were feeling as she offered them hand sanitizer. A few people decided not to enter because they were feeling a bit "off" and it wasn't worth the risk of exposing Myrna to a potential infection.

Avoiding Infections

One of the gravest risks of hospitalization, especially with long hospital stays, is the threat of contracting a hospital-acquired infection. Being ill and elderly can reduce the body's natural immune defenses, making a person more vulnerable to a hospital-acquired infection that can significantly complicate and prolong one's hospital stay.

An important way to safeguard against a hospital-acquired infection is by choosing a JCAHO-accredited hospital that has passed rigorous tests, including inspections for cleanliness and sterile techniques. Safe hospitals have a multitude of sinks, soap, and hand-cleaning dispensers outside patient rooms, at the entryway to the hospital, and at the elevators.

Another safeguard is for you, the patient, to frequently wash your hands and make certain that physicians, nurses, other hospital personnel, and visitors do the same. Doctors' instruments, such as stethoscopes, should be cleaned before and after contact with you. Don't feel that you are insulting staff and visitors by offering reminders. You can simply say (or post a little sign) that your doctors and nurses have instructed you to remind everyone to thoroughly wash their hands for "the safety of all." Myrna's son, Corey assumed the task of communicating this. Hand washing needs to be vigorous, lasting at least fifteen seconds with soap and warm water or an alcohol sanitizing gel. Antibacterial gel is actually discouraged because it has been proven to be no more effective than soap and may lead to antibiotic-resistant bacteria strains.

Other safeguards that reduce the risk of infection include: [4]

- Keeping a supply of alcohol sanitizing gel near your bedside. Encourage its use.

- Washing your hands especially well before going to bed and after visits to the bathroom. Avoid touching the toilet lever, seat, and faucet handles unless you, or someone, disinfects them first with alcohol gel.

- Avoiding touching any surgical wound or intravenous site.

- Making sure your wound dressing, drainage tubes, and catheter sites are dry. Alert your nurse if they become loose or wet.

- All catheters—those supplying fluids and medications, draining fluids (bladder or surgical sites), or used for drawing blood—should all be antiseptically coated. Ask the nurses if they are.

- Discouraging visits from anyone who is ill or "under the weather." If your immune system is compromised, visitors may be required to wear a mask, hospital gown, and shoe coverings.

- If your surgical wound is healing, ask the doctors, "How does my wound look today?" Don't accept the common misperception that "the best way to hide something from a hospital doctor is to put it under a bandage." If necessary, ask your doctor if it would be wise to remove the bandage so the wound can be regularly examined.

- Avoiding touching the TV remote, your handheld device, or cell phone without wiping them down with sanitizing gel, as these are among the most germ-laden items in the hospital.

- Making sure your sheets and pillowcases are changed daily.

Avoiding Medication and Other Errors

On average, one mistake is made per day per patient in most hospital settings, and many of the mistakes involve errors with medications. Even though hospitals have adopted effective protocols to reduce the risk for errors, be inquisitive and hyperalert to avoid medication errors and other common mistakes [5].

Medicare has implemented a financial reward and penalty system as an incentive for hospitals to keep infections to a minimum and the rate of medication and other errors low. Medicare provides greater financial compensation to hospitals that meet these standards, while hospitals failing to meet the mark are penalized in the form of lower payments. There has been a shift in the system of financial rewards given to hospitals from those based on the quantity of procedures performed to the quality of care provided.

For example, your hospital wristband serves as a reference and an important check point for the medical staff. Your full name, date of birth, and drug allergies should be clearly visible on the band. There are also bar codes that correspond to the medications given to you, and any drug allergies that you have should be clearly visible. Typically, before being given a drug, staff will confirm that you are the correct person by asking your full name and your date of birth and will scan your wristband. If the staff member has not confirmed your identity, politely ask him/her to check that you are the correct patient. Also, periodically ask your nurse or doctor for a copy of your most current medication record so you are familiar with medication names and dosages. These safeguards will help you (and the staff) avoid unfortunate mistakes.

If you are being transferred to another area of the hospital or taken for a test or procedure, ask where you are going and why. You should know the purpose of all procedures or tests. If it is unclear to you, simply ask. You have the right to refuse any tests or procedures. In fact, the law requires that the benefits and potential risks be explained to you and you have a clear understanding of them before signing consent forms.

Know that the majority of medically related errors occurs during transition periods, such as shift changes, transfers to other areas of the hospital, or during times when the hospital is understaffed, such as holidays and weekends [6]. During these transitions, try to have a knowledgeable family member or your advocate present. During a shift change, for example, he or she can ask the nurse, "You're changing shift now; what important things do you want me and the new nurse to know?"

As you near the end of your hospital stay, you may be transferred to a specialized unit within the same hospital for rehabilitation or other services, or to a different facility. Either can be another unsettling transition. You need to mentally prepare yourself for the understandable stress of moving to another environment, which may feel like being deported to yet another strange country without a passport or map.

Preparing for a Safe Return Home

Myrna was recovering rapidly from her open-heart surgery and she was feeling pretty good, all things considered. However, it seemed quite sudden and frightening when, only four days after her surgery, she was told that she would be discharged later that day. She and her family were surprised that it was all happening so fast. Even though Myrna was feeling okay and eager to get home, she didn't feel ready or strong enough, both mentally and physically, to go home just yet. She and her family conferenced and agreed on a plan to try to extend her stay for a few additional days. Her husband called her surgeon and cardiologist and explained everyone's concerns. The two doctors listened intently, understood her apprehension, and agreed that it could be beneficial for her to stay a little longer as long as her insurance company agreed. The surgeon's assistant called her insurance company, and authorization was received to extend her stay for one additional day instead of two. Myrna never thought she would feel as happy as she did to have a longer hospital stay, until she realized that the additional day allowed her to begin physical therapy within the safety of the hospital environment and gave her more time to mentally prepare for the transition home. Before Myrna was discharged, the discharge coordinator, with the family's help, had arranged for home visits from a nurse and physical therapist, both of whom were in network and covered by her insurance. Follow-up appointments with the surgeon, cardiologist, and her PCPhys. were already scheduled. Once Myrna returned to the familiarity of her own home, she was able to relax and recuperate.

Preparing for your return home is as important as preparing for your admission to the hospital, and sometimes requires even greater planning. Because about 20 percent of hospital patients who have undergone major procedures, such as surgery, suffer a significant complication after returning home, you and your advocate need to be especially conscientious during this time.

Pressure on hospitals from insurance companies to control costs and reduce risks from lengthy hospital stays has led to shorter and shorter hospitalizations. Despite your strong desire to return home, if you or your advocate do not feel you are ready, you can ask your doctor to extend your stay. If that proves unsuccessful, don't be discouraged. Be proactive and ask to speak with the hospital's customer service representative. If your concerns are still not being addressed, ask to speak to the chief of clinical service or chief of surgery where you are a patient. You could even call your insurance company to explain your reasons and see what advice they might offer about approving additional days in the hospital. Understand that they will need direct contact with your attending physician before granting approval.

You don't want to be taken by surprise, as Myrna was, by how quickly you are discharged. Make as many preparations as possible before even being admitted to the hospital. Once in the hospital, it may become clearer what additional care you may require, so begin thinking and planning as soon as you know. In the days preceding your return home, keep a list of things that still need to be arranged before discharge. For example, maybe you'll need to set up a bedroom on the first floor of your home, or need special equipment, or you and your healthcare team decide that you will benefit from home services, such as a nurse and/or physical therapist. Ask your physician, social worker, or discharge coordinator to arrange this with a home visiting agency, preferably one accredited by the JCAHO. All of this takes time to arrange, so start the process as early as you can. Before leaving the hospital, find out who you should contact if you have questions or problems related to your discharge, such as your medications and other issues (pain, bleeding).

Before returning home, review the discharge plan with both the in-hospital physician (hospitalist) and, if possible, with your regular physician (usually your PCPhys.) who will resume overseeing your care. Everyone should be on the same page about who your principal doctor will be once you leave the hospital. Don't assume you are supposed to follow the same medication regimes as before. Make sure you are clear about which medications to continue taking and any adjustments to make to incorporate new medications. Sign all the necessary permission forms for your hospital records to be sent immediately to your PCPhys. and all other health providers. Request your own copy, or confirm it will be on your Patient Portal to print out at home, and bring it to your follow-up appointment in case your physician(s) haven't received it in time (a common problem), and be sure to add a copy to your PHR (*see Chapter 1*). Taking all these steps has been shown to help reduce potentially preventable re-admissions by 30 percent [7].

The following are some additional questions worth asking prior to discharge, if appropriate:

- What complications should I watch for and what should I do if they occur?
- What special care is required for my surgical wound and dressings?
- Which of my usual activities should be limited and, if so, when can I return to my normal activity level?
- Should I follow a special diet? What about alcohol intake?
- When may I resume driving?
- What about sexual activity?

Do not be in a rush to pay your bills until you have carefully scrutinized them for errors. Do not be surprised if there is a $20 or higher charge for an aspirin tablet, as ridiculous as it may seem. Hospitals have to figure in all the costs associated with an order for aspirin, such as pharmacy, nursing, and administration costs. The amounts billed by the hospital and doctors to your insurance company can be two or more times higher than the contracted or "approved" amount agreed upon by your insurance company, the hospital, and doctors. Depending on your particular insurance policy, up to 80 percent of the approved amount could be paid by your primary insurer after your yearly deductible has been met. If you have a supplemental insurance policy, the remaining balance may be paid by that policy, leaving you with minimal out of pocket expenses. Allow sufficient time for the hospital and your doctors to collect the maximum payment they are entitled to from your insurers before you pay your portion. Some hospital billing departments are more efficient than others, and you want them to be as conscientious and assertive as possible with insurers before you pay what is your responsibility.

If you are still recuperating when you receive the bills for the portion you owe, wait until you have sufficiently recovered before reviewing them. Some bills are so difficult to understand that you may need to meet with a knowledgeable official in the hospital and/or doctor's billing department. You may even consider enlisting the help of your accountant. If you are struggling with an outstanding balance, hospitals and doctors are often willing to work out a payment plan with you directly rather than use a collection agency or lose out on payment altogether. Another option is to hire a private company that specializes in negotiating with your providers a reduction in the amount you owe. (*see Chapter 2 for additional suggestions*).

Chapter 8 Key Points

Key Points: Preparing for a Safe Hospital Stay

- Make clear who is the "captain" of your healthcare team while in hospital.
- All your important medical records need to go to the doctor in charge during your hospital stay.
- Bring to the hospital all insurance cards, your PHR, healthcare documents, cell phone, family photo, toiletries, etc.
- Have a family member and/or patient advocate ("guardian-angel") assist you.

Key Points: Paths to Best Care Possible

- Keep an ongoing list of questions to ask during brief doctor visits.
- Have staff see you as a person rather than a diagnosis. During times of transition, you and your advocate remain hypervigilant to avoid errors.
- If you anticipate being transferred to another facility for rehabilitation or other purposes, make sure that facility and all its providers are in network to avoid "surprise" bills.

Key Points: Avoiding Risks of Hospitalization

- Have sanitizing gel nearby; wash your hands frequently and have others do the same.
- Discourage visitors who have a head cold or are feeling "under the weather."
- Prior to being given medication, undergoing a procedure, or being transferred, make sure the staff asks you to identify yourself to confirm that you are the correct patient.
- Fully understand the purpose of medications, infusions, procedures, or tests.

Key Points: Preparing for a Safe Return Home

- Make as many preparations as possible ahead of time, and get authorization from your insurance company should you need home services, rehabilitation services, or a stay at a skilled nursing facility.
- Be prepared to return home sooner than you anticipate. Work with your discharge coordinator to have all necessary equipment and personnel lined up prior to being discharged.
- Obtain copies of all hospital records (or at least a summary) prior to discharge so you can share them at your follow-up doctor appointments. Request that your records be sent to health professionals ASAP. Add a copy to your PHR.
- Wait until your insurer(s) have paid their maximum before making payments on the amount you owe.

- If you are having financial problems, work out a payment plan with the doctor or hospital. Consider a private billing company that specializes negotiating a reduction of your bill.

References

1. Centers for Disease Control and Prevention. (2016, May 27). *Healthcare-associated Infections.* Retrieved from https://www.cdc.gov/hai/

2. Torrey, T. (2017, March 24). *Who Provides Patient and Health Advocacy? Patient Advocacy from Top to Bottom – Organizations to Individual Advocates.* Retrieved from http://patients.about.com/od/caringforother-patients/a/patadvocacy.htm?utm_term=Patient%20Safety%20in%20Hospitals&utm_content=p1-main-3-title&utm_me...

3. Editors of Consumer Reports. (2015, March 8). *Consumer Reports: Path to the best possible hospital care.* Retrieved from http://www.post-gazette.com/business/money/2015/03/08/Consumer-Reports-Path-to-the-best-possible-hospital-care/stories/201503050202

4. National Center for Emerging and Zoonotic Infectious Diseases. (2017, March 13). *Getting Medical Care? How to Avoid Getting an Infection.* Retrieved from https://www.cdc.gov/features/patientsafety

5. Eustice, C. (2016, April 1). *How You Can Avoid Medication Errors.* Retrieved from https://www.verywell.com/how-to-avoid-medication-errors-188068

6. 14 worst hospital mistakes to avoid. (2012, June 25). Retrieved from http://www.nbcnews.com/id/47954577/ns/health-health_care/t/worst-hospital-mistakes-avoid/#.W5SUzOhKiUk

7. Henry, J. (2016, June 30). *7 tips for improving patient safety in hospitals.* Retrieved from http://www.healthcaredive.com/news/7-tips-for-improving-patient-safety-in-hospitals/421712/

CHAPTER 9

Preparing for Surgery – Before and After

Promote a Successful Outcome

Joe Kramer, a former semi-professional baseball player, was eighty years old when his orthopedist recommended surgery to replace with prostheses his two painful osteoarthritic knees, which interfered with his walking and tennis. His doctor suggested he look into a new clinical study at a prestigious New York City medical center that compared complication rates, time to recover, patient satisfaction, and other variables for patients having simultaneous knee replacements with those having one knee replacement and followed a month later by the second knee operation. All study participants received thorough pre-and post-surgery evaluations. Surgery was performed by experienced board-certified surgeons, and participants incurred no out-of-pocket expenses.

Given his lifelong scientific curiosity and cautious decision-making, Mr. Kramer studied the informed consent documents, the results of previous studies via www.clinicaltrials.gov, and spoke with two orthopedic surgeons knowledgeable about the study. In other words, he did his homework. In preparing for surgery, he closely followed the recommended weight reduction diet and exercise program for two months prior to, and four months after the simultaneous knee surgeries. Two months following surgery, he was back playing tennis and was complimented on his agility.

Preparing for Surgery

If you wanted to compete in the Senior Olympics or a triathlon, you know you would need months of special exercise, diet, and coaching. Likewise, preparing for elective surgery (planned in advance rather than in an emergency) similarly requires careful preparation to ensure the best possible outcome.[5].

Your surgeon, anesthesiologist, and other members of your surgical team know their best ally for a successful outcome is a knowledgeable, conscientious, cooperative patient who is comfortable and adept at asking questions.

Promoting a good outcome also includes that you and, if needed, your patient advocate, be especially observant for hospital and medical staff errors that can occur during the many transitions along the way – transfer of care from your PCPhys. to the surgeon; transfer of all your medical information to the hospital; nursing shift changes; possible transfer from surgical unit to a medical or rehabilitation unit at the same or different hospital; and transition home.

Ensuring that you have the best outcome involves searching for the best surgeon for your particular problem, selecting the best hospital, getting in the best physical, medical and emotional state, enlisting services of a "patient advocate," preparing for your pre-surgery visit with your surgeon and anesthesiologist, and planning a safe transition home. We'll be focusing on elective surgery that's planned in advance, allowing ample time for pre-surgery physical, laboratory and other evaluations, discussion with the surgeon, anesthesiologist, and other specialist as needed, and choosing the day and time for surgery.

Choosing the Best Surgeon

You want a very well trained, experienced, board-certified surgeon specialized in the operation that you are having, especially if it's a technically difficult procedure such as heart surgery. One indication of the surgeon's accomplishments is his/her being a fellow of the American College of Surgeons, as indicated by the letters FACS after his/her name. Keep in mind that you're unlikely to have a long-term, ongoing relationship with the surgeon, so bedside manner is of less importance than his/her technical skill. As an analogy, you want a car mechanic who can fix your transmission correctly the first time; his or her interpersonal manner is less important.

Finding an excellent surgeon is similar to finding the best specialist for a complicated medical problem. The search begins by asking your PCPhys. for recommendations, but you'll need to do your own investigative work to determine if he/she is the best surgeon for your particular operation, as illustrated by the following real-life story.

When John P. was sixty-four years old, he learned that he had coronary artery disease and needed cardiac bypass surgery. Fortunately, he knew the best cardiac surgeons at a nearby academic medical institution. His investigative talents led him to find not only the best heart surgeon but also the one most experienced in bypassing his two arteries that required surgery. He was calm and confident about his upcoming surgery, from which he recovered quickly.

Finding one of the best surgeons sometimes calls for an Internet search. To find the names of fellows of the American College of Surgeons (ACS) who specialize in the surgery you require, visit **www.facs.org** or call 800-621-4111.

If you have a managed care insurance plan that has in-network contracted surgeons, contact your managed care insurance company for a list of their surgeons. Then you can google their names to obtain information about their credentials and experience to help you in the selection process. If you chose an out-of-network surgeon, your insurance company is unlikely to pay the costs (see *Chapter 2 – Strategies for Keeping Costs Down*). Another way of obtaining additional opinions is by talking with a surgical nurse or an anesthesiologist at the hospital where you are contemplating surgery and asking what surgeon they would choose were they to need your particular surgery. It's helpful to mention the name of a doctor or other health professional you know who works at the hospital.

If you want to find one of the very best surgeons in the country involved in the most advanced "cutting-edge" technique in the surgery specific to your condition, go to **www.pubmed.gov**. After entering the name of the particular surgical technique (such as cardiac bypass surgery), make note of the surgeons who are authors of recent scientific papers. These are likely to be among the most experienced researchers and practicing surgeons. While carrying out this search, you may learn of some recent surgical techniques that are less invasive and have better outcomes than previous approaches [4].

Keep in mind that a "new" surgical technique doesn't necessarily mean "better." Getting a second opinion may help you feel more secure in your final decision. Share what you've learned with your PCPhys. and ask his/her opinion about obtaining a consultation regarding your problem that requires surgery. If your family, work, financial, and other responsibilities permit, consider traveling for an appointment to the city where the consultant surgeon practices. You can also obtain a consultation with a prospective surgeon who is in a distant city via telemedicine by making an appointment where he/she practices and sending all the medical records requested (see *Chapter 7, A Second Opinion Can Save Your Life*).

Choosing the Best Hospital

If the surgeon you have selected operates at only one or two hospitals, that's where you'll have your operation. The quality of the hospital is as important as the surgeon, so you want a Joint Commission (JCAHO) accredited hospital. Top surgeons only do surgery at JCAHO-accredited hospitals.

If you want reassurance that you'll be treated at a high-quality hospital, go to **www.JCAHO.org** and enter the name of the hospital to see if it is accredited. This indicates that the hospital has complied with the Joint Commission National Patient Safety goals and other standards required to maintain accreditation.

If the operation is complicated, selecting a large teaching hospital assures you of very experienced nursing, rehabilitation (if required) and other professional medical care that can effectively deal with postoperative complications, which can sometimes be more of a problem than the actual surgery. Studies have shown that patients have better outcomes if they have a specific type of surgery at a hospital and with a surgeon that has carried out a great number of such surgeries.

Get in the Best Physical, Medical, and Emotional Shape as Possible

Get advice from your PCPhys. and surgeon or their assistants. If you're not currently in an exercise program, after getting medical advice, start slowly at a nearby gym, and take walks or hikes in order to build up your stamina. Reducing or eliminating smoking, alcohol, and recreational drugs is obviously beneficial. If you are overweight and preparing for, let's say, abdominal surgery, working with a dietitian to lose weight will likewise improve your chances of a successful surgical outcome.

Have your PCPhys. or PCP get existing medical problems under the best control possible. For example, if you are diabetic, getting your blood sugar under good control before surgery will lessen chances for complications because the physical and mental stress of surgery can cause marked fluctuations of blood sugar.

The stress of daily life compounded with nervousness about an upcoming surgery can compromise your immune system, interfere with post-surgery healing, and increase post-operative pain. Although not for everyone, meditation, yoga, relaxation techniques, and guided imagery all serve to reduce anxiety.[120]

Ask your surgeon about banking your own blood at the hospital's blood bank if you plan on undergoing surgery that may require transfusions. Even though the chance of contracting HIV/AIDS or hepatitis from a blood donor is now very unlikely, a transfusion from an unknown donor still carries the risk of contracting other pathogens. So, it's safer to have several pints of your own blood available. If you set aside several units of your own blood at the hospital's blood bank in preparation for your elective surgery, it can take weeks for your body to replenish the blood cells, so discuss and plan for this with your doctor months in advance of your surgery.[121]

Rational Use of Vitamins/Supplements Before and After Surgery

Your body uses about thirteen vitamins to help keep you healthy. A balanced diet supplies most, if not all, of these vitamins and your body manufactures the others.

120 https://integrativeoncology-essentials.com/2014/02/optimize-your-body-and-mind-before-surgery/
121 https://www.drdavidwilliams.com/fast-surgery-recovery.

It's important to inform your PCPhys. and surgeon not only about all the prescription medications you are taking (and drug allergies), but also if you are taking vitamin/mineral/herbal supplements, probiotics, and fiber because some of these can affect your heart rate, blood pressure, blood clotting, and bleeding. For example, high doses of vitamin E can interfere with blood clotting, especially if you are also taking an anticoagulant medication such as warfarin (also known as Coumadin).[122]

Vitamin C is used by the body to build and repair skin and bone. Some heart surgeons recommend taking additional daily amounts in preparation for heart surgery. But extra vitamin C is not recommended if you are having gastric (stomach) bypass surgery for weight reduction because it can contribute to the development of kidney stones after surgery.

Probiotics and fiber may be beneficial weeks before and months after surgery, especially abdominal surgery or liver transplant surgery, because they may reduce the risk of post-surgical infections, decrease the need for antibiotics, improve bowel function, and protect against the serious and sometimes fatal hospital and nursing home acquired C. difficile infection (causes profuse diarrhea). So be sure to obtain advice about taking vitamins and supplements from your surgeon and PCPhys.[123] (see *Chapter 13 – Alternative (Complementary) Treatments: East Meets West*).

Consider Enlisting the Assistance of a Patient Advocate

Having a family member, friend, or a professional patient advocate serve as your "guardian angel" can be especially valuable, particularly during the first days of hospitalization when medication, nursing, and other errors (especially during periods of transition) are all too common (see *Chapter 12, Rights You Have as a Patient – Benefits of a Patient Advocate*).

Pre-Surgery Office Visit with Your Surgeon and Anesthesiologist

Not too many years ago, a patient was usually hospitalized a day before elective surgery. However, with shortened hospital stays and pre-operative tests done on an out-patient basis, patients are commonly admitted the day of surgery. Before your surgery, expect to see the surgeon and the anesthesiologist.

---

122   Veach, M., Vitamins to avoid before surgery. Livingstrong.com, Sept. 17, 2011.
123   http://drhoffman.com/article/supplements-and-surgery-what-you-need-to-know-part-2/.

Before seeing them, write down questions you and your family would like answers to. The principal surgeon and anesthesiologist may not have the time to answer all your questions, but members of their team will. The following are the types of questions to ask. Your family or advocate may think of others.

- What are the risks and benefits of having this surgery?

- Are there alternative treatments for my condition other than surgery?

- Are there newer ways to perform the surgery that are less invasive?

- What can I do to best prepare for surgery?

- Which of my medicines, supplements, and herbal products should I take on the days, weeks, and the evening before surgery?

- How long might I need to stay in the hospital after the surgery?

- What kinds of complications are most frequent, and what is done to treat them?

- What kind of anesthesia will be best for me, and are there alternatives that entail less risk?

- How soon after surgery can I get out of bed, walk around, drive, and return to work?

- How much pain may I expect after surgery, and what painkillers will I receive?

- Will I need physical rehabilitation treatment after surgery? If so, can it be in the same hospital, another hospital, or at home? Who arranges this?

- Will all services done in the hospital (medical, surgical, consultations, x-rays, etc.) be in-network so my insurance will cover the majority of the costs? What services may be out-of-network and not paid by my insurance? Who should I talk to about my approximate financial responsibility?

- After I return home, who should I call about unexpected complications?

Be frank and honest when answering the surgeon's questions. For example, if you're dependent on alcohol or pain medications, be up front about this because sudden discontinuation while you're in the hospital can cause withdrawal symptoms. Likewise, patients who regularly use pain medications, such as hydrocodone, oxycodone, or meperidine may have built up a high tolerance (lessened effectiveness) to such pain medications and therefore may require higher doses following surgery. If pain medication is stopped abruptly, withdrawal symptoms may develop.

The anesthesiologist will ask questions you may have previously answered, such as if you recall having had a bad reaction to the anesthesia you had in the past (although you may not remember this); what medications you are currently taking; if you have drug allergies, and your opinion about your tolerance of pain. The anesthesiologist may suggest more than one type of anesthesia. Understand fully the risk/benefits of each and ask why he/she recommends one particular anesthetic. Consider selecting the type of anesthesia with the least likelihood of complications.

The surgeon, anesthesiologist, or their assistants will explain all the risks and benefits associated with your surgery and ask that you sign a consent form acknowledging your understanding and willingness to proceed. As emphasized throughout this book, don't be shy about asking questions.

You can ask the anesthesiologist if he/she or a nurse anesthetist will administer the anesthesia, and, likewise, if the surgeon or a resident in training will perform the surgery or only assist the attending surgeon. It's appropriate to make your preference known. It goes without saying that most patients prefer the most experienced surgeon and anesthesiologist rather than a resident in training.

If you are admitted to a hospital in an emergency, and you lack the mental and/or physical capacity to make an informed decision or cannot sign or give verbal consent for surgery, the hospital will try to obtain consent on your behalf from your healthcare proxy, if available, or a responsible family member, according to the laws of the state where you reside. If one of these healthcare surrogates is unavailable and emergency surgery is required to save your life, the surgeon and hospital may need to proceed without your informed consent.

Dealing with Pain

Even if you pride yourself on having a high pain threshold, don't feel you have to prove it to yourself or your doctor. Make certain that you leave the hospital or outpatient surgical center with a sufficient amount of pain medication. If you are allergic to a particular type of pain medication, remind your physician. It's best to use pain medication for as short a period as possible because chronic use runs the risk of developing tolerance and psychological and physical dependency.

For mild to moderate pain, aspirin and other non-steroidal anti-inflammatory drugs (NSAIDs) such as ibuprofen are usually sufficient. NSAIDs also reduce swelling. It's best to take them with food because when taken on an empty stomach they can cause irritation and bleeding of the stomach, as well as nausea. NSAIDs can also interfere with blood clotting. Some heart and gastrointestinal surgeons recommend discontinuation of NSAIDs weeks before and after surgery. If relevant to your situation, make certain to check with your surgeon.

For severe pain, opioids such as oxycodone, codeine, meperidine, or morphine are often prescribed. It's preferable to use them for short periods unless your doctor recommends one of them for severe chronic pain and its use can be carefully monitored. Side effects of opioids include physical and psychological dependency, constipation, nausea, drowsiness, impaired coordination, slowed respiration, and difficulties with urination. When combined with benzodiazepines and other sedating drugs, breathing difficulties, oversedation, and sudden death can occur. [See *Chapter 10, Medications: What You Need to Know – Opioid Epidemic*].

N-methyl-D-aspartate (NMDA) receptor antagonists, such as Dilaudid and Ketamine work like narcotics. They also have many side effects and are very expensive. They are sometimes used for pain in the recovery room after surgery.

Preparing for a Safe Return Home After Surgery

Be prepared to be discharged from the hospital sooner than expected because shorter stays reduce the risk of hospital-related complications (for example, infections, skin ulcers) and reduce medical and hospital expenses [1]. So, begin working with your hospital discharge coordinator or social worker soon after admission to the hospital rather than later. If you'll need nursing, rehabilitation, or other medical services at home, it's often better to initially secure more services than you will need because it's easier to reduce rather than increase the frequency of at-home visits.

Because there is often a delay in your outpatient doctor(s) receiving the official discharge summary from your hospital doctor (usually a hospitalist), obtain copies of all your hospital records prior to discharge or from home downloads from your Patient Portal so you can share them at follow-up appointments with your doctors and other health professionals. Also, add a copy to your PHR.

Have your patient advocate or reliable family member by your side when your doctor (and others) explain your discharge plans. Your advocate can take notes and even use a tape recorder so everyone understands and works together to implement the plan. Among the many questions you and your advocate consider asking, prioritize some of the following:

- What are common post-surgical complications I need to watch for? Whom exactly do I need to call or leave a message with if there is a complication? Is it more efficient to text or email that person? Obtain specific names and numbers to call.

- How much pain can I expect, and what pain pills should I take and for approximately how long?

- If relevant, how do I and my helper best take care of the incision site, dressings, and drainage tubes?

- What kind of equipment and supplies have to be in place at home before I return?

- When can I expect to resume my daily activities? How gradually should I take it? When can I resume driving and if relevant, my sex life?

- How long will the wound take to heal, and what kind of scar is likely?

- Will I need physical therapy at a rehabilitation center, hospital, or at home and for how long? What rehabilitation company should I consider, and will it be in-network so my insurance will cover the major portion of the cost?

- Should my follow-up visit be with my surgeon, my PCPhys., or both? And how soon?
- What new medications started while in the hospital should I continue and which medications I was taking at home should I resume and which should I stop?

Rita, a television news reporter living with her husband and stepson in New York City, was only forty-seven years old when she noticed small hard nodules in both breasts. Her PCPhys. referred her to a breast surgeon. After extensive tests, she was diagnosed with early-stage cancer. A second opinion from a specialist confirmed the diagnosis.

She was understandably frightened and wondered how having a bilateral mastectomy, lymph node removal and medicine to curb her estrogen (and cause menopause) would affect her career, self-image, and her already strained marriage. When her husband chose to get his teenage son into a drug rehabilitation program rather than be with her during her surgery, she felt abandoned, resentful, and depressed.

The surgery was successful and was followed by breast implants two months later. She developed hot flashes and irritability. Her ambivalence about sexual intimacy was further aggravated by her husband's indifference, preoccupation with work, and his son's problems.

She finally confessed all her miseries to her oncologist. She was referred to a psychiatrist who suggested weekly psychotherapy sessions and the antidepressant venlafaxine 75 mg/day for her depression and menopausal symptoms. He also referred her to a women's support group for breast cancer survivors [124] and for marriage and family counseling. The combination of these treatment approaches, in addition to being free of cancer after five years, led to the remission of her depression, improvement in her marriage, family, and social life, and the return to her successful career.

New Hope, Better Prognosis for Patients with Cancer

New diagnostic and treatment discoveries have transformed cancer to a frequently curable or a chronic, more manageable disease. At least half of persons who contract all kinds of cancer in the United States each year are alive five years later.

Like Rita, when people first learn they have cancer, understandable psychological reactions include fear of death, disability, and disfigurement. There is also fear of abandonment, loss of independence, disruption of relationships, and worry about finances, especially with uncertainty about their insurance coverage and spiraling medical costs.

---

124 Kissane DW, Love A, Hatton A, et al. Effect of cognitive-existential group therapy on survival in early-stage breast cancer. J Clin Oncol. 2004;22(21);4255-4260.

Death rates from breast cancer have declined substantially since the 1990's, especially for women under age fifty. The prevalence of depression among patients with breast cancer, especially during the first year, is estimated at fifty-two percent. The majority of pre-menopausal women who have anti-estrogen therapy and removal of the ovaries have disturbing hot flashes, irritability, and other menopausal symptoms. A study found that sixty-one percent of women treated with the antidepressant venlafaxine 75mg to 150 mg/day had a significant reduction of depression and hot flashes.

The benefit of group therapy for women with metastatic breast cancer, as demonstrated in a study by Dr. David Siegel, showed that women who attended weekly group counseling survived an average of eighteen months longer than patients receiving routine care.

Multidisciplinary, integrated treatment of cancer patients, like Rita, that combines medical, surgical, oncological, and mental health treatment have improved the overall care and quality of life for cancer patients [2] [3].

Chapter 9 Key Points

Key Points: What You Need to Do Before Surgery

- Get in the best physical, medical, and emotional state.
- Consider meditation, relaxation techniques, yoga.
- Bank your own blood if transfusions may be needed.
- Understand all the risks versus benefits.

Key Points: Choosing the Best Surgeon & Hospital

- Ask your PCPhys. for recommendations.
- Consider an Internet search looking for a surgeon:
    - o Board certified in specialty related to your surgery; Fellow, ACS.
- Consider getting a second opinion from another surgeon and medical center.

Key Points: Pre-Surgery Visit with Surgeon & Anesthesiologist

- Discuss anesthesia options. Which is safest?
- Be candid if you have any substance abuse problems.
- Request that the attending surgeon and anesthesiologist, rather than a resident in training, perform the procedures.

Key Points: Safe Transition Home

- Anticipate discharge from hospital sooner than expected.
- Obtain a copy of your hospital records before discharge to distribute to all your outpatient health professionals.
- Consider having your patient advocate (or family member) listen and write down instructions.

References

1. Gwande, A., A Surgeon's Notes on an Imperfect Science. Macmillan, 2002.

2. Holland, JC, Breitbart WS, Jacobsen PB, Loscalzo MJ, McCorkle R, Butow PN. *Text-book of Psychooncology.* 3rd ed. New York; Oxford University Press; 2015.

3. Michelson, L.D., Be on the cutting edge of technology, in Michelson, L.D., The Patient's Playbook. Alfred A. Knopf. New York, 2015, p. 234-241.

4. Ruizen, M.F., Oz, M.C. You the Smart Patient, Free Press, New York, 2006, p. 97-123.

5. Heffernan, S.P., Alici, Y., Breitbart, W.S., et al. Psycho-Oncology, In Comprehensive Textbook of Psychiatry. 10th Edition, Sadock, B.J., Sadock, V.A., Ruiz, P., (Eds) Wolters Kluwer Press, Philadelphia, 2017, p. 2250-2287.

Medications: What You Need to Know

Jack is a fifty-six-year-old carpenter who has several chronic illnesses, including asthma, hypertension, benign prostatic hypertrophy, arthritis, and gastroesophageal reflux disease (GERD). He takes six regular medicines—and more when his arthritis or any of the other illnesses flare up. Recently he was not feeling well, and his doctor prescribed a new medication. After one week, Jack was not feeling better and, in fact, noted new discomfort in his bowel and some nausea. The doctor had described possible side effects to his new med, but Jack took no notes and forgot what was discussed. The pharmacy provided a list of possible side effects, but Jack didn't read it.

Jack returned to his doctor, who had the following therapeutic dilemma. Were the lack of response and the occurrence of new symptoms due to the new medicine not working on the condition for which it was prescribed? Or was the new drug itself causing the new symptoms as a side effect of that drug? Or was the new drug interacting with one or more of the other six drugs Jack was taking and causing the new symptoms that the new drug alone would not have caused. Or were the new symptoms due to the progression of the disease being treated?

The physician also had to consider the possibility that the initial diagnosis was incorrect and the presumed underlying condition needed further diagnostic evaluation. Situations like this occur with some frequency. Is the medicine helping (efficacious) and/or causing side effects directly or through drug-drug, drug-food, or drug-herbal interactions?

This chapter starts with a brief overview of pharmacology and drug interactions to enhance your understanding of other topics that follow. We indicate how prescribers think through a situation such as what Jack and his doctor faced so you can appreciate the professional challenges involved in prescribing your medications. We show you how doctors deal with common medication problems, how they strive to avoid medication errors, and how they deal with special medication issues with older patients. We show you two of the most pressing medication problems in the United States: increased bacterial resistance to antibiotics and the role of pain medicines and the current opioid epidemic in the United States. We suggest what to consider when choosing your pharmacy, and how to save on the cost of prescription medicines.

An Overview of Pharmacology and Drug Interactions

An overview of drug metabolism is given in *website Chapter 10 Appendix: A Brief Overview of Pharmacology*. We note that the drug absorption in the intestine occurs only when medicines are given orally. When they are given intramuscularly or intravenously, the medicines enter the bloodstream much more directly and quickly and therefore bypass the intestine. Some drug interaction effects occur when a new drug alters the metabolism of other drugs, such as increasing the blood level of a second medicine, thereby increasing the likelihood of the higher blood level causing side effects. Frequent types of drug interactions are given in *website Chapter 10 Appendix: Examples of Drug Interactions*.

How Doctors Evaluate Possible Drug Side Effects

When a doctor prescribes a drug to a patient, he or she usually discusses how long it will take the drug to become effective and also the possible side effects of the drug. When a new drug is introduced in a situation where there are multiple chronic illnesses involving multiple drugs, the doctor has to consider several issues:

- Are the new symptoms a known side effect of the new medicine? This includes known direct drug side effects or those occurring as drug-drug, drug-food, and drug-herbal interactions.

- What is the time correlation between the start of the new drug and the start of new symptoms? If the new symptoms began (perhaps subtly) *before* the new drug was introduced, this suggests this is *not* a drug-related symptom. Conversely, if they began shortly *after* the new medicine was started, this suggests a *likely* drug side effect.

- If the new symptoms decrease or stop when the new drug is either stopped or the dose is decreased, this supports a likely drug side effect.

- If the situation is unclear, it is often wise to confirm the underlying diagnosis for which the new drug was given.

- If the diagnosis is confirmed and a likely drug side effect has occurred, it is usual to consider replacing the offending drug with a different drug approved for the same disorder.

Doctors are often alerted to possible drug interactions with emergent side effects from the electronic health records (EHRs) software that many medical practices use. When doctors are working away from their office, they can check for possible drug interactions using smartphone apps such as those provided by Medscape[125] and Epocrates.[126]

Basic Approaches to Taking Medications

Common Problems

If medications are ineffective, it is often because patients do not take them properly, discontinue them prematurely, or do not take them at all. It is estimated that only half of all prescribed medications are taken properly. Improper use of medications results in more than a million Americans becoming seriously ill each year. Common causes of medication mishaps include taking the wrong medication and the wrong dose, pharmacy errors, medication side effects (adverse reactions), and drug-drug interactions.

Avoiding Medication Errors

As a conscientious patient, do not assume that all your healthcare providers regularly share with one another information about your medications and changes in your health status. You and your healthcare advocate should be active communicators with all your healthcare professionals.

Keep on your person at all times an updated list of all your current prescribed medications, over-the-counter medications, herbal remedies, drug and other allergies, and medical/psychiatric diagnoses. You may be under the care of several physicians and other healthcare professionals who are unaware of medications prescribed by others. Give an updated list of all your medications at each visit to all your healthcare professionals. Keeping your up-to-date list in your wallet or purse or on your smartphone will be invaluable if you find yourself in an emergency room.

Additional Safeguards

- Have your prescriptions filled promptly, and take medications reliably.

- Keep your medications in the original bottles rather than combining them in a single bottle because many medications look alike.

- If you are taking three or more medications daily, use a plastic pill dispenser—available at any pharmacy—to remind you to take your medications at the right time and to reveal whether or not you have taken them in the first place.

---

125 See http://www.medscape.com/public/mobileapp/features
126 See http://www.epocrates.com/products/features?cid=headerExplore

- When picking up your medications at the pharmacy, check the labels to confirm that your name, the name of the medication, the number of pills, the dosage, and the number of refills is correct, especially if you are using a busy large retail pharmacy.

- Keep a week's supply of all your pills in a safe place in case you lose some or the mail-order service is late in delivering them.

- Don't break or crush your pills or capsules because their effectiveness may be diminished. If you're uncertain about this, read the directions that came with the pills, or call your pharmacist or doctor.

- Resist pressure from a friend or family member to share your pills with them. This practice is risky, and you will be practicing medicine without a license.

- Take pain medication at the times recommended by your physician. Under his or her supervision, cooperate in reducing their use in order to decrease the risk of becoming psychologically or physically dependent on them.

- Don't abruptly stop using medicine that you have been taking for a long or even a short period of time without first discussing it with your doctor. The use of some medications needs to be slowly tapered off under medical supervision before discontinuation.

- When traveling, keep your medications on your person at all times in case your luggage is lost.

- Keep your medications in a dry, cool place rather than a hot, humid bathroom cabinet, where moisture and heat can reduce their effectiveness.

- Before undergoing a procedure requiring insertion of dyes or radioactive material into your body, make sure you remind the attending staff of any allergies you have.

- Throw away outdated medications or those you no longer use in order to avoid accidentally using inactive medications or risk someone else using them.

- Keep your medications out of the reach of children.

- Keep a careful daily record of the names of medications and the time of day they are taken to ensure that you have not missed a dose. Record suspected side effects. Show your medication record to your doctors and other healthcare professionals so they can monitor your compliance and any possible side effects.

- Call your physician in ample time before you run out of your medication to make certain that you have an adequate supply.

Requesting Medications from Your Physician

Generic versus Brand-Name Medicines: Do Some Research Before Visiting Your Physician

If you anticipate that your physician is too busy to know whether there are less costly brand-name or generic medications available, then you and/or your healthcare advocate can do some research and planning before visiting your physician. If you have a common medical condition such as diabetes, hypertension, or depression, it's almost certain that there are generic or older brand-name medications that may be equally effective but much less expensive than new brand-name drugs.

If you know your diagnosis before visiting your doctor, call your pharmacist with your prescription drug insurance card in hand and find out what commonly used drugs are available to treat your condition, what drugs are partly or entirely covered by your insurance, and if there are generic alternatives that are equally effective.

With this information in hand, when you visit your physician, before he or she writes a prescription for a brand-name medication, ask whether there is a less expensive but equally effective generic medication. Also, mention the names of one or two less expensive brand-name and generic medications you learned about from your pharmacist or on the Internet. Don't be ashamed or embarrassed to ask for a less expensive medication because physicians are sensitive to the financial strain that patients experience, especially during hard economic times.

If you have not succeeded in obtaining a prescription from your physician for a reasonably priced medication and the pharmacist tells you that the prescription is not covered or is insufficiently covered by your insurance—and will cost hundreds of dollars per month—ask your pharmacist to call your physician to inquire about a generic equivalent or a less expensive brand-name medication. Also, have the pharmacist ask whether or not a prior authorization is needed and ask if your physician will request it.

Questions to Ask Your Doctor When You're Given a Prescription

---

Don't be shy about asking some of the following questions when your physician gives you a new prescription. Your physician will likely respect your wish to be fully informed and knowledgeable. It's best to prioritize your questions; some may not apply or may have already been answered. If you're getting more than one new medication, the questions should apply to each medicine.

- What illness is this medication being used to treat?

- At what time intervals do I take the medication, and do I take it with or without food? If I miss a dose, what do I do?

- Does this new medication replace any pills I'm currently taking?

- How long should I take the medication? Don't make the mistake of stopping the medication as soon as symptoms lessen or disappear because the illness and its symptoms may return. If uncertain, check with your physician.

- About how soon can I expect the medicine to begin working?

- What are any potential side effects, and how common are they? Might they be temporary or long lasting?

- How safe is it to take this medication with my other medications, including herbal remedies, vitamins, and organic supplements?

- Is this new medication along with my other medications safe to take with alcohol and recreational drugs such as marijuana? When the physician asks how much you drink and use recreational drugs, be honest because we all tend to deny or minimize their use, which can cause potentially undesirable consequences.

- Are there any activities I should avoid? (For example, certain tranquilizers can make your skin sensitive to sun exposure.)

- Will the prescription include the number of refills, or do I need to contact you each time for a refill?

- What are the reasons for prescribing a more expensive brand-name medication—because it is more effective or because there is no generic equivalent?

If the brand-name medication is not covered by your insurance, the doctor's office may need to call the prescription benefit department of your insurance company (the phone number is sometimes on the back of your insurance card) to have a prior authorization form faxed to the doctor's office. Some physicians' offices have ready access to these prior authorization forms. Your physician then must explain on the form why it is imperative for you to have the brand-name medication. The authorization form is faxed from the doctor's office to the insurance company. If the request is approved, the insurance company notifies your physician and you can then obtain the medication at a reasonable cost.

It's usually helpful to call your pharmacy to make certain that the medication is approved and ready for pickup.

Trying to Avoid Side Effects

There are three main safeguards against the risk of medication side effects and drug-drug interactions. The safeguards are your doctor, your pharmacist, and, most importantly, *you*, the conscientious patient. Your doctor keeps a record of all your medications. Many physicians have handheld computers that warn about drug-drug interactions. You need to keep all your doctors and other health professionals in the information loop by informing them about your over-the-counter medications and medications prescribed by all your other doctors.

Another safeguard is your local pharmacist, whose computer system checks the safety of your new prescription with other medications you are currently taking. The pharmacist can inform you about possible side effects, drug-drug interactions, and unnecessary duplication with other medications that you may be taking for the same illness. Using the same pharmacy each time enables you to develop a cooperative relationship with your pharmacist, who will safeguard you against these potential problems.

The risk of medication side effects has increased because of various factors. They include increasing longevity and the greater use of multiple medications and over-the-counter meds. Also, there may be genetic factors that influence how you absorb, metabolize, and respond to drugs, and the ability of your liver and kidneys to metabolize and excrete them. Newer drugs, although FDA approved, may contribute to side effects not recognized until the drugs have been on the market for several years.

Half of all adults in the United States take two or more medications a day, and it is not unusual for persons over age seventy to be taking six or more different medications, thus increasing the risk for side effects and drug-drug interactions. There are several types of drug interactions. In *drug-drug interactions*, a drug's action can be either increased or decreased by the presence of the other drug(s), or the combination may cause unwanted effects that neither drug alone would produce. The same thing can happen in *drug-food interactions* and *drug-plant interactions* (with medicinal herbs or plants). Examples of these types of drug interactions are given in our *website Chapter 10 Appendix: Examples of Drug Interactions*.

Special Considerations Regarding the Elderly

The likelihood of side effects increases with the number of medications taken. Persons older than sixty-five are often taking five or more prescription medications (in addition to herbal remedies and over-the-counter medications), so there is a greater likelihood for side effects and drug-drug interactions. Elderly persons metabolize and excrete drugs more slowly than younger people and are prone to developing high blood levels of certain drugs; an example is long half-life benzodiazepines given for anxiety/nervousness such as diazepam and chlordiazepoxide. Overuse of benzodiazepines, especially with the elderly, can contribute to falls, memory problems, and drowsiness. Thus, it is important to use these medicines in considerably smaller doses and try to use types that don't stay in the system (that is, have shorter half-lives). Studies at large universities found that over 20 percent of older patients were taking medications with a high potential for side effects.

In addition, the elderly may be more prone to medication errors because of visual, hearing, and cognitive impairment and concomitant alcohol and drug abuse. One or a combination of these factors can impair judgment. For example, an older person may awaken in the middle of the night not remembering whether he or she had taken a sleep medication, and then mistakenly take more—with dire consequences such as a fall where a hip or limb is fractured.

These risks point to the need for a pill dispenser so a daily or weekly supply of pills can be placed in the appropriate compartment. A very frail or otherwise impaired elderly person can benefit from a dependable healthcare advocate, and sometimes from a part-time or twenty-four-hour-a-day caregiver who can oversee and monitor dispensing of pills and other aspects of healthcare.

The mismanagement of one of the author's seventy-eight-year-old Aunt Susan's medical care is a distressing example of what can happen when coordination of treatment is lacking. She was seeing several doctors who did not communicate with one another. Her psychiatrist prescribed amitriptyline (Elavil) for depression and quetiapine (Seroquel) – a major tranquilizer– for insomnia and nervousness. Her internist, not knowing the other medications she was taking, prescribed a long-acting benzodiazepine for insomnia. Within a week, she became confused, over-sedated, constipated, and agitated and was found wandering aimlessly around her neighborhood. Taken to the emergency room, she was diagnosed as having drug-induced delirium from the combined side effects of her medications. During a two-day stay in the hospital, her medications were discontinued and her confusion completely resolved.

Example of Loss of Drug Effectiveness: Bacterial Antibiotic Resistance

Infections were often lethal before antibiotics were first used in the 1940s. Now bacterial infections again are a serious threat. Consider the case of forty-two-year-old Frank. He was admitted to the hospital because of a foot infection that was slowly growing despite oral antibiotics, with the plan to give a new intravenous antibiotic. Then Frank died of the infection. The bacteria had entered his bloodstream (a condition called "sepsis") and he died of "septic shock" despite multiple antibiotics.

What Is Antibiotic Resistance?

Antibiotic resistance is the ability of bacteria to resist the effects of medication previously used to treat them. Resistance occurs in one of three ways: natural resistance in certain types of bacteria;

genetic mutation; or by one species acquiring resistance from another. Resistant microbes are increasingly difficult to treat, requiring alternative medications or higher doses—which may be costlier or more toxic. Bacteria can become resistant to multiple antibiotics; such multidrug-resistant bacteria are sometimes called "superbugs." Resistance has varyingly occurred in many bacterial "families" to nearly all antibiotics that have been developed.

The Problem

The growing number of antibiotic-resistant bacteria is a serious and worldwide problem. "Infectious disease is now the second leading killer in the world, number three in developed nations and fourth in the United States. Worldwide, 17 million people die each year from bacterial infections" [1]. According to the Centers for Disease Control and Prevention (CDC),[127] each year in the United States at least 2 million people become infected with bacteria that are resistant to antibiotics, and at least 23,000 people die each year as a direct result of these infections. The death rate may be even higher since the Infectious Diseases Society of America notes that "Nearly 2 million Americans per year develop hospital-acquired infections, resulting in 99,000 deaths – the vast majority of which are due to antibacterial-resistant pathogens." [128]

What Can Be Done to Decrease Your Risk?

At the Public Health Level

Recent reviews [2] [3] point to a number of interventions such as:

- Commercial uses of antibiotics:
  - Decrease overuse of antibiotics, such as extensive agricultural (livestock) use
- Clinical uses of antibiotics:
  - Improve prescribing practices
    - Order laboratory tests to confirm that bacteria are causing the infection.
    - Avoid unnecessary use or wrong choice of an antibiotic agent
    - Don't honor patients' expectations of receiving an antibiotic for treatment of conditions such as colds when antibiotics are not needed and will not help since viruses cause most colds.
  - Improve diagnosis and diagnostic tools.
    - Use standard or advanced molecular detection technologies to identify pathogens and their antibiotic sensitivities.

---

127 See https://www.cdc.gov/drugresistance/
128 See https://www.idsociety.org/public-health/antimicrobial-resistance/antimicrobial-resistance/facts-about-antibiotic-resistance/

- o Improve tracking methodologies
  - CDC has recently implemented the National Healthcare Safety Network for use by healthcare facilities to electronically report infections, antibiotic use, and resistance.
- o Prevent transmission of bacterial infections.
  - Be diligent about hand hygiene
  - Disinfect the healthcare environment and patient-care equipment
- o Develop and quickly deploy new antibiotics.

At the Personal Risk Reduction Level

The CDC offers ways to minimize risk when you are well and when you are sick.[129]

Maintain Healthy Habits

- Clean Your Hands
  - o Cleaning your hands is like a "do-it-yourself" vaccine you can take to reduce the spread of diarrheal and respiratory illness to others.
- Stay up-to-date with vaccines.
  - o Disease prevention is the key to staying healthy.
  - o It is always better to prevent a disease than to treat it. Vaccines can protect both the people who receive them and those with whom they come in contact.
- Prevent the spread of food-borne infections.
- Keep your water safe.
- Prevent the spread of sexually transmitted diseases.

Staying Safe When Sick

- Use antibiotics the right way.
  - o Colds, flu, most sore throats, and bronchitis are caused by viruses.
  - o Antibiotics do not help fight viruses.
- Learn when respiratory illnesses need antibiotics.
  - o Antibiotics do not fight infections caused by viruses like colds, most sore throats and bronchitis, and some ear infections.

---

129 See http://www.cdc.gov/drugresistance/protecting_yourself_family.html

- o Unneeded antibiotics may lead to future antibiotic-resistant infections.

- o Symptom relief might be the best treatment option.

- Feel better with symptom relief.

  - o Viral infections, which antibiotics cannot treat, usually recover when the illness has run its course. Colds, a type of viral infection, can last for up to two weeks.

  - o You should keep your healthcare provider informed if your or your child's illness gets worse or lasts longer than expected.

  - o Over-the-counter medicines may help relieve some symptoms.

Staying Safe While in a Hospital

- Speak up.

  - o Talk to your doctor about all questions or worries you have. Ask them what they are doing to protect you. If you have a catheter, ask each day if it is necessary. Ask your doctor how he/she prevents surgical site infections. Also ask how you can prepare for surgery to reduce your infection risk.

- Keep hands clean.

  - o Be sure everyone cleans their hands before touching you.

- Get smart about antibiotics.

  - o Ask if tests will be done to make sure the right antibiotic is prescribed.

- Know the signs and symptoms of infection.

  - o Some skin infections appear as redness, pain, or drainage at an IV catheter site or surgery site. Often these symptoms come with a fever. Tell your doctor if you have these symptoms.

- Watch out for deadly diarrhea (aka *C. difficile*).

  - o Tell your doctor if you have three or more diarrhea episodes in twenty-four hours, especially if you have been taking an antibiotic.

Example of Serious Drug Side Effects: Pain Medications and the Opioid Epidemic

You took a fall on a hike and banged your knee in which you already have some painful arthritis. There is swelling and continued pain made worse when walking or putting weight on that leg. The pain keeps you up at night. Your doctor takes X-rays and examines the knee. He determines that nothing is broken but the joint cartilage was further damaged. He tells you that the time course for improvement of the new pain adding to the chronic pain is hard to predict. The new pain from the fall could either resolve fully in a matter of weeks—or it could gradually lessen but leave you with more chronic knee pain than your pre-fall pain level. Rest and physical therapy are discussed as well as referral to an orthopedic specialist for further evaluation. Your doctor then discusses pain medicines and recommends a stronger one in the "opioid" class. He discusses new requirements for using this type of pain medicine. They include only a one-week supply of pills at a time; a special urine test that may be repeated; and completing various rating scales concerning pain assessment, opioid risk, and pain medication misuse. You are surprised—almost feeling as though your doctor doesn't trust you with this medicine—but are not sure what to ask to better understand what is the big deal about getting a strong pain medicine for strong pain! So, in this section you'll learn the answers to your unspoken questions.

The pressing issue is that death from the opioid group of *prescribed* pain medicines is currently a major national problem. This has led recently to many changes in the way the medicines are prescribed and monitored. In the following sections, we discuss what you can do to have the benefit of these medicines and do your best to avoid the problems associated with their use.

The Opioid Epidemic

Opioids are a group of narcotic medicines used when pain is severe. The United States is in the midst of a serious epidemic of prescription pain medication misuse or abuse of opioid medicines. Death is due to respiratory depression. This danger has galvanized many responses from governmental health agencies. In 2016 alone, the U.S. Surgeon General communicated directly with all doctors on the severity of the problem. The Food & Drug Administration (FDA) has issued warnings about opioid pain medications. The Centers for Disease Control and Prevention (CDC) has created new national guidelines for using and monitoring these medications. States have ramped up their electronic databases for tracking prescriptions of opioids and other controlled substances. The warnings and guidelines may make you feel as though your healthcare providers don't trust you as much as you expect they should, and the monitoring techniques may sometimes feel irritating and onerous. It will help you to understand these new guidelines so you appreciate their impact on your doctor's approach to giving you the benefit of these medications if you need them.

Pain: Patterns, Duration, and Medications

Physical pain is a great motivator to seek relief. This is particularly true when the pain is chronic (lasting more than three months). Pain occurs in patterns that include severity (mild, moderate, severe); duration (recent acute onset, longer-term chronic); body location; daily patterns (intermittent, continuous); factors that make it worse or better; association with other non-pain symptoms; and response to drug and non-drug interventions. Your healthcare professionals are trained to recognize such patterns. Optimally this leads to identifying and correcting the medical or surgical cause of the pain. Unfortunately, "correcting the cause" is not always possible (such as with osteoarthritis), but management of the pain often includes medicines to reduce the pain.

If you should need pharmacologic pain relief, it's important to understand the different pain medications available and new strategies that your doctors will use in employing the available medicines for your benefit. So, first let's see the different classes and subclasses of pain medications. [*See website Chapter 10 Appendix*: *Overview of Pain Medicines*.]

When your pain is in the milder range, the available medications are called *non-narcotic*. There are three subclasses of non-narcotics: acetaminophen (such as Tylenol), nonsteroidal anti-inflammatory (NSAID, such as Aleve), and COX-2 inhibitor (such as Celebrex). These subgroups differ in possible adverse side effects. With the acetaminophen group, be sure to stay within the maximum daily dose to avoid potential liver or kidney problems. With the NSAID group, be aware that they might not be good for people with stomach problems as they can cause stomach irritation and even bleeding. They may also increase the risk of serious adverse cardiovascular events, such as heart attack or stroke. With the COX-2 inhibitor, you might have the benefit of pain relief without it causing stomach problems often associated with other NSAIDs although the cardiovascular risks of other NSAIDs may remain.

When your pain is more severe, you may be prescribed a *narcotic* medicine. The opioids have many potential side effects, the most serious including depression of both respiration and cough reflex along with decreased motor response rate. The depression of respiration and motor activity may cause severe respiratory distress and is the cause for fatalities that are seen in the opioid epidemic. Tramadol has its own set of possible side effects, including abuse and addiction, and can also cause the respiratory depression associated with the opioid group.

Medicines in the group labeled "Other" in *website Chapter 10 Appendix: Types of Pain Medications* include anticonvulsants and antidepressants. Both groups are used in a much more limited range of painful conditions, such as diabetic neuropathy and fibromyalgia. Their side effects do not include respiratory depression. However, antidepressants have their own depressant effects on the brain and could magnify the central nervous system depressant effects of the opioids.

Opioid Epidemic: Scope of the Problem

Now that we understand the place of opioids among other prescription pain medicines, let's turn to the serious public health problem of the epidemic of opioid abuse. First, we should note that while the opioids are legal medicines, there also are illegal drugs in this class, notably heroin and cocaine. Although heroin clearly contributes to the overall opioid problem, it is the legally prescribed opioids that are widely surpassing the heroin contribution to the national problem. The severest alarm concerns the death rate associated with these legally prescribed pain medicines. Let's get an idea of the magnitude of the problem from recent reports.

- The 2016 report of the National Safety Council shows that opioids are now the number one cause of unintentional death in America driven by unintentional drug overdose, predominantly from prescription painkillers.[130]

- The 2016 report on opioid addiction from the American Association of Addiction Medicine finds that drug overdose is the leading cause of accidental death in the United States. The report further notes that women are particularly vulnerable since they are more likely to have chronic pain, be prescribed prescription pain relievers, and be given higher doses and use them for longer time periods than men. Women may become dependent on prescription pain relievers more quickly than men.[131]

Focus on Prescription Opioids: Actions at the Federal and State Levels

Given the magnitude of the epidemic, there is sharp focus at the national and state levels concerning the prescribing of opioid medicines. There was particularly heightened and coordinated activity during 2016 as follows.

- **Surgeon General:** On August 25, 2016, the U.S. Surgeon General sent a letter to 2.3 million doctors, nurses, dentists, and other clinicians urging a commitment to reviewing prescribing practices and a commitment to "turn-the-tide" on opioid misuse [4].[132]

- **FDA:** On August 31, 2016, the FDA issued a Drug Safety Communication requiring its strongest warning on drug labels about serious risks including death when combining opioid pain or cough medicines with a benzodiazepine.[133] [See *Chapter 10 Appendix: Opioid Epidemic— FDA Warnings*.].[134] This is an important warning since "of patients receiving opioid maintenance therapy, approximately 46 to 71% use benzodiazepines" and these drugs enhance the respiratory-depressant effects of opioids [5].

In 2016 the FDA also promoted the pharmaceutical development of what are called *abuse-deterrent opioid preparations*. These medicines make certain types of abuse more difficult to execute or less rewarding, such as having to crush a tablet in order to snort the contents or dissolve a capsule in order to inject its contents. It does not mean that the product is impossible to abuse or that these properties necessarily prevent addiction, overdose, or death.[135] In fact, a recent perspective indicates that the evidence supporting the benefit of abuse-deterrent opioids formulations on abuse is "a C+" or "ambiguous" [6].

- **Actions on the state level:** Prescription Drug Monitoring Programs (PDMPs) are state-run electronic databases used to track the prescribing of drugs by doctors and dispensing by pharmacies of controlled prescription drugs to patients. The programs are designed to monitor this information

---

130   See http://www.nsc.org/learn/safety-knowledge/Pages/injury-facts.aspx?gclid=COXeuc_89s4CFQOMaQodmwwJhA
131   See http://www.asam.org/docs/default-source/advocacy/opioid-addiction-disease-facts-figures.pdf
132   See (1) http://i2.cdn.turner.com/cnn/2016/images/08/25/sg.opioid.letter.pdf; (2) http://www.cdc.gov/drugoverdose/pdf/turnthetide_pocketguide-a.pdf
133   Benzodiazepines are a group of medications used to treat anxiety, insomnia, and seizures. Examples of this group are Ativan (lorazepam), Librium (chlordiazepoxide), Klonopin (clonazepam), Valium (diazepam), and Xanax (alprazolam).
134   See http://www.fda.gov/Drugs/DrugSafety/ucm518473.htm
135   See http://www.fda.gov/NewsEvents/Newsroom/PressAnnouncements/ucm492237.htm

for suspected abuse or diversion (that is, channeling drugs into illegal use), and can give a prescriber or a pharmacist critical information regarding a patient's controlled substance prescription history. This information can help prescribers and pharmacists identify patients at high risk who would benefit from early interventions.[136]

- **Pharmacists can notify doctors when they suspect that patients have access to prescriptions for pain pills from various practitioners.**

New National Prescribing Guidelines: Centers for Disease Control and Prevention (CDC)

The CDC developed the new *CDC Guideline for Prescribing Opioids for Chronic Pain*—United States, 2016 [7] to help primary care providers make informed prescribing decisions and improve patient care for those who suffer from chronic pain (pain lasting more than three months) in outpatient settings. The guideline consists of twelve recommendations. It is important to note that the guideline is not intended for patients who are in active cancer treatment, palliative care, or end-of-life care. [See details in *Chapter10 Appendix: Opioid Epidemic—CDC Guidelines*.]

What You Can Expect If You Have a Prescribed Opioid

Guidelines are extremely important. But they may seem more like a policy rather than focused on you or a loved one as the actual patient. Here are some of the things you might encounter from your healthcare prescriber concerning your pain management. You might be surprised by some of the items and feel that your doctor or their staff does not trust you enough. Please understand that the professionals are trying to respectfully comply with new national guidelines in order to lessen your pain yet avoid problems with the pain meds themselves.[137] The professionals also want to avoid medical legal problems, such as loss of their prescribing license, if the guidelines are not followed.

- If you experience a recent onset of pain:
  - Don't be surprised if the opioid prescription is for only a small number of pills (for example, a three-day or one-week supply).
- If you have chronic pain (persisting for at least three months)
  - Face-to-face treatment appointments with your physician every sixty to ninety days to reevaluate the efficacy and risks of the opioids

---

136   See http://www.cdc.gov/drugoverdose/pdmp/index.html
137   See http://www.cdc.gov/drugoverdose/prescribing/resources.html. Here you will find resources that succinctly summarize in 9 printable sheets much information that will help improve communication between yourself and your healthcare team.

- o Periodic assessments with some of the following assessment rating scales such as:
  - Pain assessment rating scale
  - Opioid risk rating scale
  - Substance misuse assessment rating scale
  - "Pain average, interference with enjoyment of life, and interference with general activity (PEG)" assessment scale
- o Urine drug testing at baseline and subsequently if there is any question of using other drugs or question of compliance with prescribed treatment
- o Reference to reviews of your state's Prescription Drug Monitoring Program (PDMP) records for avoidance of conflicting or duplicate treatments from other providers
- o Pill counts (showing your prescriber how many pills are left in your current opioid prescription)
- o Education regarding potential risk and warning signs of opioid dependence and addiction
- o Treatment agreement plan: signed by both the patient and prescribing physician to reduce pain and reduce opioid dose and to increase function and quality of life
- o Review of non-opioid treatment options [138]
  - Acetaminophen (Tylenol®) or ibuprofen (Advil®)
  - Cognitive behavioral therapy
  - Physical therapy and exercise
  - Medications sometimes used to treat depression (for example, duloxetine) or treat seizures (for example, gabapentin)
  - Interventional therapies (injections)
- The list of non-pharmacologic treatments grows with a review of complementary approaches for five painful conditions by the National Center for Complementary and Integrative Health at the National Institutes of Health [8]:
  - o Based on a preponderance of positive trials versus negative trials, current evidence suggests that the following complementary approaches may help some patients manage their painful health conditions:
    - acupuncture and yoga for back pain
    - acupuncture and tai chi for osteoarthritis of the knee
    - massage therapy for neck pain with adequate doses and for short-term benefit
    - relaxation techniques for severe headaches and migraine

---

138   See https://www.cdc.gov/drugoverdose/prescribing/patients.html

○ Weaker evidence suggests that massage therapy, spinal manipulation, and osteopathic manipulation might also be of some benefit to those with back pain, and relaxation approaches and tai chi might help those with fibromyalgia. *See Chapter 13 Alternative (Complementary) Treatment Approaches: East Meets West.*

Safe Storage and Disposal Recommendations

Taking opioids responsibly also means preventing misuse and abuse by not selling or sharing prescriptions of these painkillers. This is a major issue: <u>more than 50 percent of people misusing painkillers are getting them from family and friends</u>.[139] Sharing medications can be dangerous and contribute to overdose and addiction. Thus, opioid pain medicines should be stored securely in your home in their original bottles in a locked cabinet or lockbox or in a hidden location. Leftover or expired medication should be safely disposed of, which can be as simple as flushing them down a toilet or a sink.

If opioid dependence does occur, see information about treatment in our *website Chapter 10 Appendix: Effective Treatments for Opioid-Dependent Patients.*

Your Pharmacist—An Important Member of Your Healthcare Team

Advantages of a Small Neighborhood Pharmacy

There are advantages to using a small neighborhood pharmacy. You will be able to establish a good, long-term working relationship with your pharmacist, who:

- Has a record of all the prescriptions you have filled in the past, including those from your other doctors.
- May have a computer system that can detect potential drug-drug interactions.
- Is knowledgeable about medication side effects.
- Knows when to call your doctor with questions about your prescriptions.
- May be able to accept prescriptions that are electronically sent from your doctor's office, reducing errors from misread handwritten prescriptions.

---

139   See (1) http://commitmentsinpaincare.com/appropriate-storage-disposal; (2) https://www.fda.gov/ForConsumers/ConsumerUpdates/ucm101653.htm

If you are using your neighborhood pharmacy and value and trust one or two particular pharmacists, learn their schedules so you can bring in prescriptions or questions when they are on duty.

Advantages of a Large Countrywide Pharmacy

The disadvantages of mega pharmacies are similar to those of large discount stores, including impersonal service, longer waiting lines, and frequent staff turnover. However, there are also distinct advantages to using a large countrywide pharmacy, such as:

- Mega pharmacies are more technologically organized.
- They have larger supplies of various medications, and sometimes are less expensive.
- Some are open twenty-four hours a day, seven days a week.
- If you travel frequently and run out of medications while you're away, a big chain pharmacy's computer system can communicate with the branch pharmacy near your home to verify who you are and contact your physician to get approval for a supply of medication to last until your next office visit.
- Large pharmacy chains have more locations, so you have easier access to them.

Advantages of a Mail-Order Pharmacy

A third option is to use a mail-order pharmacy, which has certain advantages that include:

- Often are less expensive
- Are good when you will be taking certain medications over the long term
- If you need a certain medication for a long time, it may be possible, depending on your insurance company's policy, to buy a three-month or longer supply from your mail-order company.
- Will typically send alerts when your medication is due for a refill
- Many offer an option of automatic refills and will contact your physician to refill the prescription if all refills have been used.
- If you don't have automatic refills, notify the mail-order service weeks before your supply of medications runs low because mail delivery can be slow during holidays and other times.

Several Ways to Save on Drug Costs

Insurance companies and employers have shifted more of the financial burden of medical care, including medications, onto you in the form of higher co-pays and deductibles. Patients with multiple illnesses can pay thousands of dollars each year for prescription drugs. Many seriously ill patients with limited financial means are forced to choose between the necessities of life (food, clothing, and shelter) or the medications necessary for their survival.

After a pharmaceutical company's brand-name medication has been on the market for a certain number of years (usually twelve to fourteen years), other companies can make generic drugs that are often (but unfortunately not always) as effective as the brand-name drug. This may not be a serious concern for generic drugs manufactured in the United States because the Federal Drug Administration provides significant oversight. But be careful of generic drugs manufactured in Asia, Mexico, and other regions of the world where oversight and quality are often deficient. Also, unscrupulous companies make counterfeit drugs that are worthless.

Sometimes pharmaceutical companies will come out with a once-daily new version of the same medication that is taken two or three times daily. The once-daily new variant of the same medication may be much more expensive but not more effective than the multiple-dose variety, so consider the latter.

Sometimes you pay as much for a high-dosage pill as for a lower dose pill. Ask your physician or pharmacist whether the higher-dose pill, which costs the same, would have the same effectiveness if you were to divide it with a pill cutter.

If your physician wants to write a prescription for a brand-name medication, make certain that the "no substitution" box is checked on the prescription.

If you don't have prescription drug insurance, one alternative is to go to the Internet website Consumer Reports Best Buy Drugs,[140] which provides a list of reasonably priced drugs for various common ailments. With this information, you or the pharmacist can call your physician to consider the lower-cost medications. Big department stores such as Walmart[141] have a variety of generic drugs that cost about four dollars for a one-month supply. There are also drug discount companies that may save you money[142] or let you comparison shop for the best prices.[143] Sometimes your doctor's office has drug discount cards that can lower your cost.

---

140 www.crbestbuydrugs.org
141 www.walmart.com/cp/1078664
142 For example, see www.discountdrugnetwork.com/
143 For example, see www.goodrx.com/

Buying Medications on the Internet

_____

You can sometimes save substantially by buying medications from Canada.[144] However, you need to be cautious when buying medications on the Internet because some unscrupulous companies sell counterfeit pills, and many are manufactured outside the United States. Also, be wary of sites that do not require a prescription, especially for narcotic drugs. Or you may want to avoid buying any drugs on the Internet simply because it can be very risky.

Make certain that the Internet company is legitimate and has a person you can talk to on the phone. Also, make certain that the Internet company is certified by the Verified Internet Pharmacy Practice Site (VIPPS), which means it has met standards set by the National Association of Boards of Pharmacy. If you do not see the VIPPS seal and are suspicious, you can check the National Associations' Board[145] to verify that the Internet pharmacy is licensed and in good standing.

Accepting Sample Drugs from Your Physician's Office

_____

Another strategy to reduce the cost of expensive brand-name medication is to ask your physician if he or she has samples that you can try before investing in a one-month or more supply. Keep in mind that the samples are brand name rather than generic drugs, so when you eventually need to purchase them and your insurance doesn't cover part of the cost, the drugs can be very expensive.

Samples may help you save considerable charges but only if you will need this medication for a short time because your physician may have a limited supply that is dependent on the ability of the pharmaceutical representative to provide additional samples. Once generic equivalents of the brand-name medication become available, your physician may no longer be able to obtain samples of the brand-name medication. Ask your physician what you can expect if you rely on samples. If the physician's supply of sample brand-name medication is limited and unreliable and/or you will need this medication for weeks or months, you may want to use one of the other strategies described in this chapter.

---

144 Check these Internet sites: www.discountdrugsfromcanada.com (516-731-1500); www.thecanadianpharmacy.com; and www.Jandrugs.com.
145 https://rxlogic.wordpress.com/tag/vipps/

What If You Need an Expensive Brand-Name Medication

If you have a serious, rare ailment that requires an expensive brand of medication because there are no inexpensive alternatives, there are prescription assistance programs run by private companies and foundations to help lower costs. On your internet browser search "prescription assistance programs" for further information on such programs.

Many pharmaceutical companies offer discounts on their brand-name drugs for low-income individuals, such as Pfizer Friends Program[146] or Janssen Pharmaceuticals patient assistance program.[147] Find out the company that manufactures the medication you need, enter the name on your Internet search screen, and ask the company whether it offers drug discounts.

Buying Medical and Prescription Drug Insurance

Under the Affordable Care Act (ACA)

Under the ACA, at the time of this book's publication, if you are not covered by governmental insurance (for example, Medicare) or your employer's insurance, you can purchase medical and prescription drug insurance on a state or federal insurance exchange. The exchange lists all available insurance policies, dividing them into a hierarchy of levels beginning with "bronze" (least expensive), "silver," "gold," and "platinum" (most expensive). Also, only some of these insurance policies will include prescription drug insurance. In the past few years, many insurance companies have dropped out of the exchanges, limiting the number of policies from which you can choose. Compare these different policies carefully. Don't assume that because two policies are both "gold," they offer similar medical and prescription drug coverage.

It may be less expensive to first choose a medical insurance plan (for hospital and doctor visits), and then select a separate prescription drug policy that covers the drugs that you and your family take regularly. First, make a list of all the drugs that you and family members are currently taking and expect to be taking over the long term. Then check to see which prescription plan includes the drugs you will need. You can call your pharmacist or insurance company for advice on most if not all the medications. You'll want to repeat this process every year, especially if your regular medications have changed.

---

146 Cal1 866-776-3700, or go to https://www.pfizerrxpathways.com/
147 Call 1-800-652-6227 or www.janssenprescriptionassistance.com

Medicare Part D

We will be the first to admit that deciding on medical and prescription drug insurance can be confusing, frustrating, and time-consuming. We suggest enlisting the advice of your doctor's office manager, insurance agent, healthcare advocate, family, and friends who work in the healthcare industry and your employer's human resource office to help you make important insurance decisions. Given the ever-increasing cost of healthcare, put aside money in a health or flexible savings account and try to purchase the best policy you can afford to protect you and your family from a devastating and costly illness. Under the ACA, Medicare Part D was made more affordable in regard to the coverage gap (the so-called "donut hole"). The gap will be decreasing each year until 2020, at which point it will be closed.[148] Medicare itself suggests six ways to lower your coverage gap drug costs:[149]

1. Consider switching to generics or other lower-cost drugs.

Talk to your doctor to find out if there are generic or less expensive brand-name drugs that would work just as well as the ones you're taking now. You might also be able to save money by using mail-order pharmacies.

2. Choose a plan that offers additional coverage during the gap.

There are plans that offer additional coverage during the coverage gap (Medicare prescription drug coverage), such as for generic drugs. However, plans with additional gap coverage may charge a higher monthly premium. Check with the drug plan first to see if your drugs would be covered during the gap.

3. Drug assistance programs

Some pharmaceutical companies offer help for people enrolled in Medicare Part D. Find out whether there's a Pharmaceutical Assistance Program for the drugs you take.

4. State Pharmaceutical Assistance Programs.

Many states and the U.S. Virgin Islands offer help paying drug plan premiums and/or other drug costs. Find out if your state has a state Pharmaceutical Assistance Program.

---

148 In 2018 the gap (www.medicare.gov/Pubs/pdf/11493.pdf) occurred for drug expenses at $3,750. Once you've spent $5,000 out-of-pocket in 2018, you're out of the coverage gap (the so-called **Medicare doughnut hole**). Once you get out of the coverage gap you automatically get "catastrophic coverage." It assures you only pay a small coinsurance amount or copayment for covered drugs for the rest of the year. Progressive declines in the gap occur each year up to 2020 (www.medicare.gov/part-d/costs/coverage-gap/more-drug-savings-in-2020.html).

149 www.medicare.gov/part-d/costs/coverage-gap/ways-to-lower-drug-costs.html

5. Apply for extra help.

Medicare and Social Security have a program for people with limited income and resources that help you pay for your prescription drugs. If you qualify, you could pay no more than $3.30 for each generic or $8.25 for each brand-name covered drug in 2017.

6. Explore national and community-based charitable programs that can help with your drug costs:

- o National Patient Advocate Foundation
- o National Organization for Rare Disorders
- o Benefits checkup

Using Medicare Most Cost Effectively

It's best to begin studying the many Medicare options you can choose from months before turning age sixty-five or if you obtain Medicare at a younger age because of a disability. Choose plans from parts A, B, and D that will best provide the coverage you believe you'll need given your overall state of health. For example, if you are very healthy, exercise regularly, and eat nutritious food, are not taking expensive brand-name medications, and have no family history of early-onset medical conditions such as diabetes or heart disease, you'll still want to enroll in all three parts of Medicare but consider plans that are moderately priced that provide you with assurance of adequate coverage should you unexpectedly become ill. If you put off enrolling in Medicare A, B, and D months or years past the deadline (three months after turning age sixty-five), you'll be penalized with much higher premiums that will remain high as you get older. So, consider enrolling in Medicare A, B, and D and choose coverage plans compatible with your medical and medication needs. *See also information in Chapter 11 regarding Medicare Plans and their coverages.*

As you grow older, and medical problems and medication needs increase, consider changing to more comprehensive (and more expensive) plans that provide more adequate protection. Do this during the yearly open enrollment period.

For example, when the author was nearing sixty-five, he chose a relatively inexpensive Medicare Plan A, B, and D but an additional inexpensive Medicare supplemental plan that provided a fair amount of additional coverage should a serious illness occur. As the years passed, the Medicare Part D plan was gradually changed to a more expensive plan that covered all his medications. He likewise gradually changed his Medicare supplemental plan from the most inexpensive to the most expensive Plan F, which even covered the cost of medical evacuation from a foreign country back to the United States. He called his pharmacist yearly to make certain that the medications were covered. He also asked his pharmacist for the names of comparable medications that were covered, compared the cost and efficacy of alternative less expensive medications, and discussed the choices with his physician.

As our healthcare system and its therapeutic tools continue to change in complex ways, it is important to try to keep abreast of such changes. If you, a family member, or a loved one is living alone and without nearby involved family members, it is hard to keep abreast of all these relevant changes. Again, we encourage you to develop and maintain strong connections with your healthcare team. Ask them about any important changes. Go on the Internet to some of the sites we have cited in footnotes. Be your own advocate. And use other professionals as important resources to best utilize the evolving changes.

Chapter 10 Appendix

Opioid Epidemic

FDA Warnings

A number of cough medicines contain opioids such as codeine or hydrocodone. The additive effects of these medicines when combined with opioids for pain can cause serious and sometimes fatal interactions. As noted in the FDA communication, patients taking opioids with benzodiazepines, other CNS depressant medicines such as sleep medicines, antipsychotics, muscle relaxants, or alcohol, and caregivers of these patients, should seek medical attention immediately if they or someone they are caring for experience symptoms of unusual dizziness or light-headedness, extreme sleepiness, slowed or difficult breathing, or unresponsiveness.

CDC Guidelines

Although the published guidelines are intended for your healthcare professionals, it is worth reviewing the CDC website that directly addresses patients. We encourage you to review this information. We supplement this with some important perspectives from the published guidelines that are helpful to know about.[150]

- Nonpharmacologic therapy and nonopioid pharmacologic therapy are preferred

- From the outset, treatment goals should be established that include realistic goals for pain and function. Function can include emotional and social as well as physical dimensions.

- When opioids are used for acute pain, the quantity of prescribed pills can be as little as three days or less; more than seven days will rarely be needed.

- There should be an evaluation of benefits and harms with patients within one to four weeks of starting opioid therapy for chronic pain or of a dose escalation. Thereafter there should be similar evaluations at least every three months.

- Ideally, Prescription Drug Monitoring Program (PDMP) data should be reviewed before every opioid prescription or at least every three months. The purpose is to see if the patient is receiving opioid dosages or dangerous combinations that put him or her at high risk for overdose.

- Urine drug testing should be used prior to starting opioids and periodically to assess for prescribed opioids as well as other controlled substances and illicit drugs that increase risk for overdose when combined with opioids, including nonprescribed opioids, benzodiazepines, and heroin. The guidelines recommend that "before ordering urine drug testing, clinicians should explain to patients that testing is intended to improve their safety, should explain expected results (e.g., presence of prescribed medication and absence of drugs, including illicit drugs, not reported by the patient) and should ask patients whether there might be unexpected results."

---

150   See http://www.cdc.gov/drugoverdose/prescribing/patients.html

Chapter 10 Key Points

Key Points: How to Evaluate Possible Drug Side Effects

- Is the new drug known to cause the particular symptoms as a side effect (either directly or indirectly as drug-drug, drug-food, or drug-herbal interactions)?
- Did new unwanted symptoms start before or after the new drug was started?
  - o If before, this suggests it is not a drug side effect.
  - o If after, this suggests a drug side effect.
- Do unwanted symptoms decrease or disappear if the new drug dose is decreased or stopped?
- Has the underlying illness been reviewed and confirmed for which the drug was selected?
- Has using a different drug approved for the confirmed condition been considered?

Key Points: Special Problems with the Elderly

- They are often taking multiple drugs
  - o Thus, more chance of drug-drug interactions.
- They have slower metabolism and excretion of meds.
  - o Tendency to have higher blood levels of many meds with increased chance of side effects occurring.
  - o Thus, often need to use lower doses of meds to offset higher blood levels than desired
- They are more prone to medication errors and are less reliable in taking their multiple medications.

Key Points: What is Bacterial Antibiotic Resistance

- This is the ability of bacteria to resist the previously effective antibiotics used to eradicate them.
- The growing number of antibiotic-resistant bacteria is a serious and worldwide problem, including in the United States.
  - o In the U.S., some 2 million people become infected with resistant bacteria.
  - o In the U.S., some 23,000 people die each year directly due to these bacteria.
- Be familiar with both public health and personal recommendations to reduce your risk of infections with these resistant bacteria.

Key Points: How to Save Money on Drug Costs

- Generic drugs are less expensive than brand-name drugs.
- Consider buying on the Internet.

o Use caution and check reliability of manufacturers

- Review your specific drug coverages in choosing Medicare Part D plan.

- Consider obtaining drug samples from your doctor's office.

- Consider possible discounts from drug manufacturers.

References

1. Martens, E. and A.L. Demain, *The antibiotic resistance crisis, with a focus on the United States.* The Journal of Antibiotics, 2017. **70**(5): p. 520.

2. Ventola, C.L., *The antibiotic resistance crisis: part 1: causes and threats.* Pharmacy and Therapeutics, 2015. **40**(4): p. 277-83.

3. Ventola, C.L., *The antibiotic resistance crisis: part 2: management strategies and new agents.* Pharmacy and Therapeutics, 2015. **40**(5): p. 344-52.

4. Murthy, V.H., *Ending the Opioid Epidemic—A call to Action.* New England Journal of Medicine, 2016. 375(25): p.2413-15.

5. Soyka, M., *Treatment of benzodiazepine dependence.* New England Journal of Medicine, 2017. **376**(12): p. 1147-57.

6. Becker, W.C. and D.A. Fiellin, *Abuse-deterrent opioid formulations—Putting the potential benefits into perspective.* New England Journal of Medicine, 2017. **376**: p. 2103-2105.

7. Dowell, D., T.M. Haegerich, and R. Chou, *CDC Guideline for Prescribing Opioids for Chronic Pain—United States, 2016.* Journal of the American Medical Association, 2016. **315**(15): p. 1624-45.

8. Nahin, R.L., et al., *Evidence-Based Evaluation of Complementary Health Approaches for Pain Management in the United States.* Mayo Clinic Proceedings, 2016. **91**(9): p. 1292-306.

Part 4

Further Healthcare Evaluations and Choices

CHAPTER 11

Choosing the Best Insurance and Assuring End of Life Wishes

Do you know exactly what your health insurance does and does not cover? Do you know that if you don't register for Medicare when you are eligible that there are potential significant financial penalties? Do you understand the important coverage and copayment limits of Medicare when that is your only health insurance? Do you appreciate the likely unease in your family and your doctors if you are seriously ill and they do not know how aggressively you want to be treated? Do you know ways to maximize a loved one's ability to stay living safely in the community as frailties and illnesses evolve? In this chapter you will learn more about these and related issues that are best to understand and plan for.

How Good Are Your Insurance Coverages?

For those of you who are young, say in the age group of 25-40, you may feel that medical insurance is too expensive even under the ACA. You may feel that your health is good and you'll take your chances either with no insurance or one with lower cost and very high deductible. We hope that your view will turn out to be correct. However, suppose that you or a family member is suddenly seriously ill or sustains life-endangering injuries in a major accident and hospital care is necessary. Just as you will insure a home you own against small and large-scale damages unlikely to occur, you may want to re-think your health insurance to be sure you have reasonable coverage for most contingencies. For those of you in your 50's and 60's it's not too early to start to get familiar with insurance issues even though you're not yet eligible for Medicare. If you are satisfied with your own health coverage, you might be concerned about the health services available to your aging parents or friends. We want to help you in such a review.

There are, of course, many private major medical plans to choose among. In this section we will focus on the "original" current Medicare. We will not include Medicare Advantage plans since they encompass many different plans and do not promote easy comparisons with any particular private medical plan you may have or may be considering. *See Chapter 11 Appendix: Medicare Advantage Plans for further information.* **We pick Medicare as a primary health insurance for comparisons since it is a single plan that is national in scope and its benefits are often a benchmark reference for private major medical policies.**

Our discussion will help you formulate questions about your own potential or actual private health insurance in comparison with Medicare. You will learn about penalties for late enrollments; limitations in hospital coverage; limitations in Skilled Nursing Facility coverage; limitations of dental coverage; good coverage of Mental Health services, Home care and Hospice care; limitations in Respite care; good coverage for Preventive and Screening services; and limited geographic coverage of telemedicine services. If you plan to use Medicare as your primary insurance, your need to consider having secondary or supplemental medical insurance (e.g., "Medigap"), long-term care insurance and dental insurance will become clear. We understand that you or your loved ones may not be able to afford each of these insurance protections. However, when you see some of the potential financial exposures you may want to speak with a professional who can advise you on tradeoffs in risk-benefit analyses that may be within your means to consider. A quick overview of the pricing of Medicare options is available on the Medicare website[151] .

Let us begin by first understanding that Medicare has 4 Parts: A, B, C & D

- <u>Part A</u> provides inpatient/hospital coverage.

- <u>Part B</u> provides outpatient/medical coverage.

  o Most beneficiaries choose to receive their Parts A and B benefits through <u>Original Medicare</u>, the traditional fee-for-service program offered directly through the federal government.

- <u>Part C</u> offers an alternate way to receive your Medicare benefits often called Medicare Advantage plans[152] or Medicare private health plan

  o Medicare Part C is not a separate benefit. Part C is the part of Medicare law that allows private health insurance companies to provide Medicare benefits. These Medicare private health plans, such as HMOs and PPOs, contract with the federal government and are known as Medicare Advantage Plans. If you want, you can choose to get your Medicare coverage through a Medicare Advantage Plan instead of through Original Medicare.

  o Medicare Advantage Plans must offer, at minimum, the same benefits as Original Medicare (those covered under Parts A and B) but can do so with different rules, costs, and coverage restrictions. You also typically get Part D as part of your Medicare Advantage benefits package (MAPD). Many different kinds of Medicare Advantage Plans are available. You may pay a monthly premium for this coverage, in addition to your Part B premium.

  o Be aware that a Medigap policy is different from a Medicare Advantage Plan[153]. Those Advantage plans are ways to get Medicare benefits, while a Medigap policy only supplements your Original Medicare benefits. Note that You must have Medicare Part A and Part B.

- Part D provides prescription drug coverage.

---

151 See: www.medicare.gov/your-medicare-costs/costs-at-a-glance/costs-at-glance.html
152 https://www.medicareinteractive.org/get-answers/medicare-basics/medicare-coverage-overview/medicare-advantage
153 See: (1) https://www.medicare.gov/supplements-other-insurance/whats-medicare-supplement-insurance-medigap; (2) https://www.medicare.gov/supplements-other-insurance/whats-medicare-supplement-insurance-medigap/medigap-medicare-advantage-plans

In the following discussion we will use the *Original Medicare* as the basis for comparisons with other insurance policies you may be considering.

Medicare has Penalties for Late Enrollments

If you need to enroll in Medicare Part A and Part B and do not do so in a timely manner, you may be subject to financial penalties. Some people are *automatically enrolled* in Part A and Part B in certain circumstances *[See details in our website Chapter 11 Appendix: Medicare enrollments]*. However, you need to sign up for Part A and Part B if: (1) you aren't getting Social Security or Railroad Retirement Board benefits (e.g., because you're still working); or (2) you have End-Stage Renal Disease; or (3) you live in Puerto Rico and want to sign up for Part B (you automatically get Part A). You're eligible for Medicare Parts A and B when you turn 65. You can sign up during the 7-month period that begins 3 months before the month you turn 65, includes the month you turn 65, and ends 3 months after the month you turn 65. If you aren't eligible for premium-free **Part A**, and you don't buy it when you're first eligible, your monthly premium may go up 10% *[see website Chapter 11 Appendix: Premium-free Medicare Part A]*. You'll have to pay the higher premium for twice the number of years you could have had Part A, but didn't sign up.[154]

In most cases, if you don't sign up for **Part B** when you're first eligible, you'll have to pay a late enrollment penalty for as long as you have Part B. Your monthly premium for Part B may go up 10% for each full 12-month period that you could have had Part B but didn't sign up for it. Also, you may have to wait until the General Enrollment Period (from January 1 to March 31) to enroll in Part B, and coverage will start July 1 of that year.

The late enrollment penalty for **Part D** is an amount added to your Part D monthly premium. You may owe a late enrollment penalty if you go without Part D or "creditable prescription drug coverage" for any continuous period of 63 days or more after your Initial Enrollment Period is over. Creditable coverage refers to drug coverage through a current or former employer or union that is at least as good as the Medicare drug benefits. See *Chapter 11 Appendix: Medicare Part D Prescription Drug Late Enrollment Penalty* regarding the calculation of the penalty.[155]

Once you have Medicare you need to know how it coordinates with any other health insurance you may have. Is it primary (first to pay) or secondary (second to pay)? *See website Chapter 11 Appendix: Is Medicare primary or secondary?* In our following discussion we'll assume it is the primary coverage.

---

154   See also https://medicare.com/about-medicare/medicare-late-enrollment-penalties/
155   See also www.medicare.gov/part-d/costs/penalty/part-d-late-enrollment-penalty.html

Medicare has Limitations in Hospital Coverage

The limitations are based on the concepts of a "Benefit Period" and "Lifetime Reserve Days". A Benefit Period starts when you are admitted to a hospital if you have been out of a hospital or skilled nursing facility for 60 days. It lasts for a period of 90 days during which **Part A** pays hospital expenses either completely or partially. Beyond 90 days, you can draw on a total of 60 reserve days that can be used during your lifetime as additional days that Medicare will pay all covered costs except for a daily coinsurance[156]. If you go into a hospital or a Skilled Nursing Facility after one benefit period has ended, a new benefit period begins. You must pay the inpatient hospital deductible for each Benefit Period. There's no limit to the number of Benefit Periods.[157] During 2017, for each Benefit Period there is a $1,316 deductible. After this deductible, Medicare pays fully for hospital days 1-60 and no coinsurance is needed. However, for Days 61-90 there is a $329 coinsurance per day of each benefit period. For Days 91 and beyond there is a $658 coinsurance per each "Lifetime Reserve Day". As you can see, there is a substantial initial $1,316 deductible coupled with further daily accruals of costs after hospital day 60. Thus, a 90-day hospital stay could generate a deductible plus uncovered coinsurance financial exposure of **$11,186** per Benefit Period. Now that you have an idea of potential financial exposure, *it is clearly in your interest to consider having supplemental or secondary or Medigap medical coinsurance that can pay these potential expenses!* You need to be aware that there are different types of supplemental insurance. [See *website Chapter 11 Appendix: Medicare Supplemental Insurance*].

Medicare Part B pays for a brief hospital stay in the Emergency Department or in another part of the hospital. This is referred to as *Medicare Outpatient Observation Services*, also called an *Observation Stay*. Although you may be physically on an inpatient unit, you are considered to be an outpatient and in this status the hospital services are paid for by Part B (not Part A). Observation Services have three characteristics. First, they are given to help your doctor decide if you need to be admitted as an inpatient or discharged. Second, they are given in the emergency department or another inpatient area of the hospital. Third, the services usually last 48 hours or less.

Medicare has Limitations in Skilled Nursing Facility (SNF) coverage

It's important to understand the term "skill". Let's start by clarifying some basic concepts concerning *Skilled* Nursing Facility (SNF) coverage. According to Medicare[158] *"skilled care"* is provided by Nursing,

---

156   Some health insurance terminology: Deductible is what you pay each year before your insurance begins to pay. After you pay any deductibles, Coinsurance is what you pay for health care services or prescriptions usually as a percentage (e.g., 20%). Copayment is usually a set amount rather than a percentage that you pay for health care services or prescriptions (e.g. $10 or $20 for a doctor's visit or prescription).

157   See also www.medicare.gov/glossary/b.html

158   See: www.medicare.gov/HomeHealthCompare/Resources/Glossary.html

Physical Therapy, Occupational Therapy, and Speech Therapy. In addition to providing direct care these professionals manage, observe, and evaluate your care. *"Skilled nursing care"* is given or supervised by registered nurses. Nurses provide direct care; manage, observe, and evaluate a patient's care; and teach the patient and his or her family caregiver. Examples include: giving IV drugs, shots, or tube feedings; changing dressings; and teaching about diabetes care. Finally, a *"Skilled Nursing Facility"* has the staff and equipment to give skilled nursing care and, in most cases, skilled rehabilitative services and other related health services. With this understanding of "skill" we can now turn to Medicare coverage in the SNF setting.

Medicare covers up to 100 days of SNF care per spell of illness under several stringent conditions. You must enter the SNF within 30 days of a hospital stay that lasted at least 3 days. The nursing home care must be for the same condition as the hospital stay. However, it could also be for a condition that started while you were getting care in the SNF for a hospital-related medical condition. An example would be getting an infection requiring antibiotics while continuing to recover from a stroke that was originally treated in hospital. The Medicare coverage is applicable both to patients that are expected to recover or improve from their conditions as well as those where the goal is to prevent or slow deterioration and maintain the beneficiary at the maximum practicable level of function. Thus, assuming the post-hospital criteria are met, the critical additional factor is *not* the beneficiary's restoration potential but whether *skilled care* is required along with the underlying reasonableness and necessity of the specific services themselves.[159]

There are important co-payments. Medicare covers 100% of the costs for days 1-20 for each Benefit Period. For days 21-100 there is a co-payment ($164.50 per day in 2017). After day 100, you are responsible for all costs.[160] Thus, a 100-day SNF stay generates a potential coinsurance or personal financial exposure of **$13,160** per Benefit Period. With this financial exposure in mind, *it is clearly in your interest to consider having a separate Long-term Care medical insurance policy that can pay these potential expenses! [See Chapter 11 Appendix: Long-term Care Insurance]*

Medicare has Sharp Limitations in Dental Coverage

Dental care can be expensive and is largely *excluded* from Medicare coverage. "Currently, Medicare will pay for dental services that are an integral part either of a covered procedure (e.g., reconstruction of the jaw following accidental injury), or for extractions done in preparation for radiation treatment for neoplastic diseases involving the jaw. Medicare will also make payment for oral examinations, but not treatment, preceding kidney transplantation or heart valve replacement, under certain circumstances".[161] Thus, again

159 In 2013 the settlement of a federal lawsuit (*Jimmo v. Sibelius*) confirmed that skilled care may be necessary to improve a patient's current condition, to maintain the patient's current condition, or to prevent or slow further deterioration of the patient's conditions. This applies in SNF, Home Health and Outpatient Therapy settings. See details in: (1) www.cms.gov/medicare/medicare-fee-for-service-payment/SNFPPS/downloads/jimmo-factsheet.pdf; (2) www.cms.gov/Medicare/Medicare-Fee-for-Service-Payment/SNFPPS/Downloads/jimmo_fact_sheet2_022014_final.pdf
160 See also www.medicare.gov/coverage/skilled-nursing-facility-care.html
161 See www.cms.gov/Medicare/Coverage/MedicareDentalCoverage/index.html?redirect=/MedicareDentalCoverage/

it is clearly in your interest to have a separate Dental Insurance policy that can cover many routine dental services on an outpatient basis. Further information about dental insurance is available online. [162]

Medicare has good coverage for Home care

Medicare pays for home health care if: (1) you are homebound; (2) need skilled nursing care on an intermittent basis; (3) your doctor certifies that you meet these two requirements; and (4) you receive your care from a Medicare-certified home health agency. To be homebound means that: leaving your home isn't recommended because of your condition; your condition keeps you from leaving home without help (such as using a wheelchair or walker, needing special transportation, or getting help from another person); and leaving home takes a considerable and taxing effort. [163] Coverage includes skilled nursing services and home health services; skilled therapy services (e.g., speech, physical and occupational therapies); certain medical supplies (e.g., catheters); certain types of durable medical equipment (e.g., wheelchair or walker). There is no prior hospital stay requirement for home health care for Part B coverage and there is no deductible or coinsurance for these covered home services. The home services can continue as long as you continue to qualify for such care. However, a new plan of care is needed from your doctor every 60 days. Further information is available online. [164]

Medicare has good coverage for outpatient Rehabilitation services

These services include Physical Therapy, Speech-Language Pathology and Occupational Therapy [165]. In 2018 Congress permanently repealed Medicare's long-standing annual dollar caps for these services. Now vulnerable patients will be protected from an arbitrary limit on how much Medicare will pay for needed therapy [166]. Regarding Physical Therapy: "Medicare covers evaluation and treatment for injuries and diseases that change your ability to function, or to maintain current function or slow decline, when your doctor or other health care provider certifies your need for it" [167]. So-called "hard caps" are now replaced with flexible "thresholds". Just as in the previous payment system, the new system doesn't separate physical therapy from speech-language pathology in establishing thresholds. In 2018 the two annual threshold limits are $2,010

---

162   Such as: www.fairhealthconsumer.org/
163   See www.medicareinteractive.org/get-answers/medicare-covered-services/home-healthservices/the-homebound-requirement
164   See: (1) www.medicareinteractive.org/page2.php?topic=counselor&page=script&script_id=66 ; (2) www.medicare.gov/Pubs/pdf/10969.pdf
165   https://press.aarp.org/2018-2-9-AARP-Praises-Several-Health-Care-Provisions-Budget-Bill
166   https://press.aarp.org/2018-2-9-AARP-Praises-Several-Health-Care-Provisions-Budget-Bill
167   See: (1) **Medicare & You 2019** The Official U.S. Government Medicare Handbook; p. 43;(2) https://www.medicare.gov/pubs/pdf/10988-Medicare-Limits-Therapy-Services.pdf; (3) http://www.apta.org/PTinMotion/News/2018/02/16/BudgetDeal5Things/

and $3,000 for physical therapy and speech-language pathology therapy combined and the same amounts for Occupational Therapy alone. If total therapy costs reach the lower amount, Medicare requires your provider to confirm that your therapy is medically necessary. When therapy reaches $3,000, it's subject to possible targeted medical review. If Medicare denies coverage because it finds your care is not medically necessary, you can appeal. Note that this information only applies if you have Original Medicare. If you have a Medicare Advantage Plan (like an HMO or PPO), check with your plan for information about your plan's coverage rules on these therapy services.

Medicare has good coverage for Mental Health services

Outpatient coverage has no limits as long as the services are medically necessary. Inpatient psychiatric hospitalization in a general hospital is covered in the same manner as other Part A hospital admissions discussed above. If care is given in a specialized free-standing psychiatric hospital, there is a limit of 190 days over one's lifetime. Additional coverage includes Partial Hospitalization programs that offer intensive psychiatric treatment on an outpatient basis. Psychiatric patients are eligible for Home Health services if they require skilled care on a part-time or intermittent basis and are confined to the home even if they have no physical limitations. Treatment of alcoholism and substance use disorders are covered in both inpatient and outpatient settings. Medicare has a history of treating mental health services at lower levels of reimbursement than other health services and this has likely discouraged patients from seeking these services. However, this has changed and as of 2014, Medicare pays outpatient mental health services at the same 80 percent of approved charges as other Part B services. Be aware that not all psychiatrists, clinical psychologists, social workers or other mental health providers participate in Medicare. Thus, it is important to verify that your clinician does participate so your expenses will be covered for their Part B services. Additional details are available online.[168]

Medicare has good coverage for Hospice care

Hospice is not just for cancer. Rather it is a program where treatment is for *comfort and not for cure* and where life expectancy is *less than 6 months*. When a person chooses hospice care, they have decided that they no longer want care to cure their terminal illness and/or their doctor has determined that efforts

---

168   See also: (1) www.cms.gov/Outreach-and-Education/Medicare-Learning-Network-MLN/MLNProducts/Downloads/Mental-Health-Services-Text-Only.pdf; (2) www.medicareadvocacy.org/ medicare-info/medicare-coverage-of-mental-health-services/ #Clinician%20Coverage%20and%20Outpatient%20Mental%20 Health%20Services

to cure their illness aren't working. The care is usually given in the home but can also be covered in a hospice inpatient facility. In recent years there have been large increases in hospice use among patients with noncancer terminal conditions, such as heart failure and dementia, and patients living in nursing homes [1]. The same source notes that more than 25% of people dying in the United States die in nursing homes. Furthermore, a recent article [2] indicates that "The landscape of hospice providers in the United States has changed, from small not-for-profit providers to increasingly for-profit hospice chains. The percentage of persons receiving hospice care in a nursing home tripled from 14% of Medicare decedents in 1999 to nearly 40% in 2009."

The hospice care plan is constructed and implemented by a hospice team headed by a physician. The care is coordinated by a Medicare-certified hospice agency. The patient has signed a form indicating their desire for palliative care such as pain management rather than care to try to cure their condition. Details of the available services are described by Medicare.[169] The potential duration of Hospice Care is two 90-day hospice benefit periods followed by an unlimited number of 60-day benefit periods. Several situations come to mind. First, if you live more than 6 months, you can still get hospice care as long as you are still terminally ill. Second, while you have hospice, you can still get coverage for treatment of all conditions unrelated to the terminal condition. That is, there can be *curative* treatment of conditions *unrelated* to the terminal illness. Third, you can end hospice at any time and get curative care for your terminal illness. Further, you can later choose hospice care again as long as you continue to meet the eligibility requirements. Additional details of these benefits and situations are available online.[170]

Medicare has limited coverage for Respite care

Respite means a rest and that's what respite care allows the caregiver to take. Respite care is for the direct benefit of the caregivers to give them a "short break" so they can reduce the stresses of giving long-term care in the home. It is of benefit to the patient in that it can avoid or delay out-of-home placements and maintain ongoing relationships with medical providers. Medicare covers respite care for the caregiver if your loved one has a life-threatening illness *and qualifies for the hospice benefit*. Thus, Respite and Hospice care are linked. This benefit can occur in an approved hospital or skilled nursing facility for up to five days at a time. Medicare will pay 95 percent of the approved charges for respite care.[171] The important limitation here is that the patient must first be in the Hospice program. It's worth noting that when Long-term Care Insurance covers respite care it is often separated from a Hospice Care requirement.

---

169 See: www.medicare.gov/coverage/hospice-and-respite-care.html
170 See: www.medicareinteractive.org/page2.php?topic=counselor&page=script&toc_id=64
171 See: www.medicareinteractive.org/page2.php?topic=counselor&page=script&script_id=1293

Medicare has good coverage for Preventive and Screening services

Health services are more than just treatment of illness. They include wellness and prevention approaches which also address modification of risk factors for disease. We review this topic so you are aware of it if you or loved ones have Medicare Part B or so you can compare it with a different primary health insurance you may have. The coverage includes a yearly "Wellness" visit during which your doctor will develop or update a personalized prevention plan to help prevent disease and disability based on your current health and risk factors. Among the usual outcomes of the visit is a list of risk factors and treatment options for you as well as a screening schedule for appropriate preventive services. Further details are available online.[172]

In addition to the Wellness visit there are some 23 areas of specific screenings that can occur at any time. Many of these items can be done annually though for some there are multi-year intervals (e.g., cervical and vaginal cancer screening; colonoscopy screening; bone mass density). The targeted areas include four main categories.[173]

- Screenings for *early detection of cancer* such as: cervical & vaginal cancer; colorectal cancer, prostate cancer; and breast cancer.

- Screenings for *non-cancerous diseases* such as: abdominal aortic aneurysm; cardiovascular disease; alcohol misuse; depression; diabetes; Hepatitis C; HIV; sexually transmitted infections; obesity; bone density measurement; and glaucoma tests

- *Vaccinations* that include: Flu shots; Hepatitis B shots; and Pneumococcal pneumonia shots

- *Educational services* that include: Nutrition therapy: Diabetes self-management training; and tobacco use cessation counseling

Medicare has Limited Geographic Coverage of Telemedicine Services

Medicare covers telemedicine by multiple providers but with several important restrictions. The patient must reside in a medically underserved (often rural) area. The patient must receive the services at specified medical facilities but not in their home. For those who are eligible, the list of providers and services is quite broad and coverage includes robust mental health services. See website *Chapter 11 Appendix: Medicare Coverage of Telemedicine Services* for further information.

---

172 See: www.medicare.gov/coverage/preventive-visit-and-yearly-wellness-exams.html
173 For further details see: www.medicare.gov/coverage/preventive-and-screening-services.html

Medicare has Good Coverage for Second Surgical Opinions

_____

Medicare will cover a second opinion concerning non-emergency surgery. It will also cover a third opinion if the first and second opinions disagree. The surgery must be medically necessary to diagnose or treat a condition. Some surgical procedures such as strictly cosmetic surgery are not covered as they may not be viewed as medically necessary. [174]

Medicare has Excellent Coverage for End-of-Life Counseling

_____

Beginning in 2016, Medicare will cover this counseling. It may occur during an annual wellness visit or during any other visit. There are no pre-determined numbers of times the counseling may occur as it is recognized that health status may change and related counseling may be appropriate. [175]

Housing and Living Arrangements

_____

Independent Living—Aging in Place

There is the understandable desire to remain in one's home of choice for as long as possible. As infirmities or illnesses occur, the availability of Home Care services from your health insurance is critical and already discussed above. There are other threats that need attention with the most prominent one being the avoidance of falls in your home. The possibility of injuring yourself by taking a fall in or around your home can be reduced by a variety of home modifications [3] [4] such as the following:

- Indoor changes include: handrails for inside stairs; accessible light switches at both ends of stairs; grab rails for bathrooms and toilets; keeping areas free of electric cords on which one could trip; improving indoor lighting including adequate night-lights; eliminating throw rugs; fixing lifted edges of carpets and mats; nonskid flooring; non-slip bathmats; walk-in bathtubs; and electric stairlifts.

_____

174 See: www.medicareinteractive.org/planning-for-medicare=and-securing-quality-care/medicare-and-second-opinions
175 See: http://www.nytimes.com/2015/07/09/health/medicare-proposes-paying-doctors-for-end-of-life-counseling.html?_r=0; www.abcnews.go.com/Health/wireStory/medicare-cover-end-life-counseling-34863650

- Outdoor changes include: handrails for outside steps; high-visibility and slip-resistant edging for outside steps; adequate outside lighting; slip-resistant surfacing for outside surfaces such as decks; and ramps for easier entry and exit. Safety can be further enhanced with smart-home technologies for medical alert systems to call for help should an accident (including a fall) or a medical emergency occur.[176]

Assisted Living Facilities and Retirement Communities

There are stand-alone housing facilities such as Assisted Living Facilities. Their services can include: supervision or assistance with activities of daily living, administration or supervision of medication, and monitoring of resident activities as well as coordination of care by outside health care providers. Such care is appropriate if you cannot safely live independently but don't need 24-hour medical care and are too young to live in a retirement community. Be aware that Medicare will not pay for a facility that provides custodial and personal care services (such as meals and assistance with bathing and dressing) but does not provide skilled nursing or therapy services.

The most comprehensive care is the blended arrangement found in Continuing Care Retirement Communities (CCRCs). They contain all levels of care from Independent Living with occasional services if needed to Assisted Living with regular services as needed and finally to Nursing Home for highest level of ongoing assistance. As described by Medicare,[177] CCRCs "are retirement communities that offer more than one kind of housing and different levels of healthcare. In the same community, there may be individual homes or apartments for people who still live on their own, an assisted living facility for people who need some help with daily care, and a nursing home for those who require higher levels of care. Residents move from one level to another based on their needs, but usually stay within the CCRC. If you're considering a CCRC, be sure to check the quality of the nursing home. Your CCRC contract usually requires you to use the CCRC's nursing home if you need nursing home care. Some CCRC's will only admit people into their nursing home if they've previously lived in another section of the retirement community, like their assisted living or an independent area. Many CCRCs generally require a large payment before you move in (called an "entry fee") and charge monthly fees."

We have friends who are in their 60's and early 70's who are in reasonably good health but who are anticipating this won't last forever. They have entered waiting lists for Independent Living facilities in Retirement Communities—often a 5+ year wait while they remain in their community. They view this as "preparation" and creating "options" for future needs. We salute such anticipatory coping and bring it to your attention to see if their approach might also work for you.

---

176 See reviews and comparisons: (1) www.consumerreports.org/cro/2014/06/what-to-look-for-in-a-medical-alert-system/index.htm; (2) www.consumeraffairs.com/medical-alert-systems/
177 See: www.medicare.gov/what-medicare-covers/part-a/other-long-term-care-choices.html#collapse-4920

PACE (Program of All-inclusive Care for the Elderly)

PACE is a comprehensive Medicare program and Medicaid state option for older adults living with disabilities. This program provides community-based care and services to people who otherwise need nursing home level of care. It is only available in states that offer PACE under Medicaid. There are 114 PACE Programs operating in 32 states as of January 2015. You can have either Medicare or Medicaid, or both, to join PACE. To qualify for PACE, you must: be 55 or older; live in the service area of a PACE organization; need a nursing home-level of care (as certified by your state); and be able to live safely in the community with help from PACE. If you don't have Medicare or Medicaid, you can pay for PACE privately. The program is quite comprehensive. See online details of program health coverage and costs as well as to check if your state offers this program. [178]

Communicating Your Wishes if You are Seriously Ill

The Conversation Project

As we get old we face the knowledge that our life will end someday. If we are young but seriously ill we also may need to confront death. It is important that in facing end-of-life issues we are able to communicate our wishes for our care to health professionals and to our friends and family. The ***Conversation Project***, co-founded by Pulitzer Prize winner Ellen Goodman, is a public engagement campaign with the goal of making sure that every person's wishes for end-of-life care are expressed and respected. The Conversation Project offers people the tools, guidance and resources they need to begin talking with their loved ones, around the kitchen table, about their wishes and preferences. The Conversation Project does not promote any specific preference for end-of-life care; instead, it seeks to encourage and support people in expressing their own individual end-of-life wishes for care.[179] It gives guidance in terms of suggesting questions you may want to think and talk about and ways to get comfortable communicating your wishes. You can download "Your Conversation Starter Kit" where you fill out your answers to nine questions concerning your care that give you a wide degree of choices to stimulate your thinking on these issues. There is also A Starter Kit designed to help parents of seriously ill children who want guidance about "having the conversation" with their children. The Conversations may start with Health and End-of-Life issues but can also expand to conversations about Legal and Financial issues.[180]

---

178 See: (1) https://www.medicare.gov/your-medicare-costs/get-help-paying-costs/pace (2) www.npaonline.org/website/article.asp?id=12&title=Who,_What_and_Where_Is_PACE?; (3) www.npaonline.org/website/download.asp?id=2378&title=Quick_Facts_about_PACE_(CMS_Publication)
179 See: (1) http://theconversationproject.org/; (2) http:// http://theconversationprojectinboulder.org/starter-kit/
180 See: www.n4a.org/files/Conversations.pdf

Five Wishes

Five Wishes is an easy to use legal document written in everyday language that lets adults of all ages plan how they want to be cared for in case they become seriously ill. It is America's most popular *living will.* It is accepted by most states (except for eight) as a legal document. It is unique in speaking to all a person's needs: medical; personal; emotional; and spiritual. In addition to family, it is used for communication with doctors and hospitals and can be purchased online at minimal expense.[181] The five wishes are given below. Wishes 1 and 2 are legal documents in most states once the document is signed.

- **Wish 1:** The person I want to make health care decisions for me when I can't
- **Wish 2:** The kind of medical treatment I want or don't want
- **Wish 3:** How comfortable I want to be
- **Wish 4:** How I want people to treat me
- **Wish 5:** What I want my loved ones to know

The Five Wishes and The Conversation Project are complementary to each other and we recommend that *both* be used.

---

181 See: (1) https://fivewishes.org; (2) https://fivewishes.org/shop/shop

Chapter 11 Appendix

Medicare Advantage Plans

These plans are offered by private companies that Medicare approves. There are many types of Advantage Plans. Medicare identifies 6 categories of these Plans[182]:

- Health Maintenance Organization (HMO) Plans
- Preferred Provider Organization (PPO) Plans
- Private Fee-for Service (PFFS) Plans
- Special Needs Plans (SNPs)
  There are other less common types of Medicare Advantage Plans that may be available:
- HMO Point of Service (HMOPOS) Plans: An HMO Plan that may allow you to get some services out-of-network for a higher cost.
- Medical Savings Account (MSA) Plans: A plan that combines a high deductible health plan with a bank account. Medicare deposits money into the account (usually less than the deductible). You can use the money to pay for your health care services during the year

Some important differences between the categories include: can you get health care from any doctor, other health care provider, or hospital; are prescription drugs covered; must you choose a primary care doctor; do you have to get a referral to see a specialist. Further guidance on comparing costs and coverages within and across these different Advantage Plans is available from consumer groups [183] as well as from insurance consultants.

Medicare Part D Prescription Drug Late Enrollment Penalty

The cost of the late enrollment penalty depends on how long you went without Part D or creditable prescription drug coverage. Medicare calculates the penalty by multiplying 1% of the "national base beneficiary premium" ($35.63 in 2017) times the number of full, uncovered months you didn't have Part D or creditable coverage. The monthly premium is rounded to the nearest $.10 and added to your monthly Part D premium. The national base beneficiary premium may increase each year, so your penalty amount may also increase each year. The late enrollment penalty can be avoided if you: join a Medicare Prescription Drug Plan when you're first eligible; don't go 63 days or more in a row without a Medicare drug plan or other creditable drug coverage; tell your Medicare Drug Plan about your creditable drug coverage.

---

182   See: https://www.medicare.gov/sign-up-change-plans/types-of-medicare-health-plans/medicare-advantage-plans
183   For example, see: www.consumerreports.org/cro/news/2014/10/medigap-vs-medicare-advantage-consumer-reports/index.htm

Long-term Care Insurance

Long-term care is the assistance needed over an extended period of time to *manage rather than cure* a chronic condition such as arthritis, a stroke, dementia, frailties of aging, recovery from surgery or an accident. Care could be needed for weeks, months, or years. This care is often not well-covered by other health insurance policies. Long-term Care Insurance is quite variable in coverage features. Costs for similar coverages may vary considerably between different insurance companies. Coverage may typically include Home & Community-based care benefits (e.g., Home care; Adult Day Care Center); assisted living; respite care; hospice care; nursing home and Alzheimer's facilities. Other services covered may include Caregiver training and Care management (i.e., designing a Plan of Care meeting long-term care needs). There may be coverage for durable medical equipment such as: walkers; wheelchairs; hospital beds; infusion pumps; grab bars; ramps to permit movement from one level of residence to another. Two typical clinical requirements to activate covered benefits include: (1) a person is chronically ill or has a loss of functional capacity that is expected to last at least 90+ days; (2) assessment shows an inability to perform 2 or more Activities of Daily Living (ADLs) or that the disability is due to Severe Cognitive Impairment. ADLs include: Bathing; Continence; Dressing; Eating (Feeding); Toileting; Transferring (in/out of chair or bed). Not all long-term care insurance policies cover all of these services nor do they all pay the same for similar services. It is best to study several different plans with a professional advisor who can help you understand the costs, services, benefits and limits of different available coverages. Keep in mind that the younger you purchase this particular insurance the less expensive it will be. It is important to assess the value of such a policy to fill healthcare gaps left by other insurances such as Medicare. Further information is available online. [184]

Chapter 11 Key Points

Key Points: Insurance Penalties & Coverage Limitations

- Are there penalties for later adding coverage options that were available earlier?
- What limitations are there concerning:
    - Hospital inpatient days
    - Skilled Nursing Facility days
    - Home care services
    - Dental services
    - Prescription drug coverage
    - Mental Health services
    - Outpatient Rehabilitation services (Physical Therapy; Speech & Language; Occupational Therapy)
    - Respite Care
    - Hospice Care
    - Prevention & Screening services
    - Telemedicine services

---

184 For example, see helpful discussions in: (1) American Association for Long-term Care Insurance (www.aaltci.org/); (2) www.consumeraffairs.com/insurance/ltc.html; (3) www.guidetolongtermcare.com/whatisltc.htmlml; (4) http://member.aarp.org/health/health-insurance/info-06-2012/understanding-long-term-care-insurance.html ; (5) www.guidetolongtermcare.com/whatisltc.html

o Second Surgical opinions

o End of Life counseling

- If Respite and Hospice care covered

  o What are the limitations on number of days for these services?

Key Points: Potential Medicare Uncovered Institutional Expenses

- If your only insurance is Medicare, there are substantial financial exposures. For example:
- Hospital: A 90-day stay exposes you to $11,186
- Skilled Nursing Facility: A 100-day stay exposes you to $13,160

Key Points: Independent Living

- Are you safe in your home?

  o Fall prevention modifications

  o Medical alert systems

  o Is transportation available

- Do you have Home Care services if needed?
- Are you eligible for the Programs of All-Inclusive Care for the Elderly (PACE) in your state to help you to continue living in the community?

Key Points: Communicating Your Wishes

- Have you downloaded, read and completed the Conversation Project starter kit?
- Have you considered the other important topics beyond health issues?

  o End-of-life issues

  o Legal issues

  o Financial issues

- Have you started the conversations?
- Have you expressed your Five Wishes?

References

1. Hamel, M.B., *Investing in better care for patients dying in nursing homes.* New England Journal of Medicine, 2015. **372**(19): p. 1858-9.

2. Gozalo, P., et al., *Changes in Medicare costs with the growth of hospice care in nursing homes.* New England Journal of Medicine, 2015. **372**(19): p. 1823-31.

3. Robinovitch, S.N., V. Scott, and F. Feldman, *Home-safety modifications to reduce injuries from falls.* Lancet, 2015. **385**(9964): p. 205-6.

4. Keall, M.D., et al., *Home modifications to reduce injuries from falls in the home injury prevention intervention (HIPI) study: a cluster-randomised controlled trial.* Lancet, 2015. **385**(9964): p. 231-8.

Your Rights as a Patient

David, a bright twenty-one-year-old recent college graduate, was driving alone across the country to begin a job with a high-technology company when he began acting strangely while having lunch in a diner. The owner observed him talking to imaginary objects on the ceiling. Emergency medics were called. David was evaluated at a nearby emergency room and admitted to the hospital's psychiatric unit, where, of course, no one knew him. He was frightened, reclusive, and paranoid. But his doctors thought he was competent when he adamantly refused to give the hospital staff permission to contact his parents (their information was in his wallet) or to cooperate with a urine drug screen test for drug abuse. David had never completed a Health Insurance Portability and Accountability Act (HIPAA) form.

His doctors' diagnosis was either paranoid schizophrenia or drug-related psychosis. While being observed for the following two days and awaiting the results of a urine test, he finally cooperated and his parents learned about his hospitalization. They were understandably frustrated when David's doctor explained that he could not verify that David was in the hospital or discuss his condition because of the HIPAA rules. Fortunately, there was no restriction that prevented David's parents from revealing that their son had been hospitalized once before from an overdose of cocaine. David's successful treatment finally began on the fourth hospital day. He was discharged two days later under his parents' care. If David had a HIPAA form stored in his smartphone that permitted information to be shared with his parents, or if he had given verbal permission for his doctors to talk with his parents, his treatment and recovery would have proceeded more quickly.

Moral of this true-life story: Although HIPAA forms are usually filled out by those in their forties and fifties, and even later in life, it's reassuring to have even younger family members complete this document and store it in their smartphones or other electronic device along with their personal health record (PHR). This information can be carried on their person and be easily accessible in emergency situations.

It's been estimated that 75 percent of adult Americans have never filled out a simple document, such as HIPAA, to permit their doctors to talk with family members should they become ill. Most Americans haven't completed a healthcare directive (living will) that provides direction to their doctor and other health professionals regarding how they would wish to be treated or not treated were they to become terminally ill. Without such documents, doctors can be left perplexed and struggling to figure out what their patients' wishes/preferences are [1]. Family members can become mired in arguments and conflict trying to second guess end-of-life preferences when this could be avoided if four crucially important legal documents are completed. We will discuss these documents in detail.

The main reason for putting off completing the four essential documents is an understandable tendency to avoid coming to grips with being mortal and accepting the fact that our lives are time-limited [2]. When we're middle-age we're reminded of our mortality when observing our parents and grandparents aging and our friends looking older. Denial of our own aging may make us more vulnerable to undue risks and accidents.[185] Nonetheless, we tell ourselves there's ample time to get our late-life affairs in order. Those of us fortunate to reach our seventies and eighties realize how much more quickly time is passing and how it is imperative to get our late-life responsibilities in order. But it's not easy to deal with such emotionally-laden issues.

A second reason for procrastinating is because some of us put complete faith in our health professionals and assume they know what we would want done if seriously ill even though we've never discussed it or completed the necessary documents. When we need medical care, we assume and trust that the hospital, doctor, and other health professionals will always act in our best interest. This is illustrated by the following situation. Susan, a sixty-four-year-old retired journalist, experienced abdominal pain, dizziness, and weakness while visiting family and friends in California. She was admitted to a nearby hospital and was asked to sign reams of legal forms – agreement to be admitted and consent for diagnostic tests and specific treatments. She had never bothered to fill out the four central legal documents to be discussed shortly or a PHR. She figured that her illness was serious enough to warrant hospitalization. And she assumed that her doctor and other hospital staff knew what was best for her, so she didn't ask any questions. She was frightened, not clear headed, and nervous about what was going to happen next. Susan felt pressured to sign all the forms quickly so her doctor and nurses could get on with things. And she assumed that what she signed was in her best interest.

Susan's rights as a patient entitled her to a complete explanation of the consent forms, one of which was for exploratory abdominal surgery (a laparotomy). Fortunately, she took the time to ask her trusted family member and advocate, who accompanied her to the hospital, for her opinion about surgery. She knew she had the right to ask questions and have her doctor explain and summarize the forms, but she was understandably upset and preoccupied. Her advocate encouraged Susan to ask questions of the doctor, and the advocate also posed questions until both were satisfied that they fully understood all the benefits and risks of surgery and anesthesia. The surgeon removed an early stage colon cancer, and Susan recovered quickly and is alive and well five years later.

In this chapter, we'll discuss beneficial and constructive ways to complete each of the four important legal documents, ways of ensuring that your end-of-life wishes will be respected and carried out, and how to help your family accept and carry out your wishes. *Sample documents are available in this chapter's website appendix.* We discuss the rights we all have as patients, the benefits of having a healthcare advocate, strategies for preventing an impaired elderly parent from driving, and the ongoing controversy of a terminally ill patient's right for physician-assisted aid in dying.

---

185   350,000 Americans fall and break a hip: M. Gillick, The Denial of Aging: Perpetual Youth, Eternal Life, and Other Dangerous Fantasies (Harvard University Press, 2006).

The Four Important Legal Documents

The four legal documents that are crucially important to complete include:

- The HIPAA – Health Insurance Portability and Accountability Act of 2003.
- The POLST – Physician Orders for Life-Sustaining Treatment or the MOST – Medical Orders for Scope of Treatment (or similar form specific to your state).
- Healthcare Directive (also called living will).
- Power of attorney for making healthcare decisions (healthcare proxy) and financial decisions (financial proxy).

Please keep in mind that the state where you live has variations and different titles for some of these four documents. Although the POLST (used in California) and the MOST (used in New Mexico and Colorado) may be similar to forms used in your state, we suggest using documents specific to your state because the healthcare and legal systems are more familiar with your state's documents. Documents specific for your state can be downloaded from the Internet.[186]

Suggestions for Filling Out These Four Documents and Follow Through

See examples of the forms on our website Chapter 12 Appendices.

- It's best to complete all these documents when you are healthy and clearheaded.
- After reviewing the instructions for filling out these documents, discuss questions you have with your doctor, especially the POLST, MOST, or similar form. Most states require the POLST to be filled out and signed by both you and your physician.
- Consider reviewing all the forms with your lawyer, even though it is not required.
- Most importantly, sit down with your family, healthcare and financial teams, and your proxies to explain what your true wishes are regarding end-of-life medical, financial, and other decisions so they can work together effectively should they one day need to make decisions on your behalf. Encourage your family to express their feelings about your wishes, be patient in answering their questions and possible objections, and help them understand how important it is for your wishes to be respected. If some family members have strong opposing views, it's far better to have these feelings expressed in the present so you can explain your reasons rather than have family members bicker and quarrel in front of your doctor and hospital staff while you're coping with a serious illness. If a face-to-face meeting with everyone is impractical, send everyone a letter with the pertinent documents and encourage their reactions and questions. For more suggestions about these family issues, *see "The Conversation" in Chapter 11.*

---

186   https://www.everplans.com/articles/state-by-state-polst-forms.

- Make certain that there is consistency among the various documents to avoid misunderstanding among your doctors, lawyer, and those you've given responsibility for carrying out your wishes.

- When all the legal forms are completed, make certain that everyone involved receives a copy.

- Review these documents every two to three years, or sooner should your late-life preferences change as you get older (and wiser!), or you decide to change the person(s) serving as your proxies (for healthcare and financial decisions), or you make other changes.

- If you make changes in one or more of these documents, make sure that everyone involved replaces the old documents(s) with the new one(s).

- Completing these documents sets a good example for your family and friends to carry out advance planning for themselves.

- Helping your doctor, family, and proxies understand and faithfully carry out your wishes lightens the burden on them and helps them work together as a team. It also alleviates potential guilt on your family's part wondering if they made the wrong decision because they are really honoring your wishes rather than having to figure out, without guidance from you, what your wishes are.

- Should you decide you want "comfort measures only" during the last phase of life, rather than aggressive measures to keep you alive at all costs with little likelihood of returning to a reasonable quality of life, you can avoid spending tens of thousands of dollars for days or weeks of emotional and physical discomfort in an intensive care unit [2] [3] or other medical setting.

- Should you decide on "comfort measures," learn about the benefits of palliative and hospice care [4].

- If you move to another state, you'll need to use state-specific forms and, if necessary, review documents with an attorney knowledgeable about state laws.

- Consider making a copy of all four documents and add them to your PHR in the electronic device you carry on your person in case of emergency situations. Figure out a way for only specified family members and your healthcare team to access your information.

Let's now discuss the first of these four crucially important documents – the HIPAA.

HIPAA – Health Insurance Portability and Accountability Act of 2003

This Congressional Act protects the privacy and confidentiality of your healthcare records. You can list on the HIPAA form to whom you give permission to review your medical records, such as your spouse and patient advocate, and specify what you don't want revealed (for example, past substance abuse). Please see our website for the HIPAA form. Doctors are very careful about disclosing medical information about you unless your HIPAA form lists persons who have permission or you've given permission verbally to your doctor [5].

John, a doctor, visited his long-time friend Mary, who had just been hospitalized. Mary's doctor looked rushed as he was leaving her hospital room when John asked for information about her condition. The doctor immediately darted back into her room to obtain verbal permission to talk with John because John was not listed on her HIPAA form. Had she not verbally given permission, either because she chose not to or was too incapacitated, her doctor would not, by law, have been able to discuss her condition. Also, recall twenty-one-year-old David's story at the beginning of this chapter.

HIPAA also allows you to inspect your past and current medical records. If you discover errors, you can request that your doctor consider making corrections.[187] HIPAA officially begins when you sign the form. You can specify the date you want your permission to end and periodically add or remove persons from the list who have permission to review your records and talk with your doctor(s). If you make changes on the HIPAA form, replace your previous one with the new document and distribute the new one to your doctor(s) and everyone involved.

The "Omnibus Rule" in 2013 extended protection of your health records under HIPAA in today's digital age, to the business associates of your doctors and medical facilities, such as software and computer company employees who have access to your confidential information.

The POLST – Physician Orders for Life-Sustaining Treatment

The POLST was originally developed in Oregon for patients to discuss with, and receive guidance from their physician about the extent of medical intervention they wanted or did not want should a patient become terminally ill. Please see our website for the POLST.

The POLST is much more than an order from; it should reflect diligent, individualized conversations between medical professionals and patients and their families. For each patient, a POLST is only as good as the conversation that precedes and accompanies its completion.[188]

All fifty states have documents similar to the POLST. In Colorado and New Mexico, for example, a document similar to the POLST is called the MOST (Medical Orders for Scope of Treatment). Other states refer to it as the MOLST, POST, COLST, and other names.

You can indicate on the form whether or not and to what extent you want extensive and aggressive medical measures instituted to keep you alive, such as cardiopulmonary resuscitation (CPR) and respiratory assistance on a ventilator, or selective treatment such as treating medical conditions but avoiding burdensome

---

187 https://www.hhs.gov/hipaa/for-professionals/privacy/guidance/access/.
188 Steinberg, K. On my mind. The Power of POLST in Caring for the Ages, Volume 18, p. 1-2, July, 2017.

measures such as CPR, or simply "comfort measures" such as pain meds, fluids for hydration, or suctioning for airway obstruction to ease the dying process.

Most states require that you discuss and complete the POLST (or similar form) with your doctor because, in essence, you are sharing and discussing ideas about what you want done or not done if you become seriously ill. If you never completed the POLST and currently lack the mental capacity to complete it, your legally recognized healthcare decision maker, such as your proxy or other designated person (depending on what state you live in) who is knowledgeable about your end-of-life wishes, can complete and sign the form on your behalf or verbally explain your wishes to your doctor. In most states, if you previously completed the POLST when you were younger and indicated that you wanted aggressive and extensive measures to keep you alive (for example, CPR) but are now much older, and let's say terminally ill and lack the mental capacity to change your POLST, your proxy or a legally qualified healthcare decision-maker who knows what your current wishes are (for example, "comfort measures") can complete a new POLST or verbally convey to your doctor your current preference.

Make a copy of the HIPAA and POLST (or similar document for your state) and keep a smaller size version in your wallet or as part of your PHR in your smartphone so you can carry it with you in case of an emergency. If you haven't executed an advance directive (living will), the POLST or similar document is a perfect option. You can type "POLST" or "MOST" into your Internet browser to obtain more information about the form used in your state.

If you have a valid, current POLST reflecting your current preferences, you can take it with you when you're discharged home from a hospital, nursing home, or other facility. Your POLST should also accompany you if you have to be re-admitted to the hospital where it is usually honored. You can display it in your home on your bedpost or your refrigerator door in case you are visited by an EMT following an acute medical event so the EMT knows your wishes. Also, send a copy to your PCPhys. You can also consider purchasing a metal bracelet or necklace with the letters DNR or DNI.

If you have never filled out an advance directive or POLST and are admitted to some type of medical facility, your doctor or staff member may give you a form similar to the POLST to specify whether or not and to what extent you want life-sustaining measures, such as CPR, should your heart or breathing suddenly stop. These forms are routinely given to all patients who are admitted without an advance directive or POLST, so don't perceive this as preparation for a dire outcome.

You have the prerogative of changing your POLST at any time because your preferences may change as you get older, but the new form has to be signed by you (and, in most states, your doctor).

Healthcare Advance Directive (Living Will)

This document is very similar to the POLST (or MOST) regarding your end-of-life preferences. In many states, you also designate who serves as your PCP and alternate in case your PCP is unavailable. The directive may also include a section to indicate whether or not you want to make an anatomical gift of some of your organs for transplant to a suitable recipient, for research or for medical student teaching. It's advisable, although optional, to have two witnesses indicate that they were present when you sign the advance directive.

Just as with the other two documents, you can revoke or change certain parts of your directive by completing a new form and distributing it to your PCPhys., lawyer, hospital, and proxies with instructions to replace your previous directive with the new one. Your preferences and wishes expressed in your advance directive and other two documents should concur with one another.

An excellent example of the importance of having an advance directive is demonstrated by Mrs. Simmons, a ninety-year-old retired college professor. At age eighty-six she suffered a stroke, causing an inability to express herself. Four years later, she was admitted to the hospital with a fractured hip, advanced cancer, and an inability to eat. Because she could not speak, her hospitalist misdiagnosed her as "demented." Her family pressured her doctor to insert a feeding tube, which she didn't want. A few days later, her advance directive (completed five years before her stroke) was found. It stated: "I do not want to be fed artificially if two physicians certify that I have an incurable illness, determine that death is imminent, and life-sustaining procedures would only artificially prolong the dying process." A physician consultant specializing in geriatrics was able to use hand signs to communicate with her and discovered she was not demented and had full capacity to make her own medical decisions. She was adamant about not wanting a feeding tube. Because she not only had an advance directive and was also capable of making decisions, her wishes were respected. Please refer to our website for an example of a healthcare directive.

Healthcare Power of Attorney (or Proxy)

This document, often part of the healthcare advance directive, designates the person and an alternate to make all healthcare decisions on your behalf should you lack the capacity to make these decisions. Your proxy will be responsible for making all healthcare decisions on your behalf unless you specifically limit the scope of decision-making (for example, not permitting your proxy to replace your PCPhys.). Should you regain the capacity to make healthcare decisions, you can revoke the decision-making role of your proxy.

States vary in their procedures for appointing and challenging default surrogates, the attributes they require of such persons, their priority ranking of possible decision makers, and dispute resolution [6]. In some states, if you haven't filled out the healthcare directive, you can simply tell your doctor who you've selected. But if you've never indicated your proxy either in writing or verbally and currently lack that capacity, laws in most states allow persons in somewhat the following order to make decisions on your behalf: 1) spouse; 2) significant other; 3) adult child; 4) parent; 5) adult sibling; 6) grandparent; 7) close friend. The laws about the order of persons assuming the role of your healthcare decision-maker, if you've never chosen someone, may differ in other states so use state-specific documents and consider legal advice.

You can revoke your advance directive, or change certain parts of it, at any time by completing a new form and promptly notifying and giving the new form to your PCPhys., lawyer, hospital, proxies, and all others involved. In New Mexico, you are required to sign the advance directive. It's advisable to have two witnesses sign.

The Responsibilities of Your Healthcare Proxy

Both your proxy and alternate need to be very knowledgeable about how you wish to be medically treated should you lack the capacity to make such decisions. They both need a copy of your HIPAA, POLST, advance directive, and healthcare proxy, which verifies their important role. Inform your doctor, family, and others about your proxy's role. If you haven't informed everyone and should you one day lack the capacity to make healthcare decisions, your proxy can provide the relevant documents so everyone involved understands his/her important responsibilities.

Should you become incapacitated and your proxy's responsibilities begin, he/she needs to establish good rapport with your physician(s), other health professionals, and your family and friends and keep up-to-date about your medical status so he/she can share this information with those listed on your HIPAA form.

The active role of your proxy is appreciated by your healthcare team because they can concentrate their efforts on getting you well and rely on your proxy to serve as their communicator with your family and friends.

Your proxy can be under considerable stress because he/she is dealing with his/her own emotions and reactions witnessing the ebbs and flows of your medical condition while tending to similar reactions of your family and friends. Your proxy needs to keep in mind that he/she is making decisions reflecting your wishes and not his/her own or those of your family members, especially if your family has opposing views. This may assuage some of your family's potential psychological anguish and guilt knowing that your proxy may need to make end-of-life decisions reflecting your wishes even though they may differ from those of some family members.

Who to Designate as Your Healthcare Proxy and Alternate

Even though your spouse is legally considered your next of kin and is often the person you select as your proxy, you can select anyone. You want someone who is readily accessible, stays calm and rational under stress, understands the complexity of the healthcare system, and is knowledgeable about your wishes regarding your healthcare, finances, and insurance coverage should decisions need to be made about post-hospital healthcare, such as rehabilitation, or nursing home care.

If you do not have a family member or friend to serve as your proxy, you can ask your attorney, your hospital's administrator, or a social worker for candidates (some available proxies are former health professionals) to interview. Learn about the candidate's experience and fees and determine how understanding and sensitive he/she is about your life story, values, current health problems and end-of-life preferences. In other words, determine how well he/she understands you as a person, who may have idiosyncrasies like most people! Take your time in selecting who you want as your proxy and alternate.

Consider what William, a healthy sixty-six-year-old widowed, successful estate-planning attorney did. He arranged a meeting with his attorney, financial and healthcare proxy, secretary, financial advisor, and his two sons and daughter to discuss his four healthcare and estate planning documents, as well as details of some of his financial assets and debts. The goal of the meeting was for everyone to understand and provide their input about how to best function as a cohesive healthcare and financial team should William ever become disabled.

Several constructive decisions resulted from this one-and-a-half-hour meeting. Everyone got to know one another and shared their telephone numbers and e-mails. It was decided that William's two adult sons and daughter, Nicole, would be added to William's checking account so incoming bills could be paid promptly if he became incapacitated and couldn't pay the bills. William's oldest son, Robert (also a lawyer), would serve as financial proxy and have permission to have access to William's safety deposit box. He was given keys to his father's home. Robert agreed to work closely with his father's attorney and financial advisor to assist in handling financial matters and, if necessary, his father's will. All three adult children were shown the location of their father's personal valuables, located in various places at home and a list and photographs of artwork with estimated values and advice about their disposal. William's daughter, Nicole, a medical researcher knowledgeable about the healthcare system, would serve as healthcare proxy.

William agreed to write a letter every two years or more often to his attorney, financial advisor, and his adult children that included information about any changes in his financial and health status, such as a change to a different PCPhys. or specialist, and any modifications in the four legal documents. If changes were made, all those involved would replace the former with the new documents.

Although you may think that this extensive planning is a bit over the top, compare this to John, an eighty-two-year-old retired grocery store owner who had not done any advance planning. His wife and three adult children had no knowledge of his end-of-life preferences, or the details of his finances. John's family suddenly learned that he was unconscious in the nearby hospital's ICU after suffering a massive brain hemorrhage. Since John had never completed any of the four legal documents, no one was healthcare proxy for making end-of-life decisions. Fortunately, the state where he lived had laws that permitted his spouse to make such decisions. Nevertheless, the family was in a quandary about what his wishes were. It took ten days and the assistance of the family's attorney to gain access to his bank account so bills could be paid. Family members quarreled about how aggressively they wanted the doctors to be to keep him alive. Finally, after two weeks in the intensive care unit and hospital bills over $300,000, which the family could not afford, his wife finally agreed with the doctors to institute hospice care because the extensive brain damage was irreversible.

Because there is no way of predicting when life may deal you a bad hand, is it far better for you and your family to follow some of the ways that William prepared for life's unpredictability? You may want, as William did, to have your designated healthcare and financial team work to make decisions on your behalf that best reflect your wishes.

Donation of Organs and Issue of an Autopsy

Were you to die suddenly, do you want your viable organs donated to a needy recipient? Do you want to have an autopsy? Understandably, many people, for religious and personal reasons, feel uncomfortable subjecting their bodies for these purposes.

But an autopsy can educate your medical team about possible diagnostic and treatment errors so they can save future lives and advance medical knowledge. If you donate your body to a medical school, first-year medical students can learn about anatomy.

In some states, you can indicate on your driver's license whether or not you want to donate organs in case you die suddenly. Whatever your wishes, you need to sign the appropriate documents and deliver them to the appropriate persons; for example, the Department of Motor Vehicles in your state.

Another benefit of an autopsy is to provide your children and relatives with more information about their risk of developing an inheritable disease (should you be found to have one) and about any unknown medical conditions so they can consider taking precautionary measures to avoid such illnesses.

For example, if your parents or other close relatives were found to have Alzheimer's or another type of dementia, younger family members may be able to reduce their risk and bolster their brain health by adopting a healthier lifestyle. A recent report in the British medical journal, The Lancet [7], states that 35 percent of dementia cases around the world could be delayed or even prevented by avoiding key risk factors or supporting healthier living starting in childhood that can make the brain more resilient to memory loss in old age. Nine factors identified include: 1) ensure good childhood education; 2) avoid high blood pressure, obesity, and smoking; 3) manage diabetes, depression, and age-related hearing loss; 4) be physically active; and 5) stay socially engaged in old age.

The strongest evidence that lifestyle changes help safeguard against dementia comes from a large study in Finland [189] that found that older adults at high risk for developing dementia scored better on brain tests after two years of exercise, diet, cognitive stimulation, and social activities.

Confirmation of these encouraging studies awaits additional research, but if you have older family members with dementia, making these suggested lifestyle changes when you are young may increase your chances of living longer, healthier, more satisfying lives.

How Patients' Rights Came About

The following is a brief history of the development of patients' rights and protections, summarizing the rights we presently have as patients and how best to exercise them. We assume you already have a will, and if relevant to your personal situation, a trust.

Confidentiality between doctor and patient is one of the oldest and most important rights we have as patients. It was first advocated by Hippocrates, the Greek philosopher and father of medicine, in about 400 BC. Confidentiality has a very long history.

In the United States, many documents have enumerated the rights we have.[190] In 1973, the American Hospital Association developed the "Patient's Bill of Rights." Subsequently, the Joint Commission on Accreditation of Healthcare Organizations (JCAHO) developed patients' rights, which hospitals and other healthcare facilities need to honor to maintain their accreditation. In 1997, the Consumer Bill of Rights and Responsibilities was established. In 2003, a major step was taken to protect patients' privacy and confidentiality when Congress passed the Health Insurance Portability and Accountability Act (HIPAA).

These documents ensure and protect your right to:

- Obtain current, understandable information from your healthcare professionals regarding your diagnosis, treatment options, progress, prognosis, and estimated medical costs.

- Have the above explained in a way you can understand if you speak another language, are disabled, or have hearing loss.

- Receive respectful, considerate healthcare.

- Know the roles and identities of all health professionals involved in your care.

- Agree to or refuse proposed tests and treatments.

- Agree to or refuse to participate in research studies.

---

189 https://www.scientificamerican.com/products/axa-research-fund/slowing-mental-decline-in-the-elderly/

190 http://www.emedicinehealth.com/patient_rights/article_em.htm#informed_consent.

- Review your medical records either in written or electronic form, have their contents explained, and propose changes if you find errors.[191]

- Have your medical information and records be kept confidential except when laws require them to be reported (for example, a communicable disease that could endanger the public).

- Have a HIPAA form, a living will and a durable power of attorney for healthcare and financial decisions (healthcare and financial proxy).

- Decide in advance what you want done or not done medically if you become terminally ill.

- Determine whether or not you want to donate your organs and/or body to benefit science.

- Have a patient advocate.

Healthcare rights continue to evolve. Take the following example in 2010 regarding hospital visitation rights. You should know that hospital visitation is a right not just for blood relatives but also for designated people such as those who are a Healthcare Proxy and/or a Patient Advocate. A true-life story[192] occurred when Lisa, who was in a same sex relationship for eighteen years, became unconscious following a brain aneurysm. Even though her partner, Janice, had a medical proxy to make medical decisions on Lisa's behalf, Janice was not even permitted to visit Lisa in her hospital room during her last hours of life because Janice was not a blood relative and because of the nurses' prejudice about lesbian relationships. However, when this heart-breaking story became national news, then President Obama responded by issuing an executive order[193] to the DHHS giving same sex couples the right to sit by their loved ones' side should one partner be hospitalized. The executive order reads, in part, that DHHS is to:

> "Initiate appropriate rulemaking, pursuant to your authority under 42 U.S.C. 1395x and other relevant provisions of law, to ensure that hospitals that participate in Medicare or Medicaid respect the rights of patients to designate visitors. It should be made clear that designated visitors, including individuals designated by legally valid advance directives (such as durable powers of attorney and health care proxies), should enjoy visitation privileges that are no more restrictive than those that immediate family members enjoy. You should also provide that participating hospitals may not deny visitation privileges on the basis of race, color, national origin, religion, sex, sexual orientation, gender identity, or disability. The rulemaking should consider the need for hospitals to restrict visitation in medically appropriate circumstances as well as the clinical decisions that medical professionals make about a patient's care or treatment."

191 https://www.verywell.com/medical-records-privacy-accuracy-and-patients-rights-2615509.
192 See: (1) http://web.archive.org/web/20140413201825/; (2) http:/patients.about.com/b/2010/04/16/new-gay-rights-healthcare-law-should-be-unnecessary.htm
193 http://web.archive.org/web/20140629033221/http://i.cdn.turner.com:80/cnn/2010/images/04/15/2010rightspatients.mem.final.rel.pdf

What is a Patient Advocate and What does a Patient Advocate Do?

Patient advocates help people deal with doctors, hospitals and insurers. They help patients deal with and navigate our complex healthcare system. Their primary responsibility is to give ongoing personalized guidance to patients as they move through the healthcare system.

An Advocate is different from a healthcare Proxy. The latter takes over making healthcare decisions on your behalf were you to become incapacitated. An Advocate, in contrast, is an advisor, helper, or supportive person who assists you in specified ways, but you are fully in charge of making your health-related decisions. It's important that your Advocate, your Proxy, and alternate are all knowledgeable about your health problems/preferences and know one another so they can fill in for one another should one of them become unavailable.

The National Patient Safety Foundation (NPSF)[194] gives a useful overview of who is a Patient Advocate and how to think about their services: An advocate is a "supporter, believer, sponsor, promoter, campaigner, backer, or spokesperson." It is important to consider all of these aspects when choosing an advocate for yourself or someone in your family. An effective advocate is someone you trust who is willing to act on your behalf as well as someone who can work well with other members of your healthcare team such as your doctors and nurses.

As discussed in *Chapter 1*, a Patient Advocate may be a member of your family, such as a spouse, a child, another family member, or a close friend.

Another type of advocate is a professional Patient Advocate. Hospitals usually have professionals who play this role called Patient Representatives or Patient Advocates. Social workers, nurses and chaplains may also fill this role. These advocates can often be very helpful in cutting through red tape. It is helpful to find out if your hospital has professional advocates available, and how they may be able to help you.

Specific examples of their assistance include: a) accompanying/participating at doctor appointments; b) scrutinizing medical bills for errors and negotiating reductions; c) finding the best medical specialists should you have complicated problem(s); d) coordinating your medical care, especially if you're seeing multiple doctors; e) communicating on your behalf with your family and health professionals; f) arranging with your social worker for medical/rehabilitation/nursing services at home should they be necessary; g) helping you get on Social Security and Medicare. You can probably add to this list. See *chapter Appendix: Interviewing a Prospective Patient Advocate.*

---

194   https://www.npsf.org/page/patientadvocate?&terms=%22patient+and+advocate%22

Getting started with your Patient Advocate

The NPSF gives further guidance on helping your Advocate to help you.

- "Decide what you want help with and what you want to handle on your own. For example, you may want help with:
    - o Clarifying your options for hospitals, doctors, diagnostic tests and procedures or treatment choices
    - o Getting information or asking specific questions
    - o Writing down information that you receive from your caregivers, as well as any questions that you may have
    - o Assuring that your wishes are carried out when you may not be able to do that by yourself.
- Decide if you would like your advocate to accompany you to tests, appointments, treatments and procedures. If so, insist that your doctor and other caregivers allow this.
- Be very clear with your advocate about what you would like them to know and be involved in— Treatment options? Any change in your condition? Test results? Keeping track of medications?
- Let your physician and those caring for you know who your advocate is and how you want them involved in your care
- Arrange for your designated advocate to be the spokesperson between you and your family and make sure your other family members know this. This will provide a consistent communication link and can help to minimize confusion and misunderstandings within your family".
- Make sure your doctor and nurses and family have your advocate's phone number and e-mail. Make sure your advocate has all the information regarding your providers, hospital, pharmacy, and anyone else you want your advocate to contact.

Once you have selected your Patient Advocate and alternate, be sure to add their names to your HIPAA forms.

What does a Patient Advocate Not do?

The American Medical Association (AMA)[195] has endorsed the role of Patient Advocates and also noted certain limitations. Limitations include "Patient navigators should refrain from any activity that could be construed as clinical in nature, including interpreting test results or medical symptoms, offering second opinions or making treatment recommendations". Ethical standards are promoted by groups such as the National Association of Healthcare Advocacy Consultants.[196]

---

195 https://www.ama-assn.org/sites/default/files/media-browser/public/patient-navigators.pdf
196 http://www.nahac.memberlodge.com/

Different types of Patient Advocates

As noted, a Patient Advocate can be a trusted family member or friend. It could also be a professional who works independently or for a specialized company. Sometimes Patient Advocates are also called Patient Navigators or Patient Health Navigators.

Is there certification for Patient Advocates?

There are several certifying agencies that can credential Patient Advocates. They include the Patient Advocate Certification Board (PACB)[197] which is focused on development and maintenance of certification for the profession of patient advocacy. There is also the Professional Patient Advocate Institute[198] that has a certificate program.

Finding and Selecting an Independent Patient Advocate

There are several websites for locating candidate Patient Advocates. One organization is Patient Advocate Foundation (PAF)[199]whose services are free. They describe their services as providing "an active liaison between the patient and their insurer, employer and/or creditors to resolve insurance, job retention and/or debt crisis matters relative to their diagnosis through case managers, doctors and attorneys. Patient Advocate Foundation seeks to safeguard patients through effective mediation assuring access to care, maintenance of employment and preservation of their financial stability." Their case management services, educational materials and live chat services are provided at no charge to patients.

Another organization offers the ADVO Connection Directory [200] to locate Patient Advocates. They also give helpful guidance in assessing and choosing a patient advocate.

Are Patient Advocate services covered by health insurance?

Patient Advocates who work privately for you are not paid by any insurer. They are paid directly by you.[201]

Other Patient Advocate resources

While there are many websites dealing with this topic, a useful one is the Patient Advocate Foundation[202] that helps solve insurance, healthcare /access, and other problems.

---

197   https://pacboard.org/bcpa-certificant-list/
198   http://www.patientadvocatetraining.com/certificate-programs/
199   http://www.patientadvocate.org/
200   https://advoconnection.com/hire-a-patient-advocate/; https://profile.advoconnection.com/search/
201   https://advoconnection.com/2017/03/23/are-health-or-patient-advocate-services-covered-by-insurance/
202   http://www.patientadvocate.org/

An example

If you are young and healthy, you probably question why you should bother reading about the benefits of having a patient advocate. The answer is that you may have a chronically ill or elderly parent, sibling, or friend living alone in a distant city and you are worried about him/her being able to navigate today's complicated healthcare system. Consider that your elderly, impaired parent, relative or friend may be hesitant to ask for your help because he/she doesn't want to burden you. When you visit him/her, you soon realize that having an advocate will not only lessen everyone's worry but may also save his/her life.

Take the case of Tom, an eighty-five-year-old architect, who lived alone in St. Louis and was chronically ill including some mild cognitive impairment. He insisted on living independently and being self-sufficient as he had been his entire life. His two adult daughters lived with their families on the East/West coasts. Tom was invited but didn't want to live with them. With some help from his daughters, Tom and a friend composed a list of seven kinds of assistance he felt he needed now, plus three additional types of assistance he anticipated needing in the next six months, such as someone to live with him half-time to make sure that he took his meds properly as well as help with housekeeping, shopping, finances, and accompanying him to doctors' appointments to make certain that instructions were carried out.

Tom and his daughters phoned several nearby specialized healthcare firms and selected one that focused on helping elderly people remain in their own home. A simple contract, which included all services presently needed as well as some for the future, was signed by Tom and his two daughters, and copies were sent with an explanatory cover letter to Tom's close relatives, his physician, attorney, the nearby hospital administrator, and his healthcare proxy, so everyone understood the agency's role. Tom added the names of the two top executives from the agency to his HIPAA form so they had permission to talk with all members of his healthcare team. The agency arranged for Tom to wear a medical alert device programmed to signal the nearby EMT and the agency should he fall or have an acute medical problem at home or in the neighborhood.

The contract with the agency was reviewed every six months as Tom's need for home services increased. All this relieved Tom and his family's worry and enabled him to live comfortably at home for eight more years (to age ninety-three), when he was willing and ready to live in an assisted living facility.

How to Stop an Impaired Elderly Parent's Right to Drive

Nothing defines personal freedom and independence in America, especially among the elderly, as does the ability to come and go at will in one's own car. Yet the realities of aging for many elderly persons often include impaired eyesight, diminished reflexes and memory, and medication side effects, to name a few, that can diminish the ability to drive, leading to accidents and lawsuits. The following remarks about aging Dad pertain as well to elderly women who drive. If you and other family members are worrying about potential accidents were Dad to continue driving, but he gets indignant and angry when it's suggested that he "turn in his car keys," there are many strategies to consider. Keep in mind that the ultimate goal may take time and patience. A good overview of these problems and dealing with them is available online[203] .

Some family members may feel guilty even discussing how to restrict Dad's freedom and independence; some may agree but have no plan in place as to how Dad will get to important doctors' appointments and get-togethers with old friends.

What Can the Family Do?

There are no easy answers to this complex problem. It's generally best to avoid being confrontational and argumentative. When talking with Dad, you don't want to be perceived as the enemy.

First, find out if most family members recognize and agree that it's dangerous for Dad to continue driving, so Dad will be less successful pitting one family member against another. Then, one or two family members whom Dad is more likely to listen to can patiently try to get him to realize it's time to give up driving. It's possible, although unlikely, that Dad was hoping someone would take the initiative to help him make this tough decision. If that approach is unsuccessful, you can explain your concern that he might seriously injure another person and question how this would make him feel. Don't be surprised if his response is: "This would never happen to me. I've been a good, safe driver before you were even born!" You might try mentioning all the money he'd save by selling his car and not needing auto insurance.

You may think it is manipulative, yet nevertheless true, to remind him that a lawsuit could ruin him financially. Be prepared to have answers to Dad's concern about being stranded at home; explain his alternative of using taxis, Uber, and a debit card to get where he needs to go. Local senior service agencies often provide transportation services for free or minimal cost.

Enlisting Help from Your Parent's Physician

Should these approaches fail, you can enlist the help of Dad's physician. Explain to his doctor the reasons for the family's worry about his impaired driving skills. In many states, a physician can send a letter to the Department of Motor Vehicles (DMV) with details about his/her patient's medical problems (for example, poor eyesight or memory impairment), and request "thorough testing", as if he were a new driver taking all required tests for the first time. This would include a written exam, vision testing, and a driving skills test. The goal, of course, is for Dad to fail, in which case the state becomes the "bad guy."[204]

In South Florida, and many other states, there are testing sites where a physician can refer a patient for a "thorough driving evaluation," as if he were a new driver. If Dad is even mildly to moderately impaired, he's likely to fail the tests. A letter then goes to the DMV, and driving privileges are revoked. The cost for the evaluation is about $200, which is much less than an accident-associated lawsuit. Find out what options exist for requesting a driving evaluation in your state by contacting the DMV. In the long run, you'll be doing your elderly parent and other drivers and pedestrians a big favor.

---

203 https://www.nhtsa.gov/road-safety/older-drivers
204 https://www.caring.com/questions/taking-drivers-license-away-senior-driver.

California law permits family members, the police, and judges to request that the DMV assess anyone suspected of impaired driving ability and requires physicians to report to the local health office[205] anyone with certain medical conditions known to impair driving.

Controversy About Physician-Aid-in-Dying

Currently, five states in the United States, as well as Canada, a handful of European countries, and two South American countries (Columbia and Uruguay), allow for some type of physician-aid-in-dying. An additional twenty U.S. states are in various stages (for example, ballot initiatives, court cases) of deciding what to do about this controversial issue.

Opponents of physician-aid-in-dying believe that life is sacred, the endurance of suffering confers its own dignity, and it's a violation of the sanctity of life to assist in the dying process. It's also argued that physician-aid-in-dying would be the first step on a slippery slope that would be hoisted on vulnerable patients by questionable doctors, money grasping relatives, miserly insurance companies, and cash-strapped states.

Supporters of physician-aid-in-dying believe that since competent adults are allowed to make other meaningful, irrevocable decisions, such as having an abortion, why prevent people from deciding to end their physical and mental suffering, which often accompanies a terminal illness. Since most people die in a medical type of facility, sometimes in an ICU under bright lights and among strangers, why can't people suffering from a terminal illness be allowed to end their lives when they are ready and surrounded by those they love in a familiar setting like home. The famous physicist Dr. Stephen Hawkins, who has a life-long debilitating neurological disease, believes that keeping someone alive against his will is the "ultimate indignity".

The Oregon Model for Physician-Aid-in-Dying

In 1997, Oregon became the first state to pass a law allowing physician-aid-in-dying if specific conditions are met. The Oregon law has been the model for similar laws passed in five other states – Vermont (2013), Montana (2015), California (2016), Colorado (2016), and Washington, DC (2017).

To qualify, Oregon patients need to have a terminal illness and a prognosis of having less than six months to live. The patient needs to write a letter to his/her physician requesting assistance in dying. Two people have to witness and sign the patient's written request. One of the two witnesses cannot be related to the patient, or be listed in the patient's will or have any other potential conflict of interest. The physician has the option of refusing the request on moral, religious, or other grounds. He/she must inform the patient of feasible alternatives to assisted dying, such as palliative and hospice care.

---

205 http://www.dmv.ca.gov/portal/dmv/?1dmy&urile=wcm:path:/dmv_content_en/dmv/dl/driversafety/dsmedcontraffic.

If the first physician approves the request, it goes to a second physician, who is required to examine the patient's medical records to confirm the diagnosis and prognosis and make certain that the patient has no mental illness that affects his/her decision-making ability. If either physician questions whether or not the patient's judgment is impaired by a psychiatric or psychological disorder, the patient is referred for psychological examination. If testing confirms that the patient has the capacity for requesting physician aid-in-dying and has no mental illness affecting the decision, the physician prescribes the self-administered lethal medication. Even at this point, the patient is under no obligation to take the medication.

In 2016, the lethal medication was prescribed to 204 Oregon residents, yet only 133 (or 65 percent), including seventeen recipients from prior years, actually took it.[206]

Despite the dire prediction of opponents of the Oregon law, those requesting physician-aid-in-dying have, in general, been well educated, had adequate health insurance, and were receiving palliative care. They reportedly were motivated by wanting relief from pain and suffering as well as a desire to preserve their own dignity, autonomy, and pleasure in their remaining life.[207]

California is the latest of the five states to pass a bill modeled after Oregon's law but with some add-ons meant to assuage opponents. California patients have to request aid-in-dying three times instead of twice, and the prescribing physician must have a one-on-one conversation with the patient to verify that no one is putting pressure on the patient. In California, the law will expire after ten years. If the law is deemed successful, Californians may vote on a similar bill, perhaps with modifications. According to a 2015 California non-partisan opinion poll, 69 percent of Californians were in favor of physician-aided dying.

But, according to Stanford Medical School's bioethicist Dr. David Magnus, the controversy over aid-in-dying is a distraction from the reality of America's faulty end-of-life care. A report titled "Dying in America,"[208] published in 2014 by the Institute of Medicine, showed that patients often can't get or don't know about underused types of end-of-life treatments, such as palliative and hospice care. They actually may prefer what palliative and hospice care provide, such as the need to be comfortable and pain-free, in their final months, days, and hours.[209]

Dr. Magnus thinks that modern medicine over-emphasizes technology, innovation, and searches for cures, and underestimates communication between doctor and patient. Clear communication about death is probably the first prescription that most terminal patients need [3]. Dr. Magnus believes many terminal patients get excessive and unnecessary treatment that doesn't help them have a more comfortable death. This can result in a vicious cycle wherein late stage cancer patients, for example, get debilitating chemotherapy, trips to surgery, to ICU, back for more chemotherapy, to home, and then back again, each time making it more difficult on the patient and family [8].

---

206 https://www.oregon.gov/oha/PH/PROVIDERPARTNERRESOURCES/EVALUATIONRESEARCH/DEATHWITHDIGNITYACT/Pages/index.aspx
207 https://www.economist.com/assisted-dying
208 http://nationalacademies.org/HMD/Reports/2014/Dying-In-America-Improving-Quality-and-Honoring-Individual-Preferences-Near-the-End-of-Life/The-Conversation.aspx%20
209 What's the difference between palliative care and hospice care. https://www.webmd.com/palliative-care/difference-palliative-hospice-care#1

Reasons for This Vicious Cycle

Patients may sense that their condition is bad, even though doctors refrain from telling them just how bad their prognosis is because doctors often find it very difficult to communicate bad news to patients and their families. It's understandable that doctors tend to focus their discussions on the positive because they have insufficient medical training in end-of-life care and find it difficult to be the bearer of bad news.

But patients can circumvent America's medical system shortcomings when it comes to end-of-life care by completing advance directives (living wills), as discussed earlier in this chapter. These and other legal documents guide the doctors treating you towards what you want done and don't want done in the event of a terminal illness. According to Nathan Kottkamp, founder of National Healthcare Decisions Day, "100 percent of us are going to die, but only a quarter of Americans have completed advance directives." The National Healthcare Decision Day website[210] has state-specific documents and instructions for drafting legal documents such as advance directives. Dr. Magnus believes that most Americans want to choose, and have control over, their final days of life not because they are terrified of having a sickness steal away their preferred choice of life but rather because of more common fears, such as dying in pain, without control, without dignity, surrounded by people they don't know and in a place they do not want to be. The choice that concerns them is not whether to die, but how to die.

---

210   www.nhdd.org.

Chapter 12 Appendix

Interviewing a Prospective Patient Advocate [211]

1. "Learn more about their credentials. Ask the following:

    a. Do you have background, training or experience providing advocacy services?

    b. Have you handled other cases similar to mine?

    c. How long have you been a private, independent advocate? What sort of advocacy work did you do prior to creation of your own practice?

    d. Do you subscribe or adhere to a Code of Professional Standards?

    e. Have you recently undergone a background check? If so, will you share the results with me?

    f. Are you a BCPA? (Board Certified Patient Advocate)

2. What do you charge for your services? (Learn about the cost of hiring an advocate.)

3. Do you have professional liability and/or Errors and Omissions Insurance? (The great majority of advocates must have insurance to protect you and themselves. There are some special cases where E&O insurance is not mandatory, but those are rare. If the advocate you are interviewing says he or she does not have E&O insurance, ask them why not. If the answer sounds plausible, then you can decide whether you want to continue with the interview.)

4. Does anyone else pay you for helping me? (Some advocates are paid a commission for placing patients in a specific nursing home or with other services. They may be less objective, so you'll want to know more about any potential conflicts of interest.)

5. Do you have an idea of the approximate amount of time it will take you to handle the services I need? If not, how can I get an estimate?

6. What is your caseload? Do you have time to handle the work I need to have done?

7. Do you have references? (Advocates may understandably be reluctant to give you names and contact information for references due to privacy laws. However, it would make sense to ask them if they will ask a former client to contact you to provide a reference. Alternatively, you can check their directory profiles testimonials which may not be added by individual advocates.)

Additional, optional interview questions, depending on the services you need:

1. Are you "on call" 24/7 or do you have specific hours?

2. Is your location in proximity to the patient? (Many services do not require the advocate to be nearby.)

3. Do you provide reports on services you provide in my absence? (Important for situations where the caregiver lives in one place, but the patient – such as an elderly parent – lives somewhere else.)"

---

211 See: (1) https://advoconnection.com/hire-a-patient-advocate/; (2) https://profile.advoconnection.com/search/

Chapter 12 Key Points

Key Points: The Four Important Legal Documents

- HIPAA – Health Insurance Portability and Accountability Act.
- POLST – Physician Orders for Life-Sustaining Treatment.
- Living will or healthcare directive.
- Proxies for healthcare and financial decisions.

Key Points: Guide to Completing the Four Documents

- Use state specific forms.
- Discuss certain forms with your doctor and lawyer.
- Discuss your late-life medical and financial wishes with your family and doctors.
- All those involved should obtain copies of relevant documents and also when changes are made.
- If you move to another state, re-do the documents with state-specific forms, discard old forms, and inform everyone.

Key Points: Healthcare Power of Attorney (or Proxy)

- Designates the person (and an alternate) to make all healthcare decisions on your behalf should you become incapable of making these decisions unless you limit their scope in specific ways (for example, cannot replace your PCP).
- Should you regain the capacity for making healthcare decisions, you can revoke your proxy's role.
- If you've never chosen your proxy in writing or verbally and currently lack decision-making capacity, some states permit persons in the following order to make decisions on your behalf: 1) spouse; 2) significant other; 3) adult child; 4) parent.

Key Points: Stopping an Impaired Elderly Parent from Driving

- It's not easy; takes time and patience.
- Choose one or two family members to sit down with Dad for "the talk."
- If the above fails, enlist Dad's physician to write a letter to the state's DMV listing Dad's medical problems and requesting a "thorough" testing. The goal is for Dad to fail.

Key Points: Controversy About Physician-Aid-in-Dying

- Supporters argue that since competent adults are allowed other meaningful, irrevocable decisions, such as an abortion, Americans should have the right to end physical/mental suffering accompanying a terminal illness.

- Oregon, in 1997, was the first state to pass a law allowing physician-aid-in-dying if specific conditions are met. Several other states and Washington, DC have passed similar laws.

References

1. Gordon, M. and G.-A. Perri, *Conflicting demands of family at the end of life and challenges for the palliative care team.* Annals of Long-Term Care: Clinical Care and Aging, 2015. **23**(1): p. 25-28.

2. Gawande, A., *Being Mortal.* 2014, New York: Metropolitan Books, Henry Holt and Company, New York. p. 191-230.

3. Gawande, A., *Overkill: America's epidemic of unnecessary care*, in *The New Yorker.* 2015: New York. p. 42-53.

4. Connor, S.R., *Hospice and Palliative Care-The Essential Guide.* Vol. Chapter 9. 2018, New York: Routledge.

5. Sadock, B.J., *Psychiatric report, medical record, and medical error.*, in *Kaplan and Sadock's Comprehensive Textbook of Psychiatry, 9th Edition,* 2009
Wolters Kluwer, Lippincott Williams and Wilkins: Philadelphia, Penn. p. 913-914

6. DeMartino, E.S., et al., *Who Decides When a Patient Can't? Statutes on Alternate Decision Makers.* New England Journal of Medicine, 2017. **376**(15): p. 1478-1482.

7. Livingston, G., et al., *Dementia prevention, intervention, and care.* Lancet, 2017. **390**(10113): p. 2673-2734.

8. Michelson, L.D., *The Patient's Handbook.* 2015, New York: Alfred A. Knopf.

Alternative (Complementary) Treatment Approaches: East Meets West

Healthcare practices that are not an integral part of conventional or Western-style medicine are called *complementary and alternative medical practices* (CAM). Other terms sometimes used for CAM treatments are holistic, non-traditional, and integrative treatment approaches. Integrative treatment can also refer to the combined coordinated use of traditional Western medical treatment with CAM approaches.

Examples of frequently used CAM treatments include hands-on types such as acupuncture, chiropractic, and massage. Treatments taken by mouth include various herbal remedies, food supplements, special diets, and vitamins. Inconsistent research findings make it difficult to distinguish benefits of CAM treatments greater than that of placebos (sugar pills). Nevertheless, CAM treatments are used by an increasing number of people in the United States. The majority of CAM users are well educated, committed to personal growth, and satisfied with the conventional care provided by their physician. They often use prescriptions from physicians, over-the counter medications, and CAM approaches simultaneously for the same problem. More than one third of Americans use one or more forms of CAM treatment each year, but surprisingly, less than 20 percent of those using a CAM treatment inform their regular physician.[212]

Many People are Reluctant to Discuss CAM Treatments with Their Doctors

Reasons for not discussing a CAM treatment with your physician include the belief that your doctor may frown on such approaches, or that CAMs interfere with your prescription medications, or that it's not necessary to inform one's doctor, or simply "forgetting" to inform. Busy physicians and their assistants may forget to ask, so it's important for you to keep your doctor informed.

The majority of people who use CAM, herbal, and other remedies to self-treat a mental health problem, such as depression, take prescription psychiatric medicine concurrently from their PCPhys. or psychiatrist, but don't inform their physician. This trend is alarming in view of potentially serious side effects when

212   Lake, J.H. Complementary, Alternative, and Integrative Approaches in Mental Health Care. In: Comprehensive Textbook of Psychiatry, 10th Edition, Sadock, B.J., Sadock, V.A., Ruiz, P., (Eds) Wolters Kluwer Press, Philadelphia, Pa, 2017, p. 2542-2545.

combining certain herbal remedies or other over-the-counter CAM products, often available at grocery and health-food stores, with prescribed medication [2]. More than half of people who self-treat depression by using a CAM product together with a prescribed antidepressant believe that they are equally effective. But if both are taken at the same time, how is it possible to conclude they are equally effective?

The use of St. John's wort, the most frequently used herbal remedy to self-treat depression, is a good example of the risk if it's not first discussed with your physician. St. John's wort is a serotonin reuptake inhibitor and a weak monoamine oxidase inhibitor. When taken together with an SSRI antidepressant, such as citalopram or fluoxetine, side effects of each medication, such as sedation, restlessness, and nausea can worsen. Pregnant women should not take St. John's wort, and it should not be taken with Coumadin (an anticoagulant) or digoxin. St. John's wort should not be taken with oral contraceptives because it can decrease their effectiveness.[213]

The safety of imported herbal remedies and other natural products from Asia and India is difficult to assess because of the absence of strong import controls, inferior testing for efficacy and safety in that part of the world, and because imported products are sometimes adulterated with barbiturates, steroids, and acetaminophen. When taken with prescription medication, serious side effects as well as toxic reactions can occur.

You also want to have a comprehensive medical assessment by your PCPhys. or PCP to make certain you don't have a medical problem requiring treatment *before* seeing a CAM practitioner. For all the above reasons, it's advisable to first discuss with your healthcare provider whether or not an herbal remedy or some other over-the-counter CAM product is safe and right for you.

Consequences When Doctor Forgets to Ask – Patient Doesn't Tell

---

Susan is a 36-year-old widow, living with a part-time maid and her six-year-old daughter in Los Angeles. She has a history of multiple drug abuse, major depression, and fibromyalgia. Since she was a teenager she had unsuccessful treatment at two drug rehabilitative programs. For the past three years she was taking high doses of a serotonergic antidepressant along with a benzodiazepine anti-anxiety medication and gabapentin for her chronic fibromyalgia pain and depression. She was reluctant to admit to her psychiatrist how she was "really" using her medications. Without informing her doctor, she visited a health food store and complained about her nervousness and difficulty sleeping. Without asking Susan the names of prescribed medications she was taking, the saleswoman recommended four different CAM products (two of which were euphemistically named "Tranquil Sleep" and "Anxie". Each of these had ingredients with sedating and serotonergic side effects.

---

213   Freeman MP, Fava M, Lake J, et al. Complementary and alternative medicine in major depressive disorder: the American Psychiatric Association Task Force report. J Clin Psychiatry. 2010;71(6):669-681.

As in the past, Susan began experimenting with different doses of these CAM products without informing her psychiatrist. Her doctor never thought to ask Susan if she was using any over-the-counter products. After self-medicating with varying doses of CAM products while continuing her usual four psychiatric medicines, she complained of diarrhea, fever, and confusion at her next psychiatric appointment. She was agitated, sweating, with tremor and rigidity of her hands and legs. These were classical signs of a serotonergic syndrome caused by the combination of psychiatric medications and CAM products with serotonin side effects. Fortunately, she recovered after five days of intensive treatment in the hospital.

If you see a CAM practitioner, such as a chiropractor or an acupuncturist, who recommends some herbal or other CAM product without first inquiring what prescribed medicine(s) you take, make certain to first obtain your doctor's opinion. Also, ask your prospective CAM practitioner if he/she is willing to work collaboratively with your PCPhys. or PCP. If you don't get satisfactory answers, consider finding another CAM practitioner. Another reason to discuss with your doctor your interest in seeing a CAM practitioner is because traditional, Western-trained physicians have become more knowledgeable about the potential benefits and risks of CAMs, and sometimes make referrals to, and work collaboratively with, reputable CAM practitioners. Many academic medical centers have departments of complementary, alternative, and integrative medicine where traditional physicians work collaboratively with CAM practitioners and carry out research together. Discussing your interest in a CAM approach with your PCPhys. or PCP facilitates coordination of your healthcare (so everyone is on the same page). Also, some insurance companies require a referral from your PCPhys. or PCP in order for the CAM treatment to be paid by your insurer.

Several reasons account for the increasing popularity of CAM treatments. A small number of CAM treatments have been scientifically proven to be effective; many have been used for centuries. Also, CAM practitioners may spend more time and listen more attentively to patients than do busy PCPs. And patients may be dissatisfied when traditional treatment can't affect a cure. Faith and hope may be major factors that contribute to the success of these treatments (the placebo effect), and some treatments may be helpful for patients with chronic problems, such as the ubiquitous neck and low back pain, when conventional treatments fail [1].

The increasing use of CAM treatments led to the establishment of the National Center for Complementary and Alternative Medicine (NCCAM) to evaluate the effectiveness and safety of these non-traditional healing practices, to understand scientifically the reasons for their possible effectiveness, and to inform the public about their findings. A NCCAM study found that the most commonly used forms of CAM used in the United States were praying for one's own health or the health of others (more than 60 percent of those using a CAM approach), using natural products [such as St. John's wort, L-tryptophan, Gingko biloba (19 percent), deep breathing exercises (12 percent), meditation (8 percent), and chiropractic treatment (8 percent)]. Many Americans use two or more CAM treatments simultaneously. Another NCCAM study found that the most common conditions treated were back, head, and neck pain and that the majority of those using CAM believe that the greatest benefits were achieved when a CAM treatment is combined with conventional medical treatment. [214]

214 Complementary and Alternative Medicine in Psychiatry. In: Synopsis of Psychiatry, Eleventh Edition, Sadock, B.J., Sadock, V.A., Ruiz, P. (Eds.), Wolters Kluwer, Philadelphia, 2015, pgs. 791-792.

Other NCCAM studies have found that acupuncture is beneficial for those with disabilities that impair certain activities of daily living and osteoarthritic knee pain. Combined use of glucosamine and chondroitin sulfate benefits a small group of patients with severe osteoarthritic pain and impaired mobility.

However, the vast majority of CAMs are not based on scientific studies, and many physicians view most of these non-traditional treatments with skepticism. On the other hand, more than half of U.S. medical schools currently provide some education about CAM treatments, and some carry out research to determine which approaches may have scientific merit.

Some health maintenance organizations (HMOs) and other types of insurance have approved some CAM treatments for reimbursement, such as acupuncture and chiropractic treatment, and patients can visit CAM practitioners without a referral from their PCPhys. We suggest checking this out beforehand with your insurance company.

Finding an Alternative Practitioner

Although most alternative (CAM) practitioners are trained in their respective fields and are dedicated to patient care, many lack the skill and knowledge about diagnosing and treating patients with medical and/or psychiatric illnesses. They may not be thoroughly familiar with possible interactions of medical and psychiatric drugs and frequently used herbal remedies such as St. John's wort, ginkgo, and ginseng, to name a few. CAM practitioners sometimes give patients advice about medications prescribed by the patient's physician without collaboration with the physician, which can lead to serious side effects, risk of relapse, and delay in proper diagnosis and treatment. That is why it's so important to first have a comprehensive medical evaluation to identify a possible medical problem before beginning work with a CAM practitioner.

Learn about the benefits and risks of the alternative treatments you are considering by discussing them with your physician. You can also learn about the CAM treatments by contacting NCCAM's Internet site (www.nccih.nih.gov); click on *Health Information, Safety Information,* and then select *Safe Use of Complementary Health Products and Practices.* The NCCAM website also has directories of professional societies for many CAM therapies. In the final analysis, after much thought and investigation, you need to decide if a CAM treatment can be worthwhile for you. The following is a summary of just a few of the more common CAM approaches.

Chiropractic

Chiropractic is concerned with the diagnosis, treatment, and prevention of disorders of the musculoskeletal system, especially disorders of the spine and the effects of these disorders on general health. Chiropractors diagnose illness by X-rays and clinical examination. Treatment involves manual manipulation of the spine, bones, musculature, and joints to restore biomechanical function.

Chiropractic is the largest alternative health profession in the United States, with over 50,000 practitioners. Four or five years of study at one of eighteen chiropractic colleges in the United States is required, followed by passing a four-part exam. Chiropractors need to be licensed in the state where they practice. Some states and insurance companies give chiropractors more leeway (to be a PCP and to receive insurance payments) than others. Some research suggests that chiropractors are just as effective as traditional physicians at helping back pain sufferers. A good source of information about chiropractors is the Federation of Chiropractic Licensing Boards (www.fclb.org).

There are some absolute and relative contraindications to the use of spinal manipulation at any level of the spine, even though complications and adverse effects are rare. Contraindications include the following:[215]

a. Serious causes of back pain, such as cancer involving the bone; metabolic conditions affecting bone strength; use of anticoagulants or having a blood clotting disorder.

b. Acute infection or fracture of the spinal bones and associated joints.

c. Active inflammatory arthritis involving the spinal bones.

Acupuncture

Acupuncture originated as a Chinese healing technique dating back to 5000 BC and continues to be a commonly used intervention in the eastern part of the world. It is also one of the most popular and regulated CAMs in the United States. Acupuncturists insert sterilized silver or gold needles, some as thin as a human hair, into the skin at varying depths and rotate them or leave them in place for varying periods of time. It is believed that the needles stimulate the release of endorphins and enkephalins from the brain that relieve pain and alleviate symptoms of some illnesses. The benefits have been validated for pain management, fibromyalgia, headache, osteoarthritis of the knee, and postoperative nausea and vomiting. Acupuncture may also have some benefit for smoking cessation, for reducing relapse rate in recovering alcoholics, and for helping patients with insomnia and depression. Most pain management clinics in England, the United States, and other countries use acupuncture in their arsenal of treatment approaches. Thousands of traditional physicians in the United States have taken acupuncture-training courses and use it as part of their practice.

Computer controlled electroacupuncture (CCEA) uses computer-guided modulations (adjustment of electrical current delivered through acupuncture needles). In a large multi-center study of very depressed hospitalized patients treated for six weeks with electroacupuncture, a significant number showed improvement. Patients had elevated plasma norepinephrine levels, suggesting that electroacupuncture stimulates norepinephrine release, which may account for improved mood.

---

215 http://patient.info/doctor/complementary-and-alternative-medicine

To become licensed to perform acupuncture, about eighteen states and the District of Columbia require a degree from a school for acupuncture and Oriental medicine accredited by the Accreditation Commission for Acupuncture and Oriental Medicine (ACAOM). The degree is vastly different from a traditional medical degree. States differ in their licensing requirements.[216] Acupuncturists practice other modes of CAM medicine, such as the use of herbal remedies. Information about what your state requires for licensing and other information can be found at the National Certification Commission for Acupuncture and Oriental Medicine (NCCAOM). [217]

Some states require your PCPhys. or PCP to refer you to an acupuncturist before your insurance will consider paying for treatment, so check with your insurer. As with other CAMs, discuss your interest with your physician before considering treatment so your treatment is coordinated.

Here's one acupuncture success story: A ninety-four-year-old woman suffered a hairline fracture of her lower spine ten years ago. Surgery was recommended by a young, enthusiastic orthopedic surgeon who became impatient when she questioned the need for surgery; she refused to sign the consent form. By using acupuncture treatments four times a year up to the present, she has been symptom free.

Naturopathy

Naturopathy is based on the belief that the body has the power to heal itself. Naturopaths advocate some combination of healthy nutrition, pollution-free air and water, regular exercise, hot/cold compresses, colonic irrigation (such as enemas), massage therapy, herbs, and rest therapy.

There are only a few naturopathic colleges in the United States that are accredited by the Council on Naturopathic Medical Education (CNME). Four years of postgraduate training is required followed by passing a board examination known as the Naturopathic Physicians Licensing Exam (NPLEX). Currently, twenty states, the District of Columbia, the U.S. Virgin Islands, and Puerto Rico have state-specific laws that license graduates of American naturopathic schools to practice. Some states that license naturopathic practitioners allow them to serve patients as their primary care practitioner.[218] You can find out your state's licensing requirements at the American Association of Naturopathic Physicians (AANP) website.[219]

Because no standard regulations for the field of naturopathy exist, persons with minimal or no special training can set up a practice in some states and call themselves doctors. Traditionally trained physicians think it is confusing to the public when naturopathic practitioners call themselves doctors because they don't have the same rigorous training, education, and licensing requirements.

Homeopathy

Homeopathy is based on the concept that self-healing is a basic characteristic of human life. Extremely small doses of derivatives from plants (such as ergot fungus) and minerals (such as silver and iodine) are

---

216   https://www.naturalhealers.com/acupuncture/acupuncture-licensure/
217   www.nccaom.org.
218   https://aanmc.org/resources/licensure/.
219   www.naturopathic.org.

believed by homeopathic practitioners to help the body build defenses against particular diseases. Medications are prepared as tinctures (that is, sometimes mixed with 95 percent grain alcohol) or as pills. Research has shown that such highly diluted substances probably have no greater benefit than a placebo and are too dilute to cause adverse effects. However, rare cases of toxicity have been reported when dilutions of arsenic, cadmium, and other heavy metals are used. Homeopathic medications are used throughout the world and are prescribed by other CAM practitioners. Patients' strong belief in the healing aspects of these treatments may contribute to their apparent usefulness.

One of the authors knew a physician in Maine who "poopooed" homeopathy for years. He himself became so uncomfortable with a medical condition that traditional medicine could not improve that he gave in to a friend's urging and tried homeopathy. It worked so well that he now practices homeopathy as part of his traditional medical practice.

Only a few states offer licensing for homeopaths, but there are over 6,000 practitioners in the United States. Most practice in another field, such as chiropractic, and incorporate some aspects of homeopathy into their own work.

Homeopathic medicines are sold over-the-counter in the United States and around the world. As with other CAM treatments, talk with your PCPhys. or PCP before using homeopathic medications to make certain they don't interfere, or have potentially harmful effects, if combined with prescription or over-the-counter medications you are taking.

Massage Therapy

Some believe that massage therapy affects the body by improving circulation of blood and lymphatic flow, improving the tone of the musculoskeletal system, and producing a tranquilizing effect on the mind. Some studies have shown that massage therapy can reduce pain perception and generalized anxiety, especially when anxiety is related to test-taking or work stress. There are many different types of massage, such as Swedish, Oriental, Shiatsu, and Esalen, but they are more similar than different.

Most people find massage physically and mentally rejuvenating, but it's not been shown to cure any illness. Credentialing requirements vary widely in the United States. About half the states require classroom education, supervised training at an institution accredited by the Commission on Massage Therapy Accreditation (COMTA), and an examination, but the other half of states have no credentialing requirements. To check on your state's status, contact the National Certification Board for Therapeutic Massage and Bodywork – NCBTMB.

Meditation

Meditation is a technique that lets you enter a trance-like state by focusing on a word, sound, object, or your natural breathing. Upon entering this state, you experience calm, reduced anxiety, and sometimes reduced blood pressure and respiratory rate. A large study found that the majority of anxious patients who successfully completed a ten-week meditation program reported significantly decreased emotional distress, improved quality of life and sense of well-being, and greater optimism.[220] Some people practice meditation daily and report that it reduces stress. Small and large workshops are given all over the United States. One of the authors has found it a pleasant and simple way of reducing tension and stress.

Prayer

For centuries, prayer and pilgrimages to religious shrines to find relief from suffering and pain support the widespread belief that spirituality helps the healing process. Some advocate the use of silent, shared, and distant prayer (praying on behalf of someone else for a specific purpose) to benefit those who are sick and suffering. A study of inner-city homeless women found that 48 percent reported that prayer significantly reduced depression and their use of alcohol and drugs.[221] Twelve-step programs for those with substance use disorders have a long history of using prayer and spirituality as an important component of treatment. Studies have shown that personal religious beliefs and regular attendance at places of worship contribute to a decreased incidence of high blood pressure and depression. Persons with a lifetime of practicing their strong religious beliefs, contrasted with lifelong non-believers, will obviously find it more beneficial to turn to their spiritual convictions during times of sickness and stress.

Diet and Nutrition

Dietary supplements are products that contain vitamins, minerals, and amino acids that are intended to supplement, rather than substitute for, a healthy diet. Multivitamins are often components of a vast array of other compounds that can be purchased from grocery and health food stores, pharmacies, and on the Internet. About 75 percent of Americans use some form of nutritional supplements. The medical benefits of these products vary greatly, as do their safety and efficacy.

Important Role of Special Diets

Special diets have an important place in modern medicine. Alternative diets, some with specific vitamin and mineral supplements, have been developed to help patients with specific diseases. For example, diets low in fat are recommended for the treatment of those with diabetes, vascular, and heart disease. The Pritikin diet is very low in fat and high in fiber and complex carbohydrates. The Atkins diet is low in carbohydrates and high in protein and may be beneficial for short-term weight loss, but there are no long-term studies about its effect on health. Low-salt diets benefit those with heart disease and hypertension. There is evidence of the health benefits of the Mediterranean diet. It may protect you against heart and vascular disease.[222] All these diets have their advocates and adversaries, and their popularity waxes and wanes over time.

220   Marchand WR. Mindfulness-based stress reduction, mindfulness-based cognitive therapy, and Zen meditation for depression, anxiety, pain, and psychological distress. J Psychiatr Pract. 2012;18(4):233-252.

221   https://www.ncbi.nlm.nih.gov/m/pubmed/8012240/.

222   https://www.mayoclinic.org/healthy-lifestyle/nutrition-and-healthy-eating/in-depth/mediterranean-diet/art-20047801?p=1.

Studies have shown that weight loss alone, for those with newly diagnosed adult-onset diabetics and those who are overweight, can decrease blood pressure and cholesterol and sometimes reduce the need for diabetic drugs.

Those following a strictly vegetarian diet may become deficient in certain vitamins and proteins, so supplementing the diet with vitamin B12 and essential amino acids is suggested. Americans leading a busy lifestyle and frequenting fast food restaurants have been shown to be missing the minimum required amount of some vitamins and minerals. Some nutritional experts recommend that most Americans can benefit from taking a high-quality multivitamin with minerals once or twice daily. Some advocate taking a multivitamin twice daily because several vitamins dissolve in water and are excreted by the kidneys within twelve hours.

With the exception of some basic vitamins (A, C, D, E, B1, B5, B6, B12, folate, and niacin) and some minerals (iron, potassium, magnesium, calcium, and selenium), there is limited information about the value of most other vitamin and mineral supplements on the market. When choosing a multivitamin with minerals for daily use, discuss it with your PCPhys. or PCP and consider one that includes most of the above ingredients. Fortunately, for many vitamins, minerals, and other supplements, the federal government has established recommended daily allowances (RDAs) necessary to meet the nutritional needs of the average middle-aged adult. For the majority of Americans, a diet rich in whole grains, lean meat, fish, and green vegetables is recommended. It is best to avoid an excess intake of fatty foods and sugar products (plentiful in breakfast cereals, cookies, and soft drinks).

The Effect of Nutrition on Mental Health

Some depressed patients benefit from reducing or eliminating refined sugar and caffeine from their diet. Foods rich in folate and vitamins B6 and B12 may also help some with depression. These vitamins are co-factors in the synthesis of serotonin, dopamine, and norepinephrine, which are believed to beneficially affect mood [3]. Increased consumption of fish high in omega-3 essential polyunsaturated fatty acids, such as salmon and halibut, and flaxseed oil may provide a protective effect against depressed mood. Greater intake of omega-3 fatty acids is correlated with lower C-reactive protein levels, increased brain serotonin, and reduced risk of inflammatory disorders that are believed by some to play a role in reducing depression.

Several studies have shown that when one to two grams of omega-3 fatty acid was added to the daily diet of depressed patients, along with a conventional antidepressant, treatment response was significantly greater than in patients treated only with an antidepressant.[223] Persons predisposed to panic and other anxiety disorders may benefit from gradually reducing and eliminating caffeinated beverages because caffeine increases serum epinephrine and cortisol resulting in feelings of nervousness.

---

223 Sarris J, Murphy J, Mischoulon D, et al. Adjunctive nutraceuticals for depression: a systematic review and meta-analyses. Am J Psychiatry. 2016;173(6):575-587.

Vitamin Deficiencies

Vitamin deficiencies can develop in malnourished individuals and those who abuse alcohol and drugs. For example, alcoholics are often deficient in vitamin B1 (thiamine), which can lead to delirium, eventual brain damage, and even beriberi disease. Symptoms of beriberi include loss of appetite, weakness, pain and swelling of legs and feet. If thiamine deficiency is diagnosed early, these conditions can improve with thiamine pills, abstinence from alcohol, and improved diet. Deficiency of vitamin B12 or folic acid can cause depression, anemia, and delirium that can progress to dementia if not readily diagnosed and treated.[224] Deficiency of vitamin D and calcium can cause osteoporosis and bone fractures, especially in post-menopausal women. Exercise, supplemental vitamin D, and special medications can reduce the risk.

Precautions About Dietary Supplements

In contrast to prescription drugs, which are subjected to rigorous scientific studies and years of scrutiny by the Food and Drug Administration (FDA) before they are approved to be marketed, manufacturers of nutritional products can simply package and sell their products. Since 1994 the Dietary Supplemental Health and Education Act (DSHEA) has permitted herbal and other such remedies to be sold in the United States as "food products." The FDA has little to no authority or budget to monitor these nutritional supplements.

Fortunately, one precaution you can take when buying a nutritional supplement is to look for the label on the container that indicates the product is "USP-verified." This signifies that the U.S. Pharmacopeia, a nonprofit organization, has confirmed that the product contains what the manufacturer claims it has, although it doesn't make a judgment as to whether or not it's effective. Taking large doses of vitamins can cause adverse effects, so using them in moderation is preferable and safer. Get your doctor's opinion before trying a special diet, nutritional supplement, or one or more of the thousands of herbal products on the market. For example, some dietary supplements and herbal remedies can increase the risk of bleeding during and after surgery, so surgeons often recommend stopping these at least a week before and a period of time after surgery. Substances that can increase the risk of bleeding include glucosamine, ginseng, Ginkgo biloba, ginger, and garlic, as well as vitamin E, DHEA, EPA, and St.-John's-wort.[225] Because many herbal remedies find their way into breast milk, physicians often advise pregnant and breast-feeding women to avoid herbal medicines during pregnancy and lactation. Discuss this precaution with your doctor.

---

224 Hermann W, Lorenzl S, Obeid R. Review of the role of hyperhomocysteinemia and B-vitamin deficiency in neurological and psychiatric disorders-Current evidence and preliminary recommendations. *Fortschr Neurol Psychiatr.* 2007;75(9):515-527.
225 Veach, M., Vitamins to avoid before surgery. Livingstrong.com, Sept. 17, 2011.

For the majority of dietary supplements and herbal remedies, whether or not they work is part conjecture and part faith. A sixty-five-year-old woman suffered a brain injury from carbon monoxide many years ago and believes she benefited greatly from years of meditation. She spends $600 of her $2,000 monthly income on dietary supplements and herbal remedies and is absolutely convinced that they help. Faith and hope probably play a significant role in her improvement.

To find out the benefits and risks of vitamins, dietary supplements, and special diets, enter the specific supplement into your Internet browser, and look for sites ending in ".edu" or ".gov." These suffixes indicate an education or U.S. government site, respectively, which are more credible than ".com" sites, which are usually commercial sites wanting to sell you something. As with other CAMs, first discuss your thoughts about using them with your physician so you can make a more informed decision and ensure that your treatment is coordinated.

Chapter 13 Key Points

Key Points: Popular CAM Treatments (There are Many)

- Chiropractic; Acupuncture; Naturopathy; Homeopathy; Massage; Meditation; Prayer; Diet/Nutrition/ Vitamins.

Key Points: Complementary, Alternative, and Integrative Treatments

- Differ from traditional medicine.
- Important to first discuss your interest with your PCPhys. or PCP for possible referral to a CAM practitioner to understand the risks/benefits and to coordinate your overall healthcare.
- Before embarking on a CAM treatment, make certain that a suspected medical problem is ruled out.
- Benefits/safety of most CAM treatments have not been proven scientifically.
- Check credentials and licensing of CAM practitioners (some are not licensed).

Key Points: Reasons for Increasing Popularity

- Many CAMs have been practiced for centuries.
- Many CAM practitioners spend more time with patients than PCPhys. or PCP.
- Dissatisfaction with the results of traditional, Western medical treatment.
- Faith and hope to find alternative symptom relief.
- Establishment of National Center for Complementary and Alternative Medicine (NCCAM) to study effectiveness/safety.

Key Points: Results of Some NCCAM Studies

- Acupuncture may be beneficial for functional impairment, chronic pain, and osteoarthritis of the knee.
- Glucosamine and chondroitin sulfate may benefit osteoarthritic pain.
- St. John's Wort is not effective for moderate to severe depression. Has adverse effects if used with some antidepressants and over-the-counter products.

Key Points: Finding a CAM Practitioner

- Ask your PCPhys. or PCP for referrals/suggestions.
- Ask both your PCPhys. and CAM practitioner if they are willing to work collaboratively.
- Check the website – www.nccih.nih.gov.

References

1. Davies RD. Wading through the flood of nontraditional therapies. Journal of Nervous and Mental Disease. 2013;201(7):636-637.

2. Lake JH, Spiegel D, eds. *Complementary and Alternative Treatments in Mental Health Care*. Washington, DC: American Psychiatric Publishing; 2007.

3. Lake JH. *Textbook of Integrative Mental Health Care*. New York, NY: Thieme Medical; 2006.

The Future of Healthcare:
Take Advantage of New Technologies

There are many forces shaping and changing our healthcare system. The evolution of digital technologies and the rapid growth of the Internet of Things (IoT)[226] are powerful agents of change. But there are other dominant factors also at work. In this chapter we will discuss changes already visible and refrain from undo speculation. Thus, we will discuss Mergers occurring in health insurance companies, in pharmaceutical companies, and in hospital systems; growth of Direct Patient-Physician Payment mechanisms; various changes in Clinical Care; increased use of Robotics; new technologies for Outpatient Monitoring; advances in Electronic Health Exchanges; and the possible impact of pending federal Legislation.

Each category of change concludes with a section on *How this might affect you* so you can be prepared to assess and react to the coming healthcare system changes. Any and all of these changes may directly affect you and loved ones and it is important to know in broad brushstrokes what changes are coming so you can be prepared to evaluate their impact and react in your particular best interest. We also track pending healthcare legislation and possible budget cuts on our website (www.qualityaffordablehealthcare.net). Visiting it regularly for Chapter updates will help you keep track of changes in healthcare insurance, healthcare delivery systems, and new advances in treatments.

Rapid Health Industry Consolidations

Consolidation of Insurance Companies

The reduction of four of the largest health insurance companies in the United States into two giant companies was challenged in federal court. Aetna was to buy Humana[227] and Anthem was to buy Cigna [1]. The outcome was that both mergers were separately blocked in early 2017 on antitrust grounds.[228] [229] Anthem

---

226 The IoT is a network of various devices such as smart phones, smart homes, home appliances, cars and trucks that contain embedded electronics, software, sensors, actuators and connector-capacities. They are uniquely identifiable and able to connect and exchange data using the internet.
227 https://news.aetna.com//aetna-to-acquire-humana/
228 https://www.justice.gov/opa/pr/us-district-court-blocks-aetna-s-acquisition-humana
229 https://www.justice.gov/opa/pr/us-district-court-blocks-anthem-s-acquisition-cigna

has appealed its case to the U.S. Supreme Court where it is pending. [230]

Physicians were clearly concerned about any negative effects of such mergers on doctors and patients. Mergers need to be approved by the Justice Department. The American College of Physicians sent a letter to the Justice Department [231] urging close scrutiny of the company claims that savings from the merger would be passed on to consumers or result in higher quality of care. Instead, the reduction of competition in the health insurance market could result in decreased choice and increased cost for patients and employers, reduced access due to the changing and narrowing networks of physicians and hospitals, and the limited ability of physicians to negotiate over the provision of health services with those insurers.

> ***How this might affect you:*** If such mergers should eventually occur—and if physician concerns are accurate—you might find you cannot stay with your present providers as they may no longer participate in your present insurance networks. You might also notice increased premiums due to less competition, which otherwise tends to moderate cost increases.

Merger of Health Insurer Companies with Pharmacy Benefits Manager (PBM[232]) Companies

The attempted consolidation of insurance companies just discussed is an example of a "horizontal" merger where two companies in the same line of business, such as two insurers, combine. Now we turn to "vertical" integrations where companies in two different stages of a supply chain join up. Two recent examples are the joining of Aetna (a health insurer) with CVS Caremark [a PBM and a retail pharmacy and provider chain (CVS stores and Minute Clinics)]. Another very recent example is the Cigna (a health insurer) acquisition of Express Scripts (a PBM). United HealthCare has already owned OptumRX, the number-three PBM which it combined with Catamaran, then the industry's number-four player.

> ***How this might affect you:*** Predictions are mixed [233]. Positive views suggest that you could experience lower healthcare costs of drugs and of providers due to increased use of retail clinics and more integrated convenience of retail clinics and pharmacies in the same location. Negative possibilities include the demise of small drugstores. Other negatives could include competition with other rival insurers such that the insurer could refuse to offer PBM services to other insurers or might decline contracts to fill prescriptions for other insurers' enrollees in geographic areas where Aetna or Cigna might want to defend or strengthen its market share [2].

230 See: (1) http://www.modernhealthcare.com/article/20170505/NEWS/170509919; (2) https://www.forbes.com/sites/brucejapsen/2017/05/05/anthem-seeks-scotus-review-of-cigna-deal/#2b1eab8925f1

231 See: www.acponline.org/newsroom/insurance_company_mergers.htm?hp

232 A PBM is a third-party administrator of prescription drugs. They develop and maintain the formulary, contract with pharmacies, arrange discounts with drug manufacturers and pay prescription drug claims.

233 See: (a) https://www.washingtonpost.com/business/economy/what-the-cvs-aetna-deal-means-for-the-future-of-health-care/2017/12/05/e14a8d18-d907-11e7-a841-2066faf731ef_story.html?noredirect=on&utm_term=.3a23ab85637a; (b) https://www.healio.com/hepatology/practice-management/news/online/%7B844fcd28e-58fd-43e6-80a6-45f214d7a407%7D/cigna-acquires-express-scripts-plans-to-expand-health-services-portfolio; (c) https://slate.com/business/2017/12/the-arguments-for-and-against-the-cvs-aetna-merger.html

Consolidations in the Pharmaceutical Industry and in Retail Pharmacies and Their Health Clinics

In late 2015 the pharmaceutical company Pfizer announced plans to buy Allegan,[234] a move that would create the world's largest drug maker. This acquisition was largely to slash tax costs in the United States by reincorporating overseas. However, the merger was terminated in 2016 due to changes in the United States tax code.[235] Had the deal gone through, implications for consumers are not clear. It is possible that greater corporate size could result in less competition and higher drug prices. However, other mergers of retail pharmacies and their health clinics already have clearer healthcare implications. For example, in late 2015, CVS Health bought Target's on-site pharmacies and clinics.[236] This purchase included Target's 1,672 pharmacies across forty-seven states, and seventy-nine Target clinic locations will be rebranded as MinuteClinic, with CVS Health opening up to twenty new clinics in Target stores within three years of the close of the transaction.

In 2015 Walgreens announced plans to buy Rite Aid in its entirety [3], but by mid-2017 it changed the purchase to buying from Rite Aid some 2,186 of its stores, along with three distribution centers and related inventory.[237] On the pharmacy side, the increase in size and purchasing power of the retail pharmacy chains may lead to higher prescription drug prices. On the retail health clinic side, CVS Health will expand its commitment to having more MinuteClinic on-site clinics. The services at retail clinics may also evolve toward more primary care services. For example, Walmart is testing a new model (the Walmart Care Clinic), which will offer services expected from a primary care provider with referrals to specialists as needed [4]. Thus, we see the distinct possibility of more choices in primary healthcare services from either your PCP or a retail health clinic.

> *How this might affect you:* These consolidations in retail pharmacies and retail clinics might contribute to an increase in your health expenses if you use these health store pharmacy chains. However, you could see more comprehensive services in the retail clinics that would give you the option of getting primary care services on a walk-in basis.

---

234 www.reuters.com/article/us-allergan-m-a-pfizer-idUSKBN0TB0UT20151124#1zHUAS0jPp38Of3O.97
235 http://www.cnbc.com/2016/04/05/pfizer-allergan-will-mutually-terminate-merger-over-inversion-rule-changes-sources-say.html
236 See (1) www.cvshealth.com/content/cvs-health-and-target-sign-agreement-cvs-health-acquire-rebrand-and-operate-target%E2%80%99s; (2) www.cvshealth.com/content/cvs-health-and-target-announce-completed-acquisition-target%E2%80%99s-pharmacy-and-clinic-businesses
237 http://www.cnbc.com/2017/06/29/walgreens-scraps-rite-aid-deal-to-buy-some-stores-instead.html

Increased Hospital Mergers and Purchases of Medical Practices

Physician Ownership of their Practices

Data from a 2016 survey conducted by the American Medical Association[238] show that less than half (47.1 percent) of practicing physicians own their own practice. This is the first year in which physician practice ownership is no longer the majority arrangement.

Hospital and Health System Mergers

Mergers and acquisitions (M&A) have continued at a brisk pace with over a hundred transactions in 2015 that included well-known health centers such as Robert Wood Johnson and Barnabus in New Jersey and Penn State and Pinnacle in Pennsylvania.[239] The M&A trend continued in 2016 and is expected to remain strong throughout 2017. [240] The M&As have included a full range of types of facilities: nonprofit; for-profit; rural; urban; academic; faith-based organizations; and publicly owned nonprofit hospitals.[241]

Hospitals Buy Medical Practices

Hospital ownership of physician practices is on the rise, with an average of 38 percent of U.S. physicians now employed by hospitals and health systems. As of mid-2015, one in four medical practices was hospital owned. This is occurring in every region of the country but is greatest in the Midwest, where some 50 percent of physicians are employed by hospitals. A 2016 study by the American Medical Association[242] showed that for the first time less than 50 percent of physicians (47.1 percent) had an ownership stake in their practice. It also highlights that despite the continued trend toward larger practices, the majority of physicians nationwide still work in small practices. In 2016, 57.8 percent of physicians worked in practices with ten or fewer physicians. The hospitals purchase the physician services through employment contracts and typically also purchase the practice's physical building and equipment.[243]

> *How this might affect you:* The shift toward hospital ownership of physician practices has implications for both physicians and patients. For physicians, the trend can address government and private payer payment policies that increasingly favor integrated and large healthcare systems and make it challenging for physicians to maintain independent practices. For patients, this trend may affect where they receive care and also how much they pay in cost sharing. Overall system costs can increase as well.[244]

238 https://wire.ama-assn.org/practice-management/first-time-physician-practice-owners-are-not-majority
239 http://www.healthleadersmedia.com/leadership/hospital-consolidation-2016-forecast-more-same
240 http://www.beckershospitalreview.com/hospital-transactions-and-valuation/3-healthcare-m-a-predictions-for-2017.html
241 http://www.beckershospitalreview.com/hospital-transactions-and-valuation/hospital-m-a-continues-to-accelerate-in-first-half-of-2016-7-findings.html
242 https://www.ama-assn.org/about-us/physician-practice-benchmark-survey
243 http://www.fiercehealthcare.com/practices/1-4-physician-practices-now-hospital-owned
244 http://www.physiciansadvocacyinstitute.org/Advocacy/Hospital-Health-System-Physicians

Increased Direct Patient-Physician Payment Contracting

There is a trend toward an increase in physician practice models where the practice contracts with patients to pay directly for some or all services. There are many variations in these models, which are often called cash-only, retainer, boutique, concierge, or direct primary care practices. In Chapter 4 we discussed concierge and direct primary care payment models. The American College of Physicians (ACP) in 2015 published a policy position paper on this subject [5] that gives a very helpful overview of this complex trend.

All these payment models as a group are referred to as direct patient contracting practices (DPCPs). DPCPs may have monthly or annual administrative service fees (retainer or concierge fees) in addition to or instead of some of their usual fees for billable services. The growth trend of these payment models is seen in a 2013 survey that showed some 6 percent of doctors were in DPCPs (up from 4 percent in 2012) while a survey in 2014 found some 9.6 percent of "practice owners" were planning to convert to concierge practices in the next one to three years. This growth trend is largely driven by physician frustration with reimbursement and billing problems with payers and the desire to spend more time with their patients. In the fall of 2017, an estimated six hundred plus Direct Primary Care clinic physicians were operating in almost (but not all) states across the United States.[245]

The direct primary care type of DPCP is specifically authorized by the Affordable Care Act (ACA). The ACP position paper notes that the ACA "authorizes direct primary care to be included in the insurance exchanges as long as they are paired with a wraparound insurance policy covering everything outside of primary care (that is, direct primary care combined with a low-cost high-deductible plan). It is the only noninsurance offering to be authorized in the insurance exchanges." The ACP paper also discusses issues of ethics and nondiscriminatory access to the care of lower-income patients who may find the out-of-pocket fees a barrier to care.

> *How this might affect you:* More providers may discuss their newer payment options and suggest how you can benefit from them. You may want to set up a health savings account if you decide the payment arrangements make sense and you can afford it. If affordability is a concern or an obstacle, you may want to see if you can stay with the health provider without any change in your present insurance-based payment structure.

---

245 https://directprimarycarejournal.com/2017/02/04/number-of-dpcs-nationally-2016-2017/

Clinical Care Changes

_____

Increased Telemedicine and Online Services

Telemedicine has been discussed in Chapter 4. Growth estimates in market size vary considerably although market research shows strong global growth with particular strength in North America. As noted in a recent market report [246], "Telemedicine services are applied in several medical areas including consultation, surgery, diabetes, psychiatry, radiology, pathology, cardiology, dermatology and others…Hospitals, Clinics, and Residential (Homecare) with telecommunications technology are end-users of this market… The market for North America telemedicine is segmented based on type, technology and geography. Based on the type, the North America market is divided into telehospitals & teleclinics and telehome. The market is further categorized by technology as hardware, software, telecom and services."

Projections, often expressed in dollar terms, assess global and regional markets where North America is the largest market globally (about 40+ percent of global market size). Some of the estimates indicate near-term growth rates to $34 billion globally by 2020[247]—or a compound annual growth rate of 18.4 percent by 2020.[248] Driving forces for this growth include an increasing elderly population, increasing incidences of chronic diseases, and cost containment efforts to reduce hospital admissions and hospital length of stay resulting in the trend for patients to be monitored in their homes and to have virtual medical visits.

Telemedicine sites charge for their services (see Chapter 4). Given the sites' anticipated growth rate, finding the best telehealth service is in your long-term best interest. Since you may not get the same telemedicine doctor each time, you might want to become more aware of your possible health problem and possible treatments. This would be a way to supplement your use of in-person or telemedicine health services. Thus, you should know there are reputable sites that offer health information and are free to use. They are not a diagnostic tool but can help you narrow your search for information about current symptoms you may have and possible diseases or conditions that can cause such symptoms and how they might be treated. With this information, you can have a more informed conversation with your healthcare professional. Several sites to consider using are (1) "symptom checker" from the Mayo Clinic[249]; (2) familydoctor.org "Search by symptom,"[250] operated by the American Academy of Family Physicians; and (3) WebMDsymptomchecker,[251] from WebMD Health Corp, which is a reliable provider of health information services to consumers, physicians, and other healthcare professionals.

How this might affect you: There will be an increasing number of twenty-four-seven communications and health information available from your home or smartphone. Urgent "middle of the

246 See: North America Telemedicine Market - Growth, Trends and Forecasts (2016 - 2021) [https://www.mordorintelligence.com/industry-reports/north-america-telemedicine-market-industry]
247 http://www.healthcareitnews.com/news/telemedicine-poised-grow-big-time
248 https://www.researchandmarkets.com/reports/3615944/global-medical-cartsworkstations-market-outlook#pos-2
249 www.mayoclinic.org/symptom-checker/select-symptom/itt-20009075
250 www.familydoctor.org/familydoctor/en/health-tools/search-by-symptom.html
251 http://symptoms.webmd.com/#introView

night" assessments and guidance will be easy to obtain as "at home" services when physical discomfort or weather or distance might make travel to medical offices difficult.

Increased Personalized Medicine

Personalized medicine is described as making the treatment as individualized as the disease. It involves identifying genetic, genomic,[252] and clinical information that allows accurate predictions to be made about a person's susceptibility to developing a disease, the course of disease, and its response to treatment.[253] A more formal definition is given by the National Cancer Institute: "Personalized medicine is a form of medicine that uses information about a person's genes, proteins, and environment to prevent, diagnose, and treat disease." In cancer, personalized medicine uses specific information about a person's tumor to help diagnose, plan treatment, find out how well treatment is working, or make a prognosis. Examples of personalized medicine include using targeted therapies to treat specific types of cancer cells, such as HER2-positive breast cancer cells, or using tumor marker testing to help diagnose cancer.[254] For several years the federal government, through the National Institutes of Health and the Food and Drug Administration, has been promoting personalized medicine [6]. It is significant that in 2018 the company called **23andMe**, a leading personal genetics company, received the first-ever FDA authorization for a direct-to-consumer genetic test for cancer risk. The authorization allows the company to provide customers, without a prescription, information on three genetic variants found on the BRCA1 and BRCA2 genes known to be associated with higher risk for breast, ovarian and prostate cancer. The FDA included a warning about limitations of the test regarding cancer risk.[255]

Since genetic/genomic studies are very important in personalized medicine, it is useful to understand the basic areas of application. They include pharmacologic (matching a drug to the patient[256]); diagnostic (genomic profiling for disease and disease risks—see Chapter 14 Appendix: *Genomic Detection of Disease Risk*); and genetic testing for cancer [257] (where the focus is on genomic variations only in the cancer cells of a person, not in the genes of the healthy cells). Because of the growing importance of genomic studies, further information is given in Chapter 14 Appendices: *Genetic Testing and Pharmacogenomics*.

---

252 *Genetic* refers to particular genes whereas *Genomic* refers to the complete genetic information of an organism.
253 http://health.usnews.com/health-conditions/cancer/personalized-medicine/overview
254 www.cancer.gov/publications/dictionaries/cancer-terms?cdrid=561717
255 The three BRCA1/BRCA2 hereditary mutations detected by the test are present in about 2 percent of Ashkenazi Jewish women, according to a National Cancer Institute study, but rarely occur (0 percent to 0.1 percent) in other ethnic populations. All individuals, whether they are of Ashkenazi Jewish descent or not, may have other mutations in BRCA1 or BRCA2 genes, or other cancer-related gene mutations that are not detected by this test. For this reason, a negative test result could still mean that a person has an increased risk of cancer due to gene mutations. Additionally, most cases of cancer are not caused by hereditary gene mutations but are thought to be caused by a wide variety of factors, including smoking, obesity, hormone use and other lifestyle issues. For all of these reasons, it is important for patients to consult their health care professional who can help them understand how these factors impact their individual cancer risk and what they can do to modify that risk.; see: https://www.fda.gov/newsevents/newsroom/pressannouncements/ucm599560.htm
256 www.cnbc.com/2015/12/04/personalized-medicine-better-results-but-at-what-cost.html
257 https://www.cancer.org/cancer/cancer-causes/genetics/understanding-genetic-testing-for-cancer.html

How this might affect you: Initial visits to PCPs or specialists may routinely include some genomic profile "baseline" measures. You will more frequently hear "let's check your genome" or related genetic-oriented measures as your treatment plan is evolving or being revised.

First Gene Therapies Approved

In 2017 the FDA approved gene therapies for two types of blood cancers (B-cell acute lymphoblastic leukemia; and Non-Hodgkin lymphoma) [258]. These are personalized treatments that engineer a patient's own immune system to hunt down and kill cancer cells. In 2018 the FDA approved a third gene therapy for a rare retinal disorder that can lead to blindness[259]. It works by a different mechanism by supplying a third normal gene that functions in the retinal cells to correct vision problems even though the two defective mutated genes remain in place.

New Views of Cancer as a Chronic Disease

Significant life-extending advances have occurred in a number of cancer treatments. This is leading to a new view of cancer as a chronic disease rather than a terminal illness. While the cancer may not be cured, the newer treatments can add years to life expectancy as patients are living much longer with the disease.[260] Organizations such as the University of Texas M.D. Anderson Cancer Center [7] in 2008 and the American Cancer Society[261] in 2015 and 2016[262] have expressed such views. This reflects advances in treatments that are more targeted to interfere with specific molecular pathways that promote cancer. Also, now there are often second- and third-line therapies available whereas just a few years ago there was only a single therapy available. Thus, when the effectiveness of a first treatment diminishes, the patient can now have a second or third treatment approach, each treatment adding increased chances for survival.

How this might affect you: Your oncology team can be more confident of its ability to significantly help you (and sometimes even cure you). Thus, their outlook is more positive as they have more sequences of treatments available, and the longer your survival, the greater the likelihood of new

---

258 See: (1) https://www.sciencenews.org/article/car-t-cell-gene-therapy-top-science-stories-2017-yir; (2) https://www.fda.gov/newsevents/newsroom/pressannouncements/ucm581216.htm; (3) https://www.fda.gov/drugs/informationondrugs/approveddrugs/ucm574154.htm
259 https://www.fda.gov/newsevents/newsroom/pressannouncements/ucm589467.htm
260 http://health.usnews.com/health-news/patient-advice/articles/2015/11/03/managing-cancer-as-a-chronic-condition
261 www.cancer.org/treatment/survivorshipduringandaftertreatment/understandingrecurrence/whenyourcancercomesback/when-cancer-comes-back-treating-cancer-as-chronic-illness
262 https://www.cancer.org/treatment/survivorship-during-and-after-treatment/when-cancer-doesnt-go-away.html

breakthrough treatments can become available. The new treatments will likely include novel gene therapies as several were recently approved.

Robotics

A robot is a machine that is computer programmable and able to automatically execute a complex series of actions. The actions can be guided by either an external or an embedded control device. Robots may or may not look like humans. There are several areas of robotics that are already contributing to healthcare and their roles will only increase with time.

Surgical Robots

The da Vinci surgical system[263] has been available since its FDA approval in 2000. It allows an on-site surgeon to do many surgical procedures in a minimally invasive way using a laparoscope for visual guidance. The small incisions for the laparoscope and instruments allow a faster recovery from the operation. The surgical instruments are remotely controlled by the attending surgeon who is present in the operating room. The system is used in Cardiac Surgery, Colorectal Surgery, General Surgery, Gynecologic Surgery, Head and Neck Surgery, Thoracic Surgery, and Urologic Surgery. Other robot systems are being used in Neurosurgery [8]. One extension of this capability will likely be the capacity to do some surgical procedures where the surgeon is at a considerable distance and operating via tele-surgery using various surgical systems [9]. This could bring surgical services to more remote healthcare sites for planned or emergency interventions. Another potential trend is reducing or eliminating altogether the surgeon's hand control of some procedures and replacing it with "supervised autonomous robotic soft tissue surgery" [10].

Medical Robots

A different application involves what is referred to as micro- and nanorobotics. A recent review is very helpful in understanding the enormous potential in this area [11]. These are very small devices that are a few millimeters in size (nanorobots are significantly smaller) which are placed and guided into the body where they can potentially do various tasks with more precision and less adverse patient effects. Their basic functions can include:

- Targeted therapy
  - targeted drug delivery to body locations or cells of interest

---

263 www.davincisurgery.com/

- - delivery of radioactive seeds near tumor cells; local delivery of heat energy to destroy unwanted cells
  - Material removal
    - removal of material such as fatty deposits in blood vessels or destroying a kidney stone or taking a local biopsy
  - Controllable structures
    - scaffolds to support regeneration of nerves, artificial organs developed and blood vessels regrown
    - stents to keep passageways open such as in clogged blood vessels
    - occlusions introduced deliberately such as to clog a blood vessel that feeds a tumor
    - Telemetry to transmit from a specific location information that otherwise would be difficult or impossible to obtain
    - Remote sensing such as the time pattern of oxygen concentration or location of an object of interest such as cancer or blood
    - Marking and transmitting the microrobot's position in the location of phenomena such as internal bleeding

Rehabilitation Robots

The scope of rehabilitation robots includes "devices to train (robot-aided therapies), support (exoskeletons), or replace (prosthesis) impaired activities or impaired body functions and structures are covered in rehabilitation robotics [12]". Robotic arms, hands, fingers, legs and feet are becoming increasingly sophisticated and clinically available. Their robotic components typically include biosensors, controllers, and actuators. Efforts are clearly underway to improve the inclusion of robotics in the general field of rehabilitation medicine and in particular for the neurorehabilitation of the upper limb.

Other Healthcare Use of Robots

Some further examples of robotics in healthcare are found in hospitals. For example, **Hospital Robots** are being developed for cleaning areas of potential hospital-acquired infection. One type of robot, the Xenex LightStrike™ Germ-Zapping™ Robots,[264] uses high intensity ultraviolet light to disinfect any space in a healthcare facility quickly and efficiently. **Receptionist Robots** are being tested to give clear and accurate information about where a patient should go and when. **Pharmacy Robot** systems are found in the filling, monitoring and stocking of prescribed medicines. An example here is ScriptPro[265] which since its initial product in 1997, the SP 200 Robotic Prescription Dispensing System, has pioneered the use of robotics in

---

264 https://www.xenex.com/our-solution/lightstrike/
265 https://www.scriptpro.com/About/; https://www.scriptpro.com/products/robotic-prescription-dispensing-systems/

community pharmacies. The company states that it now has over 200 pharmacy automation and management system products. Many hospitals and large chain pharmacies have standardized operations around their ScriptPro robotic model.

> *How this might affect you:* **Surgical Robots** may speed your recovery from surgery and also have treatment available in more remote settings where tele-surgery is available. **Medical Robots** have the potential for enormous improvement in localized applications such as cancer treatment and cardiovascular disease. **Rehabilitation Robots** can speed recovery of lost or diminished bodily functions. **Hospital Robots** can reduce the serious problem of hospital-acquired infections.

New Technologies

Outpatient Monitoring

Medical and fitness monitoring are growing in popularity. An increasing number of devices and apps are contributing to this substantial new trend in healthcare. *Wrist and clothing monitors*[266] can track blood pressure, heart rate, and sleep activity level with headsets that can monitor brainwaves. *Ear monitors*[267] can monitor blood pressure, respiration rate, oxygen saturation, heart rate, number of steps taken, and calories burned. *Sweat sensor strips*[268] can measure metabolic substances secreted in your sweat and can also track glucose, electrolyte balance, hydration level, muscle exertion, and physical performance.

Other technologies include *smartphone case devices.*[269] Their capabilities include monitoring blood glucose levels; mobile breathalyzer for blood alcohol level; and reading and recording single-channel electrocardiogram (ECG) measurements (ECG tests measure the electrical activity of your heart, and can help monitor and detect many issues with the heart). This is only a sample of some current ambulatory monitoring devices that generate medical data. Many devices can be purchased online, such as on Google Play or iTunes. Some of these apps may soon require FDA approval and a prescription. As technology advances and new capacities are blended with new communication technologies, from home to medical facilities, use of such data may become routine.

> *How this might affect you:* You may be trained to incorporate the new monitoring capabilities that are personalized to your health issues. There will likely be more routine data communication from your monitors with your physician offices via secure health networks so your doctors will know how to respond to the medical data and how best to guide your health care.

---

266 e-patients.net/archives/2014/12/hot-trends-in-health-care-for-2015.html
267 www.cnn.com/2014/12/19/tech/partner-digital-health-trends/
268 See: (1) https://www.wired.com/2014/11/sweat-sensors/; (2) https://www.sciencedaily.com/releases/2016/10/161013150512.htm
269 www.allthingsd.com/20130703/house-call-five-smartphone-accessories-that-help-monitor-your-health/

Role of "Big Data"

Big Data refers to an accumulation of data that is too large and complex for processing by traditional database management tools.[270] Such extremely large data sets are analyzed for trends and associations, especially relating to human behavior and interactions. "Big Data in healthcare is being used to predict epidemics, cure disease, improve quality of life and avoid preventable deaths." [271] Sources of healthcare Big Data include:[272]

- Physicians' notes

- Patient-generated health data

- Genomics

- Physiological monitoring data, including data from wearable devices

- Medical imaging data

- Publicly available data

- Credit card and purchasing data

- Social media data

Here's an example of how Big Data analysis can be applied. In a hospital setting, special attention can be paid to a targeted group of patients at high risk for sepsis (a life-threatening condition when the body is overwhelmed with an infection). The hospital's electronic health record capacities can be programmed to continuously monitor key clinical indicators to recognize potential septic patterns and to notify the healthcare team of the early signs of possible sepsis for a given patient.

The types of Big Data require a different type of cloud computing.[273] This reflects that Big Data is not arranged in the traditional relational database of table and column format. The data can be used for **real time alerts,** as in the case of sepsis, above. The data can also be used for **predictive analytics,** such as comparing the details of the clinical trajectory of a particular patient with many other patients having the same or similar condition. Once predictive analytics find that the patient is in a known clinical group, **prescriptive analytics** and **genomics** can be used to therapeutically intervene and change the potential course of that illness. The progression in computing to analyzing Big Data clusters is in its relative infancy.

How this might affect you: You may hear references to Big Data or "cloud computing," which are helping your healthcare team to refine and individualize their treatments for you or your loved ones.

---

270 https://www.merriam-webster.com/dictionary/big%20data
271 https://www.forbes.com/sites/bernardmarr/2015/04/21/how-big-data-is-changing-healthcare/#58528b6f2873
272 https://www.eiseverywhere.com/file_uploads/9b7793c3ad732c28787b2a8bc0892c31_Elena-Sini_How-Big-Data-is-Changing-Healthcare.pdf
273 https://www.slideshare.net/healthcatalyst1/big-data-in-healthcare-made-simple-where-it-stands-today-and-where-its-going?next_slideshow=1

Electronic Health Exchange Advances

National Data Exchange System (eHealth Exchange)

The eHealth Exchange [274] is a rapidly growing health information exchange network for securely sharing clinical information over the Internet nationwide. The eHealth Exchange spans all fifty states and is the largest health information exchange infrastructure in the United States. Current eHealth Exchange participants include some 50,000 medical groups; four federal agencies— Department of Defense (DoD); Veterans Administration (VA); Centers for Medicare and Medicaid Services (CMS); and the Social Security Administration (SSA)—65 percent of U.S. hospitals; 3,400+ dialysis centers; and some 8,300 pharmacies. Together the eHealth Exchange supports more than 100 million patients.

Access to Your Health Records and How to Use Them

Having the eHealth Exchange in place is a major benefit to you and all patients. The most direct effect is allowing all of us to directly access and download our medical records and to use them in a variety of helpful ways. As America's healthcare system rapidly goes digital, healthcare providers, insurance companies, and others are starting to give patients and consumers access to their health information electronically through the "Blue Button," [275] whose logo is:

Health information about you may be stored in many places, such as doctors' offices, hospitals, drugstores, laboratories, and health insurance companies. The Blue Button symbol signifies that an organization has a way for you to access your health records electronically so you can:

- Share them with your doctor or trusted family members or caregivers
- Check to make sure the information, such as your medication list, is accurate and complete
- Keep track of when your child had his/her last vaccination
- Have your medical history available in case of an emergency, when traveling, when seeking a second opinion, or when switching health insurance companies
- Plug your health information into apps and tools that help you set and reach personalized health goals.

---

274   See: (1) https://www.healthit.gov/topic/health-it-basics/health-information-exchange; (2) http://sequoiaproject.org/ehealth-exchange/about/
275   See: (1) https://www.healthit.gov/topic/health-it-initiatives/blue-button; (2) https://www.healthit.gov/resource/blue-button-faqs

Blue Button capacities were originally a federally sponsored initiative. Healthcare organizations who participate in Blue Button, including Medicare,[276] display the logo as a symbol that you can easily access your health records here! The Blue Button enables you to securely access your personal health data online by clicking on a "Blue Button" icon. You can use the Blue Button Connector[277] search function to find out which healthcare providers and health companies offer electronic access to your health records. You can also use the iBlueButton[278] mobile app or similar ones for portability on your smartphone. You may have access to your claims and personal health information that is maintained by your doctors, hospitals, health plans, and others, depending on the tools and data they offer. Patients can securely access their health data and then choose to download that data to their computer, thumb drive, or smartphone without using any special software, or they can share that data with individuals they trust—whether it's their other physicians or family members. Protection of health data and compliance with HIPAA privacy requirements is a major challenge, especially with data being downloaded and stored on many laptops that have been lost or stolen. Key components of such HIPAA security compliance is discussed in a helpful online overview.[279]

While the organization of the downloaded data may be somewhat different from the organization discussed in Chapter 1 concerning your personal health record (PHR), the data can be reorganized or merged after you have downloaded it if you wish. Blue Button information can be lifesaving in an emergency situation, can help prevent medication errors, and can improve care coordination so everyone who is caring for you is on the same page.

New Ways to Use the Health Data

Once the data is downloaded, it can interact with a variety of other electronic tools and apps. Here's an example. There's an app that can graph your blood glucose levels if you are a diabetic so you can see your trends over time and tell if you are progressing and in proper control of the levels. There are currently some 14,000 apps related to health and medicine. In addition to managing health conditions, some of the apps can help you get a handle on your medical bills, access wellness resources, and support yourself and your loved ones as a family caregiver. A list of high-quality apps[280] includes those where you do not need to input the data since they can interact with the health data you have already downloaded. These listed apps use a group of nationally recognized standards that enables them to access information directly from your healthcare providers' records or another data source.

How this might affect you: These apps speed communications among your providers and allow them to be more reliable. Medical records that you wanted your provider to see used to take weeks or longer to transmit. Now your provider can routinely say, "Yup, I got those records the next day—

---

276 If you go to the Medicare site (https://www.mymedicare.gov/) you will see reference to the Blue Button download option on the initial page. After you log in you will see the Blue Button icon in the upper right corner.

277 https://www.healthit.gov/how-to-get-your-health-record/

278 http://www.ibluebutton.com/about.html

279 https://www.healthcatalyst.com/HIPAA-security-compliance-culture-technology

280 http://www.openhealthnews.com/tagged/blue-button-apps

thanks. As a result, I want to make the following changes in your treatment . . . ." You are now much more in active shared control of your health and healthcare.

Federal Legislation and Budget Cuts

New American Health Care legislation

It is too early to evaluate the impact of recent legislation on the cost and quality and availability of health services availability. We will keep you updated about future events that will be tracked for you on our website (www.qualityaffordablehealthcare.net).

Home Health Planning Changes

Several changes in home care services are presently under consideration. A roadmap of needed changes is found in a paper from The Alliance for Home Health Quality and Innovation (May 2014) entitled "The Future of Home Health Care Project." [281] The review discusses the bias toward office-based and institutional care with growing concerns that there is not enough space in facilities to meet the growing needs of an aging population. Hence the need to promote services at home. Recommendations include (1) payments revised to focus on outcome value (rather than volume); (2) a focus on continuous long-term care support not requiring the recipient to be homebound; and (3) a broader array of non-skilled services (such as transportation; personal care services and care giving supports; housing and meals/nutrition). Clearly there is both a need and an opportunity for home health care to evolve in the coming years.

A second area of improved home care services may flow from the Home Health Care Planning Improvement Act of 2017 (S.445), which was reintroduced in Congress on February 27, 2017. [282] This new area is meant to improve care planning for Medicare Home Health Services. It would allow a nurse practitioner (NP), a clinical nurse specialist working with a physician in accordance with state law, a certified nurse-midwife, or a physician assistant (PA) under a physician's supervision to sign home health plans of care and to certify Medicare patients for the home health benefit. These professionals would no longer have to find a physician who would document the NP's or PA's assessment for this care.

> *How this might affect you:* Home services would start more quickly after your need for them is established. You would see more NPs and PAs involved in your care. Home services would be broader to include non-skilled support components and could be more continuous with adjustments as needed whether you are homebound or not.

---

281 www.ahhqi.org/images/pdf/future-whitepaper.pdf
282 See: (1) https://report.nahc.org/?s=home+health+care+planning+improvement+act; (2) www.aanp.org/press-room/press-releases/166-press-room/2015-press-releases/1686-nurse-practitioners-applaud-introduction-of-the-home-health-care-planning-improvement-act-of-2015

Federal Budget Cuts

Budget cuts that were occurring in 2017 had a disproportionate impact on the elderly and the poor: reduction of Meals on Wheels[283]; low-cost and free legal services[284]; and the low-income Home Energy Assistance Program.[285] With such cuts there may be many implications for the health and healthcare of the affected population: adequacy of nutrition; protection from abuse and neglect; and choices between heating and cooling versus food and medicine.

Track Annual Changes in Your Insurance Coverage

If you have Medicare, we recommend two useful websites. You can sign up for alerts from Medicare Watch: Your Weekly Medicare Consumer Advocacy Update.[286] Or you can use the www.medicare.gov site, which is the official U.S. government site for Medicare that is both comprehensive and user-friendly.

If you do not have Medicare but have health insurance from your employer, be sure to keep in touch with your employer regarding any changes in coverage, and be sure you update to your employer any changes in your own status that could affect your coverage, such as marriage or the birth of a child. If you have or need health insurance from a state exchange, you can use www.healthcare.gov (a federal government website managed by the U.S. Centers for Medicare and Medicaid Services) to connect to your state insurance marketplace ("exchange") website. You can track changes and alternative health plans and decide whether to stay with your plan or move to a different one during defined enrollment periods each year. For example, if you had 2016 Marketplace coverage and didn't act to renew or change your health plan by mid-December 2016, you were probably automatically enrolled in the same plan for 2017 (or a similar one if your old plan wasn't available). This means you had coverage starting January 1, 2017. Alternatively, you could either call customer service at your healthcare company or go to their website to answer questions about your coverage and any changes that are to be implemented.

How this might affect you: Your pharmacy coverage may change annually if drugs you use are deleted from formularies. Your insurance company may withdraw some of its plans from the marketplace or modify them in a way that may make you look for new health coverage plans. New services or modified services may present opportunities that interest you to promote your best health.

---

283   http://www.usatoday.com/story/news/politics/2017/03/18/meal-on-wheels-trump-budget-proposal-cuts/99308928/
284   http://www.abajournal.com/news/article/trump_budget_eliminates_funding_for_legal_services_corp
285   See (1) https://assets.aarp.org/rgcenter/consume/fs138_liheap.pdf; (2) https://thinkprogress.org/trump-budget-could-mean-fatally-cold-winters-for-some-of-americas-poor-8bbb53a8e7f4#.l5ym51lxf
286   www.medicarerights.org/resources/newsletters/medicare-watch

Chapter 14 Appendix

Genomic Detection of Disease Risk

Clinical research in genomic medicine is done in what are called "genomewide association studies." These study hundreds of thousands of gene-related components [called single-nucleotide polymorphisms (SNPs)] that are associated with a disease in hundreds or thousands of persons who have the disease. As discussed by Manolio, [13] these studies have revolutionized the search for genetic influences on complex traits. These complex conditions, unlike single-gene disorders, are caused by many genetic and environmental factors working together, each having a relatively small effect. And few if any are absolutely required for the disease to occur. See the reference for further details.

Genetic Testing

The following overview is taken from "Frequently Asked Questions about Genetic Testing." [287]

What is genetic testing?

Genetic testing uses laboratory methods to look at your genes, which are the DNA instructions you inherit from your mother and father. Genetic tests may be used to identify increased risks of health problems, to choose treatments, or to assess responses to treatments.

What can I learn from testing?

There are many different types of genetic tests. Genetic tests can help to

- Diagnose disease
- Identify gene changes that are responsible for an already diagnosed disease
- Determine the severity of a disease
- Guide doctors in deciding on the best medicine or treatment to use for certain individuals
- Identify gene changes that may increase the risk of developing a disease
- Identify gene changes that could be passed on to children
- Screen newborn babies for certain treatable conditions

Genetic test results can be hard to understand. However, specialists such as geneticists and genetic counselors can help explain what results might mean to you and your family. Such specialists can be located at several online sites.[288] Because genetic testing tells you information about your DNA, which is shared with other family members, sometimes a genetic test result may have implications for blood relatives of the person who had testing.

---

287 National Human Genome Research Institute (www.genome.gov/19516567)
288 (1) National Society of Genetics Counselors (www.nsgc.org/); (2) https://ghr.nlm.nih.gov/primer/consult/findingprofessional

What are the different types of genetic tests?

Diagnostic testing is used to precisely identify the disease that is making a person ill. The results of a diagnostic test may help you make choices about how to treat or manage your health.

Predictive and pre-symptomatic genetic tests are used to find gene changes that increase a person›s likelihood of developing diseases. The results of these tests provide you with information about your risk of developing a specific disease. Such information may be useful in decisions about your lifestyle and healthcare. For example, if you have a family history of diabetes, it may influence your diet and involvement in physical exercise.

Carrier testing is used to find people who "carry" a change in a gene that is linked to disease. Carriers may show no signs of the disease; however, they have the ability to pass on the gene change to their children, who may develop the disease or become carriers themselves. Some diseases require a gene change to be inherited from both parents for the disease to occur. This type of testing usually is offered to people who have a family history of a specific inherited disease or who belong to certain ethnic groups that have a higher risk of specific inherited diseases. For example, sickle cell trait (also known as being a carrier) occurs when a person has one gene for sickle hemoglobin and one gene for normal hemoglobin. Approximately one in ten African Americans carries sickle cell trait. People who are carriers generally do not have any medical problems and lead normal lives.

Prenatal testing is offered during pregnancy to help identify fetuses that have certain diseases.

Newborn screening is used to test babies one or two days after birth to find out if they have certain diseases known to cause problems with health and development.

Pharmacogenomic testing gives information about how certain medicines are processed by an individual's body. This type of testing can help your healthcare provider choose the medicines that work best with your genetic makeup.

Research genetic testing is used to learn more about the contributions of genes to health and to disease. Sometimes the results may not be directly helpful to participants, but they may benefit others by helping researchers expand their understanding of the human body, health, and disease.

Pharmacogenomics

The following overview is taken from "Frequently Asked Questions about Pharmacogenomics." [289]

What is pharmacogenomics?

Pharmacogenomics uses information about a person's genetic makeup, or genome, to choose the drugs and drug doses that are likely to work best for that particular person. This new field combines the science of how drugs work, called pharmacology, with the science of the human genome, called genomics.

What might pharmacogenomics mean for you?

Until recently, drugs have been developed with the idea that each drug works pretty much the same in everybody. But genomic research has changed that "one size fits all" approach and opened the door to more personalized approaches to using and developing drugs.

Depending on your genetic makeup, some drugs may work more or less effectively for you than they do in other people. Likewise, some drugs may produce more or fewer side effects in you than in someone else. In the near future, doctors will be able to routinely use information about your genetic makeup to choose those drugs and drug doses that offer the greatest chance of helping you.

---

289 'National Human Genome Research Institute (www.genome.gov/27530645)

Pharmacogenomics may also help to save you time and money. By using information about your genetic make-up, doctors soon may be able to avoid the trial-and-error approach of giving you various drugs that are not likely to work for you until they find the right one. Using pharmacogenomics, the "best-fit" drug to help you can be chosen from the beginning.

How is pharmacogenomic information being used today?

Although doctors are starting to use pharmacogenomic information to prescribe drugs, such tests are routine for only a few health problems. However, given the field's rapid growth, pharmacogenomics is soon expected to lead to better ways of using drugs to manage heart disease, cancer, asthma, depression, and many other common diseases and conditions.

One current use of pharmacogenomics is with the human immunodeficiency virus (HIV). Before prescribing the antiviral drug abacavir (Ziagen), doctors now routinely test HIV-infected patients for a genetic variant that makes them more likely to have a bad reaction to the drug.

Another example is the breast cancer drug trastuzumab (Herceptin). This therapy works only for women whose tumors have a particular genetic profile that leads to overproduction of a protein called HER2.

The U.S. Food and Drug Administration (FDA) also recommends genetic testing before giving the chemotherapy drug mercaptopurine (Purinethol) to patients with acute lymphoblastic leukemia. Some people have a genetic variant that interferes with their ability to process the drug. This processing problem can cause severe side effects and increase the risk of infection unless the standard dose is adjusted according to the patient's genetic makeup.

The FDA also advises doctors to test colon cancer patients for certain genetic variants before administering irinotecan (Camptosar), which is part of a combination chemotherapy regimen. The reasoning is that patients with one particular variant may not be able to clear the drug from their bodies as quickly as other patients, resulting in severe diarrhea and increased infection risk. Such patients may need to receive lower doses of the drug.

What other uses of pharmacogenomics are being studied?

Much research is under way to understand how genomic information can be used to develop more personalized and cost-effective strategies for using drugs to improve human health.

In 2007, the FDA revised the label on the common blood-thinning drug warfarin (Coumadin) to explain that a person's genetic makeup might influence response to the drug. Some doctors have since begun using genetic information to adjust warfarin dosage. Still, more research is needed to conclusively determine whether warfarin dosing that includes genetic information is better than the current trial-and-error approach.

The FDA also is considering genetic testing for another blood thinner, clopidogrel bisulfate (Plavix), used to prevent dangerous blood clots. Researchers have found that Plavix may not work well in people with a certain genetic variant.

Cancer is another very active area of pharmacogenomic research. Studies have found that the chemotherapy drugs gefitinib (Iressa) and erlotinib (Tarceva) work much better in lung cancer patients whose tumors have a certain genetic variant. On the other hand, research has shown that the chemotherapy drugs cetuximab (Erbitux) and panitumumab (Vecitibix) do not work very well in the 40 percent of colon cancer patients whose tumors have a particular genetic variant.

Pharmacogenomics may also help to quickly identify the best drugs to treat people with certain mental health disorders. For example, while some patients with depression respond to the first drug they are given, many do not, and doctors have to try another drug. Because each drug takes weeks to take its full effect, patients' depression may grow worse during the time spent searching for a drug that helps.

Recently, researchers identified genetic variations that influence the response of depressed people to citalopram (Celexa), which belongs to a widely used class of antidepressant drugs called selective serotonin reuptake inhibitors (SSRIs). Clinical trials are now under way to learn whether genetic tests that predict SSRI response can improve patients' outcomes.

Can pharmacogenomics be used to develop new drugs?

Yes. Besides improving the ways in which existing drugs are used, genome research is aimed at developing better drugs. The goal is to produce new drugs that are highly effective and do not cause serious side effects.

Until recently, drug developers usually used an approach that involved screening for chemicals with broad action against a disease. Researchers are now using genomic information to find or design drugs targeting subgroups of patients with specific genetic profiles. In addition, researchers are using pharmacogenomic tools to search for drugs aimed at specific molecular and cellular pathways involved in disease.

Pharmacogenomics may also breathe new life into some drugs that were abandoned during the drug's development process. For example, development of the beta-blocker drug bucindolol (Gencaro) was stopped after two other beta-blocker drugs won FDA approval to treat heart failure. But interest in Gencaro revived after tests showed that the drug worked well in patients with two genetic variants that regulate heart function. If Gencaro is approved by the FDA, it could become the first new heart drug to require a genetic test before prescription.

Chapter 14 Key Points

Key Points: Health Industry Consolidations

- Major insurance companies try to merge
- Consolidation within the pharmaceutical industry
- Hospitals merge and buy private medical practices
- Less marketplace competition
- More corporate influence on governments and regulators
- Less physician influence on corporations
- Less ability to negotiate
- Probable increased consumer costs
- Probable reduced choice of doctors and hospital networks
- Larger presence of retail health clinics
- Perhaps more primary care services

Key Points: Non-insurance Medical Payments

- More frequent occurrence of direct patient contracting practices
- Direct primary care model
    - Only non-insurance authorized by ACA

      o Needs to be paired with wraparound insurance policy for all non-primary care services

- Many other variations of direct payments
  - Cash only; retainer; boutique; concierge
  - Issues of ethics, affordability, and nondiscriminatory practices

Key Points: Changing Clinical Care Trends

- Growth of telemedicine
  - Particularly in underserved and rural areas
  - "Convenience" in urban areas
- Growth of personalized medicine
  - Particular focus on one's genes and genome
  - Disease risk assessment
  - Treatment guided by various genomic indicators
- New views of cancer as a chronic disease
  - Multiple therapy sequences now often available; each prolongs survival
  - Longer survival allows newer treatments to emerge and be used

Key Points: New Technologies

- New wearable monitors
  - Wrist and clothing; ear; sweat sensor strips
  - New smartphone case medical applications
- Increased use of Robotics
  - Surgical
  - Telesurgery
  - Microrobots
  - Robots in hospitals
  - Robots in pharmacies
  - Reception robots
- Improved communication with doctors
  - Using the Internet to see what diseases may be causing your symptoms
  - Using the Internet to better understand your disease and treatment options
- Growing role for "Big Data" analyses
  - Real-time alerts to monitor patient data

  o Predictive analytics to chart clinical trajectory of illness

  o Prescriptive analytics and genomics to intervene in clinical trajectory

- National Health Data System

  o Known as the eHealth Exchange

  o Faster reliable communication between providers and hospitals

  o Avoids needless duplication of tests

  o Provides chance to download personal health records from various providers

Key Points: Improved Home Care Services

- Less red tape; faster startup when needed
- More non-skilled and support services
- More flexibility when patients are homebound
- Services can be more continuous

References

1. Mattioli, D., A.W. Mathews, and C. Dulaney *Anthem agrees to buy Cigna for $48.4 billion: Deal, which needs regulatory approval, would help reshape health insurance industry*. The Wall Street Journal, July 24, 2015.

2. Dafny, L.S., *Does CVS-Aetna spell the end of business as usual?* New England Journal of Medicine, 2018. **378**(7): p. 593-95.

3. de la Merced, M.J. and H. Tabuchi. *Walgreens to buy Rite Aid for $9.4 billion*. Oct. 27, 2015 [cited 2015 December 2015]; Available from: http://www.nytimes.com/2015/10/28/business/dealbook/walgreens-rite-aid-deal.html?_r=0.

4. Iglehart, J.K., *The Expansion of Retail Clinics—Corporate Titans vs. Organized Medicine.* New England Journal of Medicine, 2015. **373**(4): p. 301-3.

5. Doherty, R., *Assessing the Patient Care Implications of "Concierge" and Other Direct Patient Contracting Practices: A Policy Position Paper From the American College of Physicians.* Annals of Internal Medicine, 2015. **163 (12)**:949-942.

6. Hamburg, M.A. and F.S. Collins, *The path to personalized medicine.* New England Journal of Medicine, 2010. **363**(4): p. 301-4.

7. Witter, D.C. and J. LeBas, *Cancer as a chronic disease.* OncoLog: A publication of M.D. Anderson Cancer Center, 2008. **53**(4): p. 1-3.

8. Ahmed, S.I., et al., *Robotics in neurosurgery: A literature review.* Journal of Pakistan Medical Association, 2018. **68**(2): p. 258-263.

9. Nisar, S. and O. Hasan, *State of the art and key design challenges of telesurgical robotics.*, in *Encyclopedia of Information Science and Technology*, M. Khosrow-Pour, Editor. 2018, IGI Global; Information Science Reference (an imprint of IGI Global): Hershey, Pennsylvnia. p. 6872-6881.

10. Shademan, A., et al., *Supervised autonomous robotic soft tissue surgery.* Science Translational Medicine, 2016. **8**(337): p. 337ra64.

11. Nelson, B.J., I.K. Kaliakatsos, and J.J. Abbott, *Microrobots for minimally invasive medicine.* Annual Review of Biomedical Engineering, 2010. **12**: p. 55-85.

12. Oña, E.D., et al., *A Review of Robotics in Neurorehabilitation: Towards an Automated Process for Upper Limb.* Journal of Healthcare Engineering, 2018. **2018**(Article ID 9758939): p. 1-19.

13. Manolio, T.A., *Genomewide association studies and assessment of the risk of disease.* New England Journal of Medicine, 2010. **363**(2): p. 166-76.

Conclusion

Having read our book, we'd like to summarize the most important take-home messages. Most important is the need to take more control and responsibility for your healthcare decisions and for staying healthy. That's because America's healthcare system has become more impersonal; doctors are pressured to see more patients for shorter visits. There's a shortage of doctors; fewer are taking new patients, especially those with Medicare, Medicaid, and other government insurance. And, your out-of-pocket medical costs continue to spiral out of control. Healthcare bills continue as the number one cause of personal bankruptcy.

Assuming more responsibility requires overcoming our natural tendency to believe we're not vulnerable to illness so you can be fully prepared if you or a family member needs medical care. Planning includes: choosing the best doctor who's skilled at taking responsibility for being the "captain" (coordinator) of your healthcare team; selecting the right person, if needed, to be your patient advocate ("guardian agent"); preparing and updating your personal health record; evaluating yearly your health insurance; choosing the best hospital and emergency department to use should misfortune strike. Advance planning also includes: being mindful of how to avoid frequent doctor, hospital, and medication errors – especially during periods of transition (e.g. changing to a new doctor; admission to, and discharge from, a healthcare facility).

Protecting yourself from medical debt includes: using health professionals and facilities that are "in-network"; understanding the "inside" story about how medical billing really works; using strategies to negotiate medical bills before and even after they're incurred; carefully reassessing your insurance choices as you get older (e.g. studying Medicare plan options). Even though the December 2017 tax law ended the mandate for all Americans to have health insurance, which increased insurance premiums especially for the middle aged and the self-employed, maintain some type of health insurance for you and your family! You are more valuable than your insured car! Find out if you qualify for a federal tax rebate or subsidy to reduce your cost for insurance. Consider an insurance plan with a high yearly deductible which is less expensive and may make you eligible for a health savings plan where you can save tax deductible money.

Should you or a family member become ill when your PCPhys. and his/her associates are unavailable, know in advance about the availability of new, innovative, outpatient facilities. These include your employer's health clinic; a local retail or urgent care center; telemedicine (especially if you live far from a medical center); and know when to use the most expensive out-patient option for a life-threatening illness – the emergency department.

Obtaining the best medical care includes knowing when and how to obtain a second and even third medical opinion: when you're not recovering from an illness; your diagnosis is not determined; you're told by your doctor "there is nothing more that can be done" but your intuition and family tell you otherwise. Thirty percent of patients who seek a second medical opinion discover that their original diagnosis was incorrect or that a better treatment is available. Consultation with an expert can not only save you money, but can save your life!

Should you become seriously ill and require hospitalization, having a trusted family member and/or patient advocate who's readily available to oversee your care can protect you from common hospital errors that especially occur during periods of transition. Risky transition periods include: when you're admitted to a hospital and the new captain of your healthcare team is a hospitalist who doesn't know you and during nursing shift changes. Bring to the hospital all your medical information and legal documents (e.g. your PHR, living will, patient advocate form, healthcare and financial proxy) and some personal items (e.g. family photos). Get to personally know the nursing staff and be known as a real person who is inquisitive, cooperative, and appreciative rather than as a diagnosis or hospital I.D. number.

Assuming more control and responsibility also extends to the medications you take. Understand the benefits and potential side effects of your medication. If you need advice, develop a constructive alliance with those health professionals you can rely on – your physicians, pharmacist, and your trusted family member or patient advocate.

Most of us find it difficult to accept that one's life is time-limited (finite), which may account for the natural tendency to put off planning for the inevitable losses associated with late life (e.g. decline in health, loss of friends and family, to mention a few). Just as you have conscientiously attended to other phases of life, as you get older you will want to discuss with your family, doctors, and lawyer your specific wishes regarding what medical treatment you want and do not want if you become seriously ill. Complete important legal documents: HIPAA, the POLST or MOST, living will, healthcare and financial proxies and patient advocate form. Make use of "the five wishes" and "the conversation" so those involved who may need to make decisions on your behalf work together as a team to respect and carry out your end-of-life wishes. By tending to these important tasks, you make it easier for your family and doctor who want to know and respect your wishes. This kind of pre-planning serves to avoid family arguments and feelings of guilt since your wishes are being honored.

Just another reminder that Drs. Lazarus and Foster have a website – **www.qualityaffordablehealthcare.net** – where we publish a monthly medical forum and chapter updates to keep you informed about important changes in our healthcare system that may directly affect you and your family. Our website is an integral extension of our book. A section of our website includes an expanded list of Key Points and important Appendices associated with each book chapter, such as legal forms and more detailed information about Medicare.

We encourage you to also use our website to ask us questions about problems accessing quality healthcare, billing issues, etc. Our answers may help others and will appear in the following month's forum or by email if you provide your address. Your identity will, of course, be kept confidential. We cannot answer questions about your medical diagnosis and treatment because they are best addressed by your doctor and because of medicolegal restrictions.

Having read our book, we hope you are more empowered to make the best healthcare decisions for you and your family. Please keep in contact with us via our website.

Dr. Larry Lazarus

Dr. Jeff Foster

About the Authors

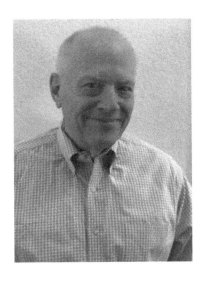

Jeffrey Foster, M.D. has spent his clinical and academic career with Geriatric Psychiatry as a prominent focus. He has worked closely with primary care physicians, nurses, social workers and various medical and surgical specialists consulting in both hospital and outpatient settings. He is a former president of the American Association of Geriatric Psychiatry and a recipient of the National Institute of Mental Health Geriatric Mental Health Academic Award. He has done federally funded longitudinal research in the long-term care setting (including Internal Medicine; Rehabilitation Medicine, and Skilled Nursing Facility areas). He is on the voluntary faculty of the Department of Psychiatry in the University of Colorado School of Medicine with the rank of Clinical Professor of Psychiatry.

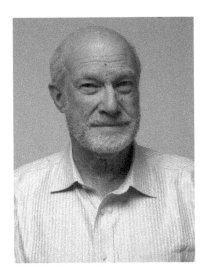

Lawrence W. Lazarus, M.D., has spent his forty-year career specializing in geriatric medicine and psychiatry, primarily at Rush Medical School and University in Chicago, Illinois. He was the founding Director of the Geriatric Psychiatry Fellowship Program at Rush University. He is a co-editor of the Comprehensive Textbook of Geriatric Psychiatry and has authored fifty medical articles for the medical and the lay public. He is a former president of the American Association of Geriatric Psychiatry and a recipient of the National Institute of Mental Health Geriatric Mental Health Academic Award. Dr. Lazarus is currently in private practice in Santa Fe, New Mexico.

Index

Made in USA - Kendallville, IN
1048279_9781733519205
02.04.2020 1019